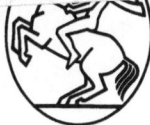

Advances in Radiosurgery

Proceedings of the 1st Congress
of the International Stereotactic Radiosurgery Society,
Stockholm 1993

Edited by
C. Lindquist, D. Kondziolka, J. S. Loeffler

Acta Neurochirurgica
Supplement 62

Springer-Verlag Wien New York

Assoc. Prof. Dr. Christer Lindquist
Gamma Knife Center, Karolinska Hospital, Stockholm, Sweden

Assoc. Prof. Dr. Douglas Kondziolka
Department of Neurological Surgery and Radiation Oncology,
Presbyterian University Hospital, Pittsburgh, PA, USA

Assoc. Prof. Dr. Jay S. Loeffler
Joint Center of Radiation Therapy, Boston, MA, USA

ISSN 0065-1419 (Acta Neurochirurgica/Suppl.)
ISBN-13: 978-3-7091-9373-0   e-ISBN-13: 978-3-7091-9371-6
DOI: 10.1007/978-3-7091-9371-6

Preface

The first congress of the International Stereotactic Radiosurgical Society convened at the birthplace of radio-surgery in Stockholm, Sweden, in June 1993. There were 345 enthusiastic participants who contributed to making the meeting a success. Radiosurgery is a multi-disciplinary speciality and it was the intention of the organizers to let this fact be reflected in the outline of the conference. Treatment modalities alternative to radiosurgery were, therefore, covered in review lectures on neuromicrosurgery, radiotherapy and radiobiology. There were also a number of panel discussions aiming at defining the proper place of radiosurgery in today's therapeutic armamen-tarium. For this volume we have, however, selected to publish mainly original contributions to reflect state-of-the-art in radiosurgery. The subspecialty is still young and subject to intense technical development. For many indications, long term follow-up of treatment effects are still lacking. New indications still need to be explored. It is encouraging to see how many centers worldwide have embarked upon this exciting new treatment avenue.

Radiosurgical developments have encouraged not only neurosurgeons but also radiotherapists into less orthodox ways of approaching treatment by ionizing radiation. Radiobiologists have quickly understood that more information is needed on the effects of single session radiation to open up roads for further developments in radiosurgery. Stereotactic radiosurgery had a breakthrough in the eighties and continues to be one of the most exciting developments of neurosurgical therapy in the nineties.

I thank the participants of the first ISRS congress for their attendance and the contributors to this book for pushing the frontiers of radiosurgery forward.

Stockholm, November 1994

Christer Lindquist, M.D., Ph.D.
Associate Professor of Neurosurgery
Director of the Karolinska Gamma Knife Center

Contents

Listed in Current Contents

Acta Neurochir (1994) [Suppl] 62: 1–4

Opening Lecture

Lars Leksell's Vision – Radiosurgery

A. Ammar

Department of Neurosurgery, King Feisal University, College of Medicine and Medical Sciences, Al-Khobar, Saudi Arabia

Dear Professor Lindquist,
Dear Friends and Colleagues,
Ladies and Gentlemen,

I am greatly honoured to be here, and to address this first meeting of the International Stereotactic Radio-surgical Society. It is an extra special honour for me, as it is being held here in Stockholm, the city in which I learned the ABC of Neurosurgery. The city where I first met Professor Leksell, a man who was to have a profound influence on me, both in the field of neuro-surgery, and in my general life. As we all know, behind every great invention is a great person, but what we often forget is that behind every great person is a great personality. This personality is what shapes the invention. None of us present must forget that the untiring striving of Professor Leksell, and his strong will and personality, are what caused us to be here today. Leksell never lost his boyish enthusiasm, and so he collected a group of willing colleagues to help him in his achievement. Among these were Professors Backlund, Steiner, Lindquist, Lunsford, Meyerson, Norén, Rähn, Forster, the biophysicist, Larsson, the neuroradiologist Greitz, and the great friend and engi-neer, Bengt Jernberg. Although we owe much to these colleagues of his, the achievement of the first radio-surgical endeavours can be firmly attributed to his determination to overcome all obstacles in reaching his goal. His determination to perfect the technique continued until his death, and he was always investi-gating technological advances in medicine, as well as other fields in order to improve the technique. I am writing a book about Leksell and whilst researching the book I have spoken to many people about Leksell in order to gain a better understanding of what drove him. Everyone I have spoken to holds different strong

opinions of the Professor, but the one undisputed opinion held by all is that he was a brilliant man with a forceful personality. This forceful personality was to play a key role in the development of the Gamma Knife. The way was not easy, but his insight, self-confidence, determination, and selfless devotion were utilised to achieve his dream, an effective method to treat cerebral disorders, in a way that inflicted the least pain on his patients. And so today we have the Gamma Knife, Leksell's vision. Although Lars Leksell left the medical profession with this great gift, he perhaps left us with something greater, an example of what all young doctors should strive for, to lessen the suffering of our patients, and to remember that all our patients are human beings, with feelings, dreams and opinions, and not merely a disease or medical number.

In order to understand the personality of Lars Leksell we must start with his early life. Professor Leksell was born into a wealthy Swedish family in Gothenburg on the 24th of November 1907[2]. From an early age he was fascinated by machines and owned a motorcycle in his teens. He was devoted to his motorbike, and it was this devotion that led by chance to his becoming a doctor. When he was not tinkering with it, he was out riding it. Until the age of 23 he believed that engineering was his destiny. However one day in 1930 all that changed. He was out riding his motorbike in Stockholm, when he had an argument with a bus. The unconscious Leksell was rushed to the Mörby Hospital where he was operated upon by a Professor Giertz. He was very impressed by the skill and discipline of the Professor, and particularly with his method of conducting grand rounds.

Being an active yound man he was bored by his hospital stay, so in order to amuse him a nurse lent him a book by Sinclair Lewis, about a boy who wanted to become a doctor. The book obviously had a profound effect on the yound Lars Leksell, as many years later, when writing his own biography, he could recall both the name of the nurse, Sister Britta, who lent it to him, as well as the names of all the characters in the plot. Leksell himself admitted that it was this book that was to broaden his horizons, and plant the seed that led him to consider a life of medicine rather than engineering, his first love[3].

After leaving the hospital he was undecided about what to read at University, literature, engineering, medicine, or for some reason that I have not been able to discover, law. The final decision again came about by chance. Whilst out walking one morning he happened to bump into a class mate of his, Knut Erik. They had a conversation that went something like this;

"Hello, Knut. Haven't seen you for a while"

"No. Where are you going?"

"Nowhere special. Just wandering."

"I'm going to Karolinska. I'm going to register to study medicine. I'm going to be a great doctor."

"Yes. That's not a bad idea. I'll come with you. I suppose I might as well register too."

We obviously owe a great debt of gratitude to Sister Britta, and of course, the luckless Knut, who was not accepted to study medicine. So it was that Leksell began his life as a doctor.

He graduated from the Karolinska Institute in 1935, and spent his time rushing between Ragnar Granit's Neurophysiology laboratory and Olivecrona's Neurosurgical Department. This was the start of his persuit of his goal. That of fighting pain and tumors. This vision was the basis for all his achievements in the field of medicine, and ultimately the Gamma Knife; to him it was not merely a distant goal to aim for, but a vision to turn into reality. His first major medical achievement was to identify the gamma-efferent system still bearing his name.

In 1945 he moved full time to the department of neurosurgery.

When I first met Professor Leksell I found him to be a very confusing man. As a young doctor I was called upon to spend many lonely hours in the hospital, but whenever I felt the need for company I could wander along to the professor's room for a conversation. This was the cause of my confusion. I loved to engage in conversation on a wide range of topics, and I found conversations with the professor to be a little difficult to follow. We would be rolling along on one subject, when out of the blue, he would switch to a completely different topic, and I would find myself striving to

make a connection. Eventually I would forget the apparent leap and just go along with him. Only days and sometimes years later would I grasp the connection. All very demoralising to a young man who considered himself to be intelligent! I think that the conversation I had with him just before I left Sweden to obtain my Ph.D. from Japan, is probably the best example of this that I can remember. I went along to say goodbye, as I was going to study microvascular surgery in Japan, and as was our habit we became involved in conversation. There we were discussing the merits of travelling and such mundane things as the weather, when all of a sudden, he started talking about microsurgery, well that was not too big a leap for me, but then came the shocker. In mid-sentence he broke off to talk about stereotaxy. Until that point I had been slightly worried about moving, but I decided perhaps it was for the best, because Professor Leksell was obviously beginning to lose his sense of reality, there just could not possibly be a connection between stereotaxy and microvascular surgery. Could there? Well about seven years later the connection was made, the stereotaxic microvascular system was produced by Ladislau Steiner and Christer Lindquist.

This extraordinary ability of Lars Leksell to make connections between two very different subjects was one of the things that led to the constant upgrading and modification of his ideas. He could look at available technology, and adapt it to perform a task that no-one else could imagine. Lars Leksell was a very tall man, and this height extended to his insight. Whilst the rest of us were struggling in the long grass, he was above it, and able to see the final goal.

Having seen his goal and decided the best path to reach it, he just ploughed on regardless of everyone else's inability to understand the scheme. He had enormous self confidence, and it was impossible to shake him once he made up his mind about something. Armed with his vision and self-confidence, it is very easy to see how his determination followed.

His first aim was to develop a technique for treating functional disorders, and following his vision, to do it in a manner that caused the least amount of suffering and pain to the patient. Of course, he met with a lot of opposition, after all everyone knows that surgery is meant to be bloody. How could anyone operate on the brain through a tiny hole? Out of this developed the Leksell Stereotaxy system.

I have asked many of his close friends and family as to whether the dropping of the atomic bombs on Hiroshima and Nagasaki had an influence on his thinking regarding the use of radiation as a method of treatment, and all said "no'. However in his biography he said "Now the world is different Einstein's equation $E = mc^2$ has set Hiroshima and Nagasaki on fire...... but now scientists must have only one great goal; to reduce the suffering of the people, and make human life happier." He decided to take Einstein's equation to reach this end, and spent a great deal of time pondering its use as a tool of medicine, until he was caught muttering to himself in a room full of people $E = mc^2$.

With his goal set and his determination in force it was inevitable that the Gamma Knife was developed. However, although its development is easy to follow in retrospect, it was not at all easy to achieve the goal at the time.

The first attempts of utilising radiation to reach deep seated areas of the brain were achieved using stereotactic frames and simple x-ray units. This however did not produce an accurate enough area of irradiation, and the hunt was on for a more accurate technique. Leksell than decided to join forces with Börje Larsson, a Biophysicist at Uppsala University, and more importantly the proud keeper of a unit capable of producing a proton beam[1]. Whilst this collaboration was an invaluable one it was to cost Leksell dearly in travelling time and inconvenience, as each time he wanted to try out a new treatment, or ultimately, treat patients, he had to make a round trip of 80 miles. This was a prime example of his not bothering with obstacles, it did not occur to him that collaboration on that scale

was unheard of, or that he had to travel so far, all he could see was his objective getting closer. At that time many experiments were carried out on animals, conveniently supplied by the would-be, part-time farmer, Lars Leksell. Once the animal experiments proved successful, Leksell decided that the inconvenience of the distance obstacle was unacceptable to patients, so he set about getting a unit set up in Stockholm. Not an easy task, as not everyone was convinced of the efficacy of this form of treatment. Here was this crazy professor back again. It was bad enough the first time, when he wanted to make brain operations virtually blood free, now he did not even want to open the Skull! Impossible, could not work!.

Eventually he managed to persuade the Studsvik Nuclear Company to build a "Gamma Unit" financed privately, (Fig. 1) as the hospital administration was still sceptical. The first case treated was in October 1967, a young boy with a craniopharyngioma, a patient of Professor Backlund. When the irradiation was complete Professor Leksell said
"There you are. All done"
"What, aren't you going to do it?"
"Yes, it's all done. We've finished."
"Well, could I have another go please?"[3]
Apparently even one so young was a sceptic! This first treatment took place on the company premises, but soon after the unit was installed in a private hospital in Stockholm.

This first unit was not enough for Leksell, and he was always looking for ways to improve the treatment. The second unit, produced in 1975 was capable of irradiating larger areas, and dose planning was no longer laboriously calculated by human beings but computer assisted.

In 1985, with the advent of MRI, the long treks back to Uppsala began again. I accompanied Christer Lindquist and the first patient to Uppsala in Christer's old white Volvo station wagon. We arrived to find Professor Leksell, and Dan Leksell already waiting and keen to proceed. The procedure took most of the afternoon, during which time, the 78 year old professor never sat down. When finally we had finished he made only one comment "Now it is perfect."

It was then for the first time that I truly realised that he was driven by some inner force, and that he would not tire or slow down until he had achieved it. His vision. Through all of the struggles, and indeed, up until the time of his death, Professor Leksell never thought of the material gains that he could receive through his work. He never counted the hours he

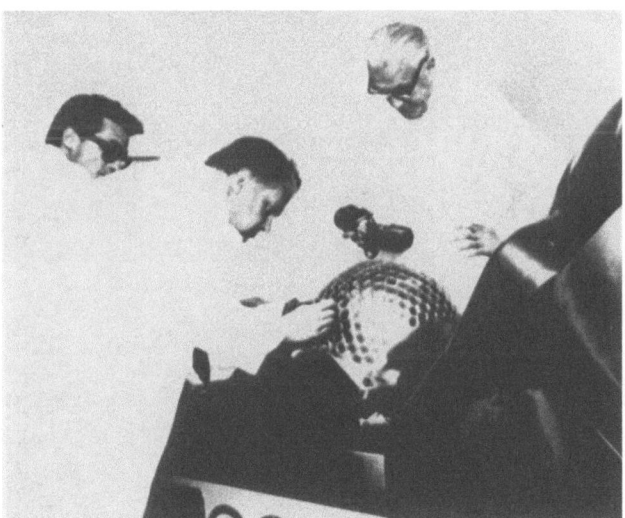

Fig. 1. Lars Leksell and Bengt Jernberg (1977) using the first Gamma Knife to treat one of the very first group of patients who were treated by radiosurgery technique

worked, or the miles he travelled. He ignored personal discomfort and fatigue. The greatest reward for him was to see the realisation of his vision, by the development and perfection of a technique to relieve the suffering of the patient. And through it all he never forgot the patient, for if he did, it would only have fulfilled half the dream. I have tried to show you a little of the man behind the machine, and what drove him. There is an example in him which all of us can follow. Today, when so many people are concerned with wealth and status, it is easy to forget the patient, but if we ever do that, we will become without feeling like the machines we use.

If he is listening now he must know how much we respect him and admire his work, but to him I do not suppose it really matters. His greatest sense of satis-faction must have come from the knowledge that his vision was turned into reality, and in his own lifetime. An achievement that most mere mortals can only dream of.

Professor Leksell, we salute you!

References

1. Backlund EO (1986) Lars Leksell – a portrait by a friend. Appl Neurophysiol 49: 173–181
2. Leksell D (1992) Lars Leksell – an historical vingnette. In: Steiner L et al (eds) Radiosurgery: baseline and trends. Raven, New York, pp 257–261
3. Leksell L (1982) Hjärnfragment. Norstedts, Stockholm

Correspondence: Ahmed Ammar, MD., Ph.D., Department of Neurosurgery, King Fahd University Hospital, P. O. Box 40040, Al Khobar, Saudi Arabia.

Acta Neurochir (1994) [Suppl] 62: 5–9
© Springer-Verlag 1994

Linear Accelerator Radiosurgery of Cerebral Arteriovenous Malformations: Current Status

F. Colombo[1], F. Pozza[2], G. Chierego[3], P. Francescon[3], L. Casentini[1], and G. De Luca[1]

[1]Department of Neurosurgery, [2]Department of Radiotherapy, and [3]Service of Medical Physic, City Hospital, Vicenza, Italy

Summary

228 patients affected by cerebral arteriovenous malformations (AVMs) underwent linear accelerator radiosurgery. Follow-up ranges from 1 to 100 months (mean 42 months).

Complete angiographic obliteration was achieved in 47% of treated patients at one year and 80% at 2 years. 17 haemorrhages were observed after treatment and 6 patients died from them. No bleeding took place after complete angiographic obliteration. 11 patients suffered for radionecrosis. In 6 patients complete recovery was obtained with corticoid medication.

The aim of this study is to present our results and to evaluate the effect of irradiation on the risk of bleeding after radiosurgery. Patients were considered at risk in the time lapse after irradiation and before angiographic obliteration or other definitive treatment or death. Patients were followed from the date of radiosurgery and the number of haemorrhages were recorded every six months. In our series the bleeding risk in patients harbouring incompletely obliterated AVMs decreases from 8% in the first year after radiosurgery to 0% starting from the 24th month of the follow-up.

Keywords: Arteriovenous malformations; linear accelerator; radiosurgery; risk of haemorrhage.

Introduction

Single session, stereotactically focused irradiation (Radiosurgery[14]) is considered an established treatment alternative for cerebral arteriovenous malformations (AVMs). The basic idea of obtaining a progressive obliteration of the diseased nidus vessels by high radiation dose has proved to be equally safe and effective, irrespective of the device employed, either Gamma Knife, Cyclothrone or linear accelerators[1,4,5,7,12,13,16,18,21,22,24,26]. On the other hand recent years, results obtained by microsurgery have progressively improved. Nowadays, impressive results are reported in large surgical series, also in small, deep seated, critically located AVMs, which were previously referred to radiosurgery[9,27,28]. Few AVMs can be defined inoperable and in most cases the choice between different therapeutic approaches is a matter for discussion. In this choice, bleeding after irradiation and before complete angiographic obliteration ("latency period") is the major shortcoming of radiosurgery in comparison with surgical removal. The aim of this report is to update our clinical experience and to evaluate the risk of bleeding in irradiated patients.

Materials and Methods

Our technique is based on multiple, non coplanar, arc irradiations focused onto the stereotactic target. The procedure has been described in previous reports[3–5].

From November 1984 to April 1992, 228 patients (111 males and 117 females) affected by cerebral AVMs were treated. At treatment, age ranged from 6 to 70 years (mean 32 years). Symptoms and signs of presentation were bleeding in 187, epilepsy in 33, neurological deterioration in 7 and exophthalmos in 1. Before radiosurgery, 35 patients underwent unsuccessful attempts at surgical removal; 15 patients underwent incomplete AVM embolization. Lateralisation of the AVMs and their location are shown in Fig. 1.

Maximum dimensions of the lesion varied from 4 mm to 40 mm in diameter (mean 16 mm). A radiation dose of 18.7 to 40 Gy (mean 28.2 Gy) was delivered in a single session at the center of the target. The borders of the target volume were encompassed by isodoses from 70 to 90%. One radiation field from 10 mm to 35 mm was utilized in 198 patients, whereas in 30, combinations of two or more (up to 4) fields were employed. While for small AVMs doses up to 40 Gy at target point were utilized, for larger AVMs doses were reduced according to the relation log dose vs log radius[12]. The entire nidus received a dose considered adequate for obliteration in 195 patients. In the other 33 patients – most of them with a large AVM – only the part of the arteriovenous malformation close to arteriolar feeders and/or draining veins was treated. In these cases, at least part of the periphery of the lesion received a dose below the optimum (Fig. 2).

Angiographic follow-up was performed at 12, 24, and 36 months. Complete obliteration, (normal circulation time, absence of former nidus vessels, disappearance or normalization of draining veins), was considered the end result of radiosurgical treatment[16,18,20]. If not attained after 3 years, further irradiation or an alternative treatment was prescribed.

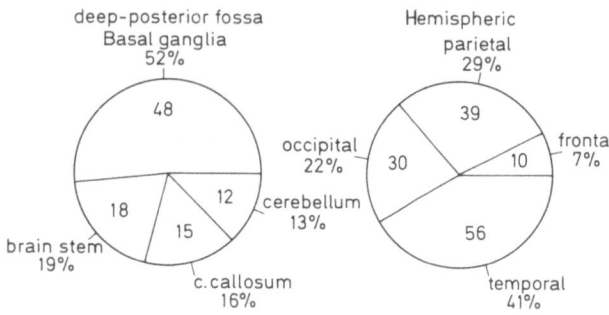

Side: 111 left   102 right   14 midline

Fig. 1. Location and site of treated AVMs

Results

Follow-up ranges from 1 to 100 months (mean 42, median 45) Up to date (April 93) clinical data are available for all 228 patients. 12 months control angiography was performed in 156 out of 170 (92%) patients with a follow-up longer than one year. 24 months control angiography is available for 113 of 142 (80%) patients with a follow-up longer than 2 years. The complete obliteration rate is 47% (74 patients) at one year and 80% (90 patients) at two years. 7 more patients showed complete obliteration at a later follow-up. Irradiation was repeated in 14 patients. Surgical

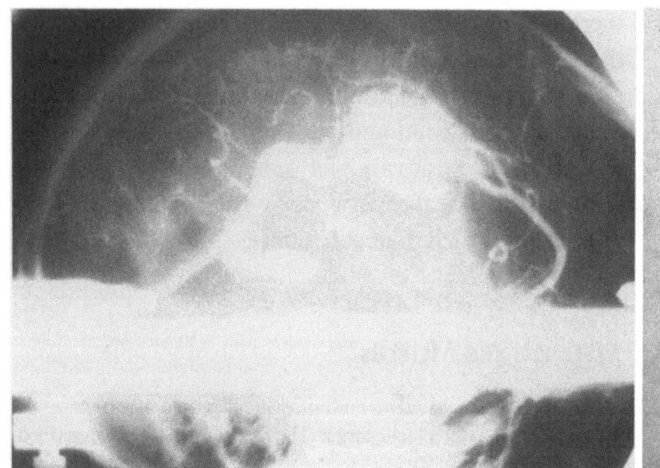
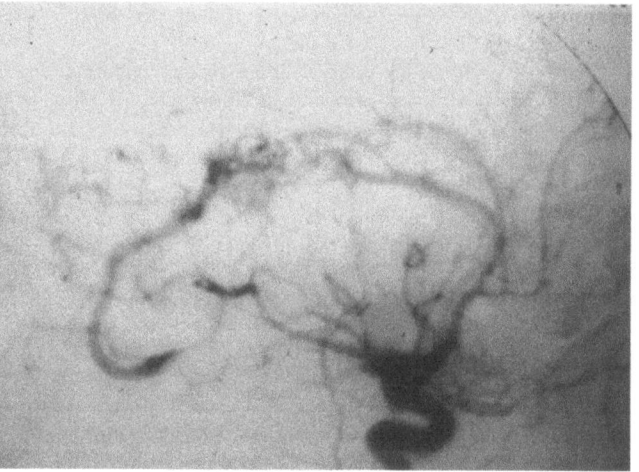

a   b

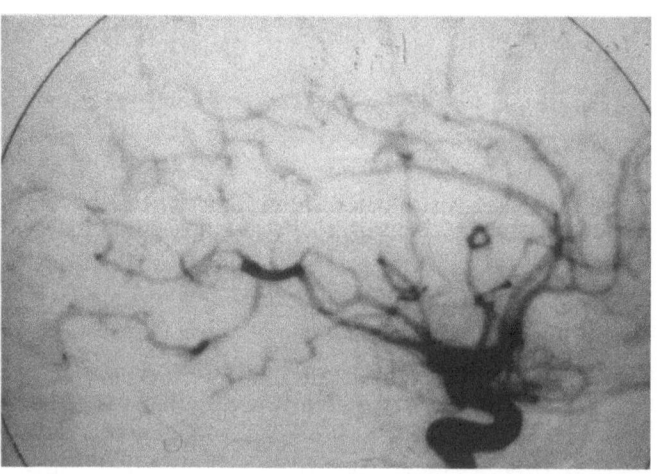

c   d

Fig. 2. Progressive decrease in AVM volume after irradiation. Patient 181: 20-year-old woman. 1 minor haemorrhage 3 months before admission. Large size (22 × 25 × 29 mm) right pericallosal AVM. At treatment (September 1988), 28.7 Gy were delivered to the center of target volume (20 Gy at 70% isodose, diameter 16 mm) with a 20 mm field. Far borders of the lesions absorbed 10 Gy. (a) stereotactic angiography at treatment, (b) at 12 months, control angiography, (c) 24 months, control angiography. At 36 months: angiography unchanged. Re-irradiation of the AVM remnant. (d) Follow-up angiography 49 months after initial treatment. Finally, complete obliteration has been obtained

removal was performed in 2, and embolization in 2 of the unsuccessfully irradiated patients.

AVMs have been subdivided into: small (S)–less than 15 mm in maximum dimension, medium (M)– between 15 and 25 mm, and large (L)–more than 25 mm. Total obliteration rate at 24 months follow-up ranged from 94% in small to 31.5% in large AVMs (Table 1).

11 patients (8 males and 3 females) suffered undue side effects of irradiation. There was a sligth preponderance of large lesions (S 3, M 3, L 4). We observed 8 sensory-motor deficits, 1Vth nerve paraesthesia, 1 hypothalamic syndrome (with weight loss and hyperthermia) and 1 confusional syndrome. On contrast enhanced CT examinations, the target volume was marked by a "ring" feature surrounded by a wide hypodense area, in 2 cases with mass effect. Symptoms appeared from 2 to 18 months after irradiation. The average duration of complaints was 4 months. All patients required corticoid medication. 6 patients recovered to a normal clinical condition. 5 patients still complain of static neurological symptoms (2%).

17 cerebral haemorrhages were observed after treatment (7 males, 10 females). 14 patients had a record of previous haemorrhages, while in 3 patients it was the first episode. AVMs dimensions were: S 4, M 6, L 7. Bleeding took place from 6 days to 2 years after irradiation. 6 patients (S 1, M 2, L 3) died as a consequence of their AVMs rupture. 3 patients required emergency surgery. 2 patients still display static neurological symptoms, and their angiographic study demonstrated an incomplete obliteration. We did not observe any bleeding after complete obliteration in 115 patients with a mean follow-up of 36 months after angiographic "cure".

We tried to investigate any possible effect of irradiation on the tendency to bleed in the latency period after radiosurgery and before complete AVM obliteration. In the evaluation were included all patients in

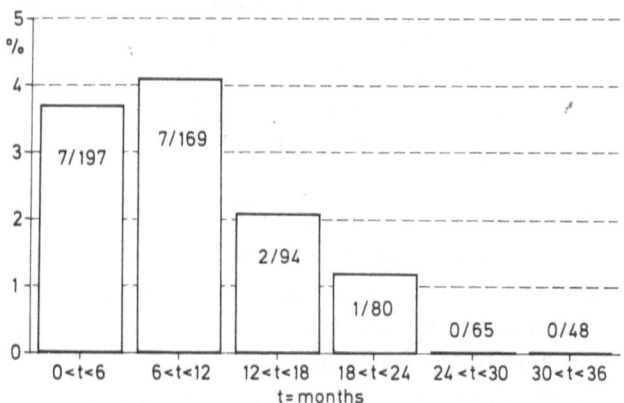

Fig. 3. Bleeding occurrences in irradiated patients harbouring still patent (not totally obliterated) AVMs

the time lapse between irradiation and either complete angiographic obliteration or other definitive treatment (surgery or embolization) or death (for haemorrhage or for unrelated disease). This group includes all irradiated patients in which the most recent angiograms showed a still non-obliterated AVM. Only these patients are considered susceptible to bleeding, while those with completed obliteration were removed from the group at risk, after angiographic "cure" was visible Patients with non-obliterated AVMs were stratified starting from 0 time (the date of radiosurgery). The bleeding risk was evaluated every six months.

197 patients have a follow-up longer than 6 months: observed bleeds from Mo 0 to 6:7 (4%),
169 patients have a follow-up longer than 12 months: observed bleeds from Mo 6 to 12:7 (4%),
94 patients have a follow-up longer than 18 months: observed bleeds from Mo 12 to 18:2 (2%),
80 patients have a follow-up longer than 24 months: observed bleeds from Mo 18 to 24:1 (1%),
65 patients have a follow-up longer than 30 months: observed bleeds from Mo 24 to 30:0 (0%),
43 patients have a follow-up longer than 36 months: observed bleeds from Mo 30 to 36:0 (0%),
(Fig. 3).

Discussion

Our results confirm those obtained with either Gamma Knife, Cyclothrone and Linear accelerator. Standard achievements of radiosurgery seem to point to 80% complete obliteration at two years, with a complication rate around 2 to 4%[16,18,24]. Bleeding occurrence after radiosurgery has been, until recently, less exhaustively investigated.

Table 1. *Linear Accelerator Radiosurgery for AVMs Angiographic Follow-up*

Max. dimension	follow-up	12 months	24 months
<15 mm (small)	patients N	92	67
	total obl	57	63
	rate	92%	94%
15 < 25 (Medium)	patients N	38	27
	total obl	14	21
	rate	37%	78%
>25 mm (Large)	patients N	26	19
	total obl	3	6
	rate	12%	32%

Bleeding risk after irradiation and before obliteration has been reported by Steiner[24,25], Kjellberg[13] and by Lunsford[18] to equal that of the natural history of the untreated AVM. However, during the latency period, a certain number of the AVMs effectively obliterates; these "cures" are detected only later on, on the occasion of the angiographic follow-up. Since AVMs are no more susceptible to bleeding from the moment (undetected) of their angiographic obliteration[18,24], observed bleedings are sustained only by those patients that still harbour non-obliterated AVMs; in the existing reports "cured" patients are not removed from population at risk. Consequently, the number of patients at risk of bleeding is overestimated and the bleeding risk is underestimated. In the complete unselected series (AVMs already obliterated together with AVMs still incompletely obliterated) "a risk equal to that of the natural history" could be sustained by an increase of bleeding occurrences in patients harbouring AVMs still not obliterated.

Our results seem to indicate a bleeding rate higher than espected in non-obliterated patients. The bleeding risk of untreated AVMs is reported to be from 2 to 5% per year, according to various authors[2,6,8,10,19,23]. In our series, in the first 12 months after treatment, the risk of bleeding varies from 7.4% to 8.2% per year (from 3.7% to 4.1% per six months).

One possible explanation of this unexpected bleeding rate is that radiosurgical treatment might induce a transitory increase in the tendency to bleed before complete obliteration is attained. Radiation induced obliteration is not an "all or nothing" instantaneous process, involving in a short time span the whole AVM nidus, but a slow progressive phenomenon that usually takes months to years to be completed. Radiosurgical dose planning requires that the nidus of the malformations is encompassed by isodoses from 50 to 70%[16,18]. In our series, even lower isodoses (30–40%) coincided with the far edge of the malformation, when a strategy of partial volume irradiation was utilized (usually in large AVMs, with the aim of decreasing the risk of radionecrosis[22]). But since "high doses provoke earlier effects than lower doses"[11] it is possible to suppose that the process of obliteration starts where the dose is higher – at the center of the radiation field – and only gradually moves to the other parts of the malformation. Also in cases in which angiographic follow-up performed year or years later demonstrated complete obliteration, for at least a brief period after irradiation, obliteration might be incomplete. But partial obliteration induces an increase in resistance through the arteriovenous shunt and consequently a parallel in-

crease in blood pressure in arterial feeders which is transmitted to that part of the AVM nidus still not protected by radiation induced obliteration. In a previous report, we examined angiograms of partially obliterated cases. In bleeding cases we noted a high frequency of increased tortuosity of the draining vein, increased blood flow velocity, appearance of aneurysms and other signs that we related to the increased pressure gradient through the malformation and to the blood flow rerouting[5]. Similar findings are described by Levy and Coworkers[15]. The hypothesis seems to be confirmed by the experimental work of Lo and Coworkers in AVM models[17]. They demonstrated that a prolonged increase in blood pressure is induced in shunt vessels in cases of large AVMs treated by non-homogeneous dose irradiation. Spetzler states that risk of haemorrhage increases with the partial embolization of an AVM[20]: a similar effect could be expected at least during the period after radiosurgery in which an AVM is only partially obliterated. The hypothesis that the increase of the bleeding risk is due to poorly syncronized obliterative effect entailed by dose inhomogeneities inside the target volume seems to be confirmed by statistical analysis of our material: among patients without a history of previous haemorrhages harbouring incompletely obliterated AVMs, the stepwise discriminant analysis with two class levels (no bleedings after radiosurgery/bleedings after radiosurgery) and 9 physical and geometrical variables, shows that the ratio between the maximum dose (at the center of the target) and the minimum dose (at the periphery of the lesion) was found to be the only significant variable to discriminate bleeding patients. Due to our dose planning, this ratio is higher in large volume AVMs: this fact probably explains the predominence of large AVMs among bleeding cases in our series. We conclude this overview of our clinical experience by emphasizing two concepts:

In the first place, the importance of dose planning affording homogeneous dose absorption throughout the entire AVM nidus as a mean of decreasing bleeding risk in the latency period after radiosurgery.

On the second place, A warning against general Indiscriminate use of radiosurgery in every case of cerebral AVM: the unique role of microsurgical removal for affording an immediate protection against bleeding should not be forgotten.

References

1. Betti O, Munari C, Rosler R (1989) Stereotactic radiosurgery with the linear accelerator: treatment of arteriovenous malformations. Neurosurgery 24: 311–321

2. Brown RD, Wiebers DO, Forbes G, O'Fallon WM, Piepgras DG, Marsh WR, Maciunas RJ (1988) The natural history of unruptured intracranial arteriovenous malformations. J Neurosurg 68: 352–357

3. Colombo F, Benedetti A, Pozza F, Avanzo RC, Marchetti C, Chierego G, Zanardo A (1985) External stereotactic irradiation by linear accelerator. Neurosurgery 16: 154–160

4. Colombo F, Benedetti A, Pozza F, Marchetti C, Chierego G (1989) Linear accelerator radiosurgery of cerebral arteriovenous malformations. Neurosurgery 24: 833–840

5. Colombo F (1992) Linear accelerator radiosurgery of cerebral arteriovenous malformations: technique and results. In: Steiner L *et al* (eds) Radiosurgery: baseline and trends. Raven, New York, pp 189–194

6. Crawford PM, West CR, Chadwick DW, Shaw MDM (1986) Arteriovenous malformations of the brain: natural history in unoperated patients. J Neurol Neurosurg Psychiatry 49: 1–10

7. Fabrikant JI, Lyman JT, Hosobuchi Y (1984) Stereotactic heavy ion Bragg peak radiosurgery for intracranial vascular disorders: method for treatment of deep arteriovenous malformations. Br J Radiol 57: 479–490

8. Graf CJ, Perret GE, Torner JC (1983) Bleeding from cerebral arteriovenous malformations as a part of their natural history. J Neurosurg 58: 331–337

9. Heros RC, Korosue K, Diebold PM (1990) Surgical excision of cerebral arteriovenous malformations: late results. Neurosurgery 26: 570–578

10. Itoyama Y, Uemura S, Ushio Y, Kuratsu J, Nonaka N, Wada H, Sano Y, Fukumura A, Yoshida K, Yano T (1989) Natural course of unoperated intracranial arteriovenous malformations: study of 50 cases. J Neurosurg 71: 805–809

11. Kjellberg RN (1979) Isoeffective dose parameters for brain necrosis in relation to proton radiosurgical dosimetry. In: Szikla G (ed) Stereotactic cerebral irradiations. Elsevier, Amsterdam, pp 157–166

12. Kjellberg RN (1979) Stereotactic Bragg peak proton radiosurgery results. In: Szikla G (ed) Stereotactic cerebral irradiations. Elsevier, Amsterdam, pp 233–240

13. Kjellberg RN (1988) Proton beam therapy for arteriovenous malformations of the brain. In: Schmidek HH *et al* (eds) Operative neurosurgical techniques. Grune and Stratton, New York, pp 911–915

14. Leksell L (1971) Stereotaxis and radiosurgery: an operative system. Thomas, Springfield

15. Levy RP, Fabrikant JI, Frankel KA, Philips MH, Steinberg GK, Marks MP, DeLaPaz RL, Chuang FYS (1992) Clinical-radiological evaluation of sequelae of stereotactic radiosurgery for intracranial arteriovenous malformations. In: Steiner L *et al* (eds) Radiosurgery: baseline and trends. Raven, New York, pp 209–220

16. Lindquist C, Steiner L (1988) Stereotactic radiosurgical treatment of malformations of the brain. In: Lunsford LD (ed) Modern stereotactic neurosurgery. Martinus Nijhoff, Boston, pp 491–505

17. Lo EH, Fabrikant JI, Levy RP, Philips MH, Frankel KA, Alpen EL (1991) An experimental compartmental flow model for assessing the hemodynamic response of intracranial arteriovenous malformations to stereotactic radiosurgery. Neurosurgery 28: 251–259

18. Lunsford LD, Kondziolka D, Flickinger JC, Bissonette DJ, Jungreis CA, Maitz AH, Horton JA, Coffey RJ (1991) Stereotactic radiosurgery for arteriovenous malformations of the brain. J Neurosurg 75: 512–524

19. Ondra SL, Troupp H, George ED, Schwab K (1990) The natural history of symptomatic arteriovenous malformations of the brain: a 24-year follow-up assessment. J Neurosurg 73: 387–391

20. Spetzler RF, Hargraves RW, McCormick PW, Zabramski JM, Flom RA, Zimmerman RS (1992) Relationship of perfusion pressure and size to risk of hemorrhage from arteriovenous malformations. J Neurosurg 76: 918–923

21. Steiner L, Leksell L, Forster DMC, Greitz T, Backlund EO (1974) Stereotactic radiosurgery in intracranial arteriovenous malformations. Acta Neurochir (Wien) [Suppl] 21: 195–209

22. Steiner L, Greitz T, Backlund EO, Leksell L, Noren G, Rahn T (1979) Radiosurgery in arteriovenous malformations of the brain. Undue effects. In: Szikla G (ed) Stereotactic cerebral irradiations. Elsevier, Amsterdam, pp 257–269

23. Steiner L (1986) Storia naturale delle malformazioni arterovenose cerebrali. In: Da Pian R *et al* (eds) Aneurismi e angiomi cerebrali. Cortina, Verona, pp 179–184

24. Steiner L, Lindquist C (1987) Radiosurgery in cerebral arteriovenous malformation. In: Tasker RR (ed) Neurosurgery: state of the art review. Hanley and Belfus, Philadelphia, pp 329–336

25. Steiner L, Lindquist C, Adler JR, Torner JC, Alves W, Steiner M (1992) Clinical outcome of radiosurgery for cerebral arteriovenous malformations. J Neurosurg 77: 1–8

26. Valentino V (1986) Stereotactic radiation therapy in arteriovenous malformations and brain tumours using the Fixter system. Acta Radiol [Suppl] 369: 608–609

27. Yamada S, Brauer FS, Knierim DS (1990) Direct approach to arteriovenous malformations in functional areas of the cerebral hemisphere. J Neurosurg 72: 418–425

28. Yasargil MG (1988) Microneurosurgery, Vol III B. AVM of the brain, clinical considerations, general and specific operative techniques, surgical results, nonoperated cases, cavernous and venous angiomas, neuroanestesia. Thieme, New York

Correspondence: Federico Colombo, M.D., Divisione di Neurochirurgia Ospedale Civile, Viale Rudolfi, I-36100 Vicenza, Italy.

Acta Neurochir (1994) [Suppl] 62: 10–12

Radiosurgery of Carotid-Cavernous Fistulae

J. L. Barcia-Salorio[1,2], F. Soler[3], J. A. Barcia[1,2], and G. Hernández[4]

[1] Servicio de Neurocirugía, Hospital Clínico Universitario, Valencia, [2] Departamento de Cirugía, Universidad de Valencia, [3] Servicio de Radiología, Hospital Clínico Universitario, Valencia, and [4] Servicio de Terapéutica Física, Hospital Clínico Universitario, Valencia, Spain

Summary

25 cases of carotid-cavernous fistulae (CCF) who underwent radiosurgery with a conventional gamma source from 1977 to 1992 are reported. 22 were low-flow, spontaneous CCFs and 3 were high flow fistulae which had undergone a previous trapping. The total dose delivered was 30 to 40 Gy. 91% to patients with low-flow CCF cured after radiosurgery in a mean time of 7.5 months, presenting improvent in a mean time of 2.3 months. Only one of the high-flow fistulae was cured. Follow-up period ranged between 14 years and 15 months (mean: 50 months). No recurrence was recorded in any case. While intravascular embolotherapy is the treatment of choice for high-flow fistulae, stereotactic radiosurgery may be the elective treatment for low-flow CCF.

Keywords: Carotid-cavernous fistulae; arteriovenous malformations; stereotactic radiosurgery.

Introduction

The close anatomical and physiological similarity between low-flow, spontaneous carotid-cavernous fistulae (CCF) and arteriovenous malformations (AVM) led the authors to apply radiosurgery, which proved to be effective for the latter, to a series of low-flow CCF[1]. Radiosurgery was also applied to high-flow or traumatic fistulae which had failed to close after previous trapping, but whose flow had been reduced by this manoeuver. This series started in 1977, and the results have been partly previously reported[2,3].

Clinical Material and Methods

Since November 1977 until November 1992, 25 low-flow CCF were irradiated. These included 22 spontaneous low flow fistulae, one of them secondary to a Gasserian ganglion percutaneous thermocoagulation, and three traumatic high flow fistulae in which a previous internal carotid trapping had reduced the flow of the CCF, but had not achieved its closure or the reversal of symptoms. We have excluded from this study one case secondary to an Ehlers-Danlos syndrome, so as to homogeneize the series. The mean interval between the begining of the symptoms and radiosurgery was 12 months (4–24 months).

The fistulae were classified according to Barrow's classification[4]:
A: high-flow fistulae.
B: low-flow fistulae between internal carotid artery branches and the cavernous sinus.
C: low-flow fistulae between external carotid artery branches and the cavernous sinus.
D: low-flow fistulae between both internal and external carotid artery branches and the cavernous sinus.

We have added type T for traumatic, high flow fistulae with flow reduction after trapping. There were 11 type B, 4 type C, 7 type D and 3 type T fistulae. The stereotactic radiosurgical technique consisted of the attachment of the stereoguide to a conventional Cobalt Unit, as has previously been reported[2]. Irradiation was performed with a 5 mm diameter collimator and a 10 mm diameter collimator in the case of dural AVMs. A total dose of 30 to 40 Gy was delivered in all cases, except one post-traumatic case in whom 20 Gy were delivered. A second irradiation with a dose of 40 Gy was performed in 2 cases, in one of the cases due to worsening of the symptoms and in the other one because there was no improvement after more than one year of follow up. Follow-up period for the entire series ranged between 14 years and 15 months (mean: 50 months).

Results

Results of spontaneous (types B, C, D) and traumatic (type T) fistulae are analyzed separately:

Of the 22 spontaneous fistulae, 20 (91%) closed completely without recurrence, with a follow-up period ranging between 14 years and 15 months. Closure occurred after a mean time of 7.5 (2–20) months after radiosurgery. Improvement began at a mean time of 2.4 months, ranging between 15 days and 14 months. It was defined as the amelioration of the main complaints of the patient (exophtalmos, diplopia, ptosis, visual disturbance or facial pain). Analyzed by types, 100% of cases of type B closed at a mean time of 6 months after radiosurgery. 75% of cases of type C

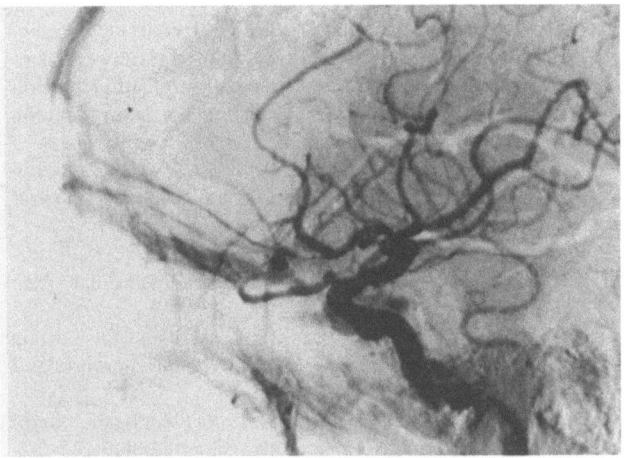

Fig. 1. Angiogram of a type D CCF in which early filling of the dilated cavernous sinus and retrograde filling of a very dilated opthalmic vein can be seen

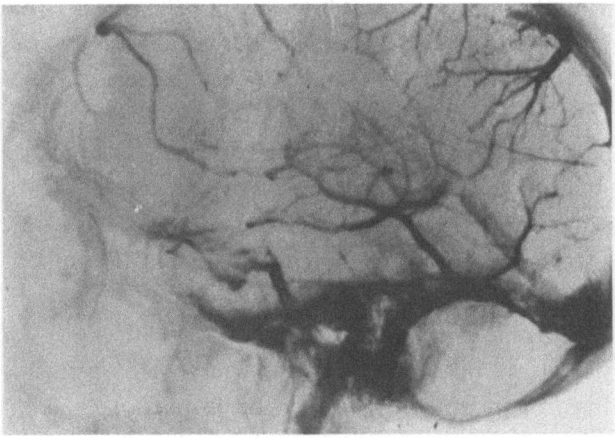

Fig. 3. Venous phase angiogram corresponding to the same investigation as in Fig. 2, showing a normal cavernous sinus

closed at a mean time of 13 months, and 86% cases of type D closed after a mean of 8 months.

In two cases, temporary reappearance of symptoms and signs occurred after mild improvement 2 and 12 months after irradiation, but they regressed and were cured in 6 and 8 months respectively. In all cured cases, a control angiogram showed total resolution. In one case of type C there was a progression of symptoms despite radiosurgery after eight months, and in other case of type D there was no cure after 15 months. These two cases were re-irradiated, but there were no clinical nor radiological modifications after three and eight years of follow-up, respectively. These patients went into other therapeutic trials (embolization, open surgery) without achieving permanent improvement.

Of the three traumatic fistulae (type T), only one was cured after six months, improvement begining two months after treatment. The other two cases did not

present and significant change after six and two years, respectively. In no case could there be found any complication attributable to irradiation.

Discussion

In contradistinction to the previous anatomical concept of the cavernous sinus, several authors described this structure as a venous plexus with its own coverings incompletely surrounding the internal carotid artery, based on anatomical studies[13]. A carotid-cavernous fistula may be produced when the internal carotid artery directly communicates with the branches of this plexus. This is frequently due to trauma to the internal carotid wall, or to a pre-existing defect in it such as an aneurysm. This situation normally leads to a high-flow communication between the two compartments, and was classified by Parkinson as a type I CCF and by Barrow as type A.

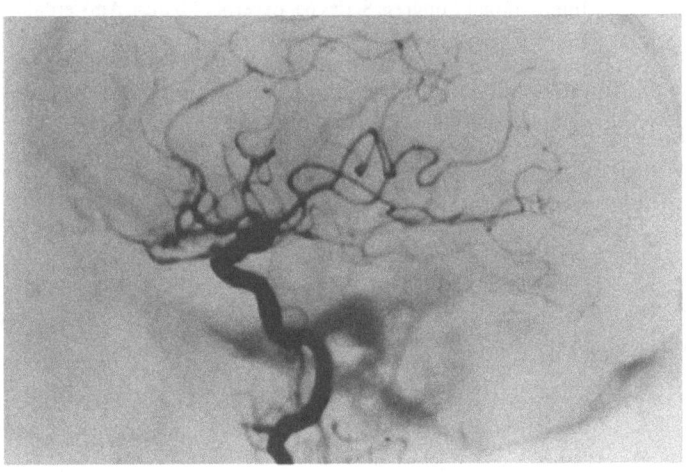

Fig. 2. Six months after radiosurgery, the intracavernous internal carotid artery is normal, and no sign of early venous filling is seen

Another possibility is that communication occurs with the intracavernous branches of either the internal (Parkinson's type II) or the external carotid arteries or both. This case is frequently produced by a pre-existing arteriovenous malformation, as Taptas described[16] or by the development of collateral circulation due to an ICA flow obstruction, and corresponds to what Barrow classified as types B, C and D. High flow fistulae can be easily closed by intracarotid embolization with detachable balloons, and some series published report a 100% rate of closures with a 80% of patency of the internal carotid artery[6]. However, this form of treatment may seem disproportionate for a relatively benign condition such as a low-flow fistula, specially when the important point in these cases is to preserve the patency of the ICA and increase morbidity. Embolization of low-flow, spontaneous CCF by different methods (external carotid or transvenous approaches) have attained a closure rate between 48 and 77% in most important series[4,6,14]. On the other hand, the complications reported include aphasia, hemiplegia, paresis of cranial nerves, intracranial haemorrage or worsening of the ocular symptoms[9,10]. Furthermore, recurrences have been reported[10,12].

One of the early effects of ionizing radiation on blood vessels is the intimal proliferation, which leads to the vessel's occlusion[8]. This is probably the mechanism which leads to the closure of low-flow CCF after radiosurgery, as it does in AVMs. In an experimental study done by our group on model arteriovenous fistula between the common carotid artery and the internal jugular vein in the rat, it was shown that there is a hyperplasia of the endothelium, greater after irradiation with doses between 30 and 40 Gy, which leads to a decrase of flow through the fistula[11].

The doses we selected for clinical use were based on those reported by Steiner[15] and later by Fabrikant[7] for AVMs (50 Gy). Other authors have also reported the application of radiosurgery[7] and of fractionated irradiated alone[5,18], or in combination with intravascular embolization[14] to CCF, achieving the begining of improvement as soon as 15 days after irradiation, and a 83% closure rate between one month and four years. These results are consistent with ours, and may help to establish stereotactic radiosurgery as the treatment of choice for low-flow CCF in the future, due to the high closure rate and the extremely low complication incidence.

References

1. Barcia-Salorio JL, Hernández G, Broseta J, *et al* (1979) Radiosurgical treatment of a carotid-cavernous fistula. Case report. In: Szikla G (ed) Stereotactic cerebral irradiation. Inserm symposium no 12. Holland biomedical press, Amsterdam, pp 251–256
2. Barcia-Salorio JL, Hernández G, Broseta J, *et al* (1982) Radiosurgical treatment of carotid-cavernous fistulae. Appl Neurophysiol 45: 520–522
3. Barcia-Salorio JL, Soler F, Hernández G, *et al* (1992) Radiosurgical treatment of low flow carotid-cavernous, fistulae. Acta Neurochir (Wien) [suppl] 52: 93–95
4. Barrow DL, Spector RH, Braun IF, *et al* (1985) Classification and treatment of spontaneous carotid-cavernous sinus fistulas. J Neurosurg 62: 248–256
5. Bitoh S, Hasegawa H, Fugiwara M, *et al* (1982) Irradiation of spontaneous carotid-cavernous fistulae. Surg Neurol 17: 282–286
6. Debrun GF, Viñuela F, Fox AJ, *et al* (1988) Indications for treatment and classification of 132 carotid-cavernous fistulae. Neurosurgery 22: 285–289
7. Fabrikant JI, Lyman JT, Hosobuchi Y (1984) Stereotactic heavy-ion bragg peak radiosurgery for intracranial vascular disorders: method for treatment of deep arteriovenous malformations. J Radiol 57: 479–490.
8. Fajardo LF, Berthrong M (1988) Vascular lesions following radiation. Pathol Ann.23: 297–330
9. Halbach VV, Higashida RT, Hieshima GM, *et al* (1987) Dural fistulas involving the cavernous sinus: results of treatment in 30 patients. Radiology 163: 437–442
10. Handa H (1984) Management of spontaneous carotid-cavernous fistulae. Neurología Col 8: 46–49
11. Joanes V, Barcia-Salorio JL, Ciudad J, *et al* (1991) Narrowbram gamma irradiation in stereotactic radiosurgery for arteriovenous fistulae. Research in Surgery 3: 67–73
12. Lasjaunias P, Berenstein A (1987) Surgical neuroangiography, Vol II. Endovascular treatment of craniofacial lesions. Springer Berlin Heidelberg New York Tokyo
13. Parkinson D (1965) A surgical approach to the cavernous portion of the carotid artery. Anatomical studies and case report. J Neurosurg 23: 474–483
14. Pierot L, Poisson M, Jason M, *et al* (1992) Treatment of type D dural carotid-cavernous fistula by embolization followed by irradiation. Neuroradiology 34: 77–80
15. Steiner L, Leksell L, Greitz T, *et al* (1972) Stereotaxic radiosurgery for cerebral arteriovenous malformations. Acta Chir Scand 138: 459–464
16. Taptas JN (1963) Arteriovenous aneurysm in pulsating exophtalmos: a new conception of the mechanism. in: Excerpta Medica International Congress Series 60. Excerpta Medica, Amsterdam, pp 98–99
17. Viñuela F, Fox AJ, DeBrun GM, *et al* (1984) Spontaneous carotid-cavernous fistulas: clinical radiological and therapeutic considerations. J Neurosurg 60: 976–984
18. Yamada F, Fukuda S, Matsumoto K, *et al* (1984) Effect of radiotherapy on dural arteriovenous malformations. Neurol Med Chir 24: 591–599

Correspondence: Juan A. Barcia, M.D., Servicio de Neurocirugía, Hospital Clínico Universitario, Av. Blasco Ibáñez 17, 46010 Valencia, Spain.

Acta Neurochir (1994) [Suppl] 62: 13–17

Radiosurgery Dose Distributions: Theoretical Impact of Inhomogeneities on Lesion Control

L. B. Marks

Departments of Radiation Oncology, Duke University Medical Center, Durham, NC, U.S.A.

Summary

Objective: To develop a mathematical model to predict the impact of dose heterogeneities on tumor/lesion control during radiosurgery. It is necessary to be able to estimate these effects in order to quantitatively and objectively assess competing treatment plans.

Methods: Target cells are assumed to be uniformly distributed throughout the lesion. The control rate for the entire lesion is assumed to be the product of the control probabilities for each subregion within the target volume. The lesion control probability (LCP) for each region is assumed to equal EXP (the number of surviving target cells within the subregion), as predicted by Poisson statistics. Subregions of variable size are assumed to receive variable doses, and the impact of this dose heterogeneity on the LCP is calculated based on the single-fraction radiation cell survival curve predicted by the single-hit multitarget model.

Results: The impact of a dose heterogeneity on LCP is related to three variables: the LCP predicted with uniform irradiation, the volume of the lesion that is irradiated to a new dose, and the magnitude of the dose change relative to the slope of the single-fraction radiation cell survival curve of ($\Delta D/D_0$). The calculations predict that the detrimental effect of underdosing regions of the lesion can, in some instances, be offset by escalating the dose to other subregions within the target volume. In this regard, the "average" dose delivered to the lesion rather than the minimum dose may be most predictive of the lesion control probability. In some situations, escalating the dose to part of the lesion may improve the lesion control rate.

Conclusion: These calculations quantify the theoretical impact of dose heterogeneities on lesion control rate and may be very useful when comparing competing treatment plans.

Keywords: Radiosurgery, treatment planning; dose heterogeneity.

Introduction

During radiosurgery, it is generally considered advantageous to irradiate the target volume with as uniform a dose distribution as possible[6,7,13]. While dose heterogeneities may be associated with an increased risk of normal tissue complications[5], their impact on tumor/ malformation control is not clear. In this article, a series of idealized calculations are presented to estimate the therapeutic implications of dose heterogeneities within the target volume during single-fraction radiosurgery.

Methods

An idealized lesion (tumor or vascular malformation) is assumed to contain M target cells that need to be damaged to control the lesion. For tumors, these target cells are tumor clonogens that need to be sterilized while the likely target cells for vascular malformations are vascular endothelial cells. The target cells are assumed to be uniformly distributed throughout the lesion and to be of uniform radiation sensitivity.

Radiation sensitivity is described by the single-hit multitarget model of cell kill where the fraction of target cells that survive a single dose of radiation (D) is given as[11]:

$$SF = \text{Surviving Fraction} = 1 - (1 - e^{-D/D_0})^N \qquad (1)$$

A typical survival curve is shown in Fig. 1. D_0 describes the straight portion of the cell survival curve and is the dose required to kill 63% $(1 - 1/e)$ of cells. N is the *y*-intercept of the survival curve extrapolated back to the *y* axis. In the straight portion of the cell survival curve, where $D/D_0 \gg 1$, the equation reduces to:

$$SF = N e^{-D/D_0} \qquad (1a)$$

The multitarget model of cell kill is used rather than the linear quadratic model since the multitarget model well describes the straight, or high-dose, region of the cell survival curve that is most relevant to radiosurgery[11].

For any lesion containing M target cells, the lesion control probability (LCP) following a radiosurgery treatment yielding a surviving fraction = SF is predicted by Poisson statistics to be[1,11]:

$$LCP_M = e^{-M \cdot SF} \qquad (2)$$

For any subvolume within the lession containing m target cells,

$$LCP_m = e^{-m \cdot SF} \qquad (3)$$

For uniform irradiation, the SF is the same throughout the lesion and,

$$LCP_m = LCP_M^{m/M} \qquad (4)$$

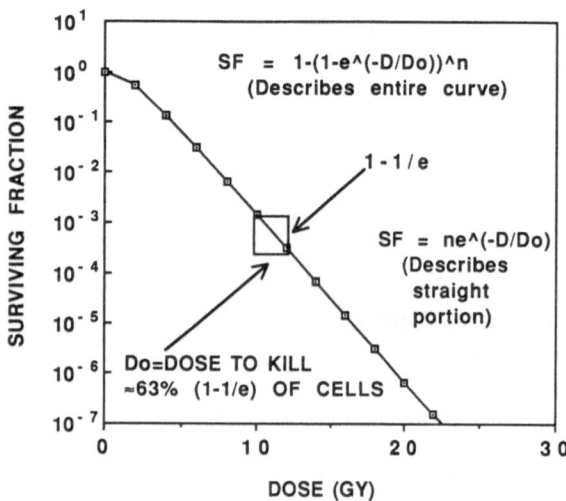

Fig. 1. The single fraction cell survival curve predicted by the multitarget model of cell kill (see text). D_0 describes the slope of the straight portion of the cell survival curve

Considering the entire lesion to be made up of multiple (i) subvolumes,

$$LCP_M = \prod^i LCP_{m_i} \qquad (5)$$

Consider the situation of heterogeneous dose delivery where one subvolume (m) receives a dose of D_2, while the remainder of the lesion is uniformly irradiation at D_1. The new LCP (denoted by subscript$_2$) is related to the LCP with uniform irradiation (denoted by subscript$_1$) by

$$\frac{LCP_{M_2}}{LCP_{M_1}} = \frac{LCP_{m_2}}{LCP_{m_1}} \qquad (6)$$

Rewriting Eq. 3 for this situation, and using the same subscript designations and rearranging,

$$LCP_{m_2} = e^{-m \cdot SF_2} \qquad (7)$$
$$= e^{-m \cdot SF_1(SF_2/SF_1)} \qquad (7a)$$
$$= [e^{-m \cdot SF_1}]^{(SF_2/SF_1)} \qquad (7b)$$
$$= [LCP_{m_1}]^{SF_2/SF_1} \qquad (7c)$$
$$= [LCP_{m_1}]^{e^{-(D_2-D_1)/D_0}} \qquad (7d)$$

By substituting into Eqs. 4 and 6, and denoting $D_2 - D_1$ as ΔD,

$$\frac{LCP_{M_2}}{LCP_{M_1}} = \frac{LCP_{m_1}^{e^{-\Delta D/D_0}}}{LCP_{m_1}} = [LCP_{m_1}]^{e^{-\Delta D/D_0}-1} \qquad (8)$$

$$LCP_{M_2} = [LCP_{M_1}][LCP_{m_1}]^{e^{-\Delta D/D_0}-1} \qquad (8a)$$

$$= [LCP_{M_1}][LCP_{M_1}^{m/M}]^{e^{-\Delta D/D_0}-1} \qquad (8b)$$

The predicted LCP with a heterogeneous dose distribution (LCP_{M_2}) is related to the LCP with a uniform dose (LCP_{M_1}), the ratio m/M (percent of the lesion that is either hot or cold), and the degree to which the dose fluctuates from the uniform dose ($\Delta D/D_0$).

Calculations are presented for a variety of clinical situations where the LCP_{M_1} is 20, 50, and 80% with uniform irradiation. The m/M is varied between 0 and 1. A wide range of values for $\Delta D/D_0$ are considered.

Results

The results of the calculations are shown in Figs. 2. and 3. In Fig. 2, the relative lesion control rate with heterogeneity/without heterogeneity (LCP_{M_2}/LCP_{M_1}) is shown for the various clinical situations. In Fig. 3, the absolute lesion control rate (LCP_{M_2}) is displayed. The highest and lowest values of $\Delta D/D_0$ shown are 4 and -4, respectively. There are minimal changes in the curves beyond ± 4.

The curves are interpreted as follows. Consider the situation where $TCP_{M_1} = 50\%$ (panel B is Figs. 2 and 3). If 20% of the lesion (m/M = 20%) is underdosed by one D_0, the LCP falls to an absolute value $\approx 40\%$ (as

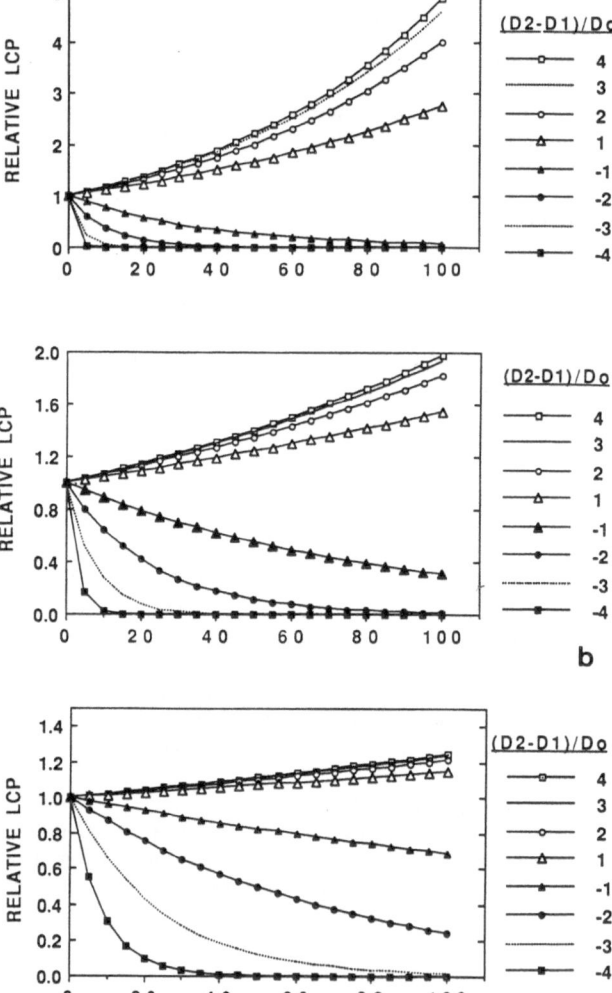

Fig. 2. Calculated results of the model are graphically shown. The relative control rate (with heterogeneity/without heterogeneity, LCP_{M_2}/LCP_{M_1}) is shown for the three clinical situations where $LCP_{M_1} = 20$, 50, and 80%, respectively, in panels a, b and c. Eight values of $\Delta D/D_0$ are shown varying from -4 to 4. Negative values are cold spots (underdosage) and positive values are hot spots (overdosage). Values beyond ± 4 show minimal further changes

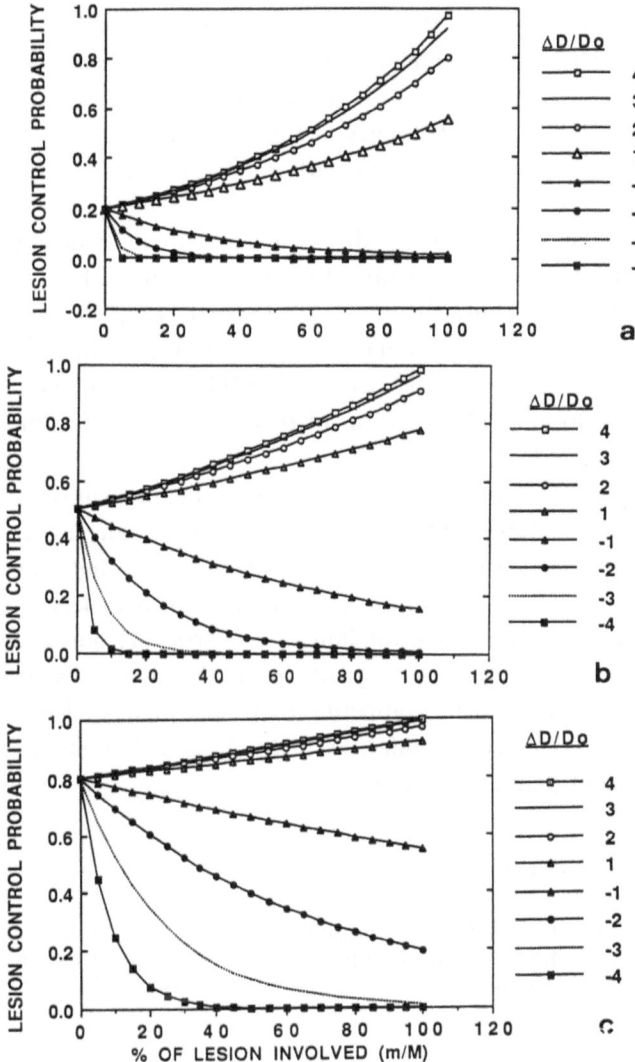

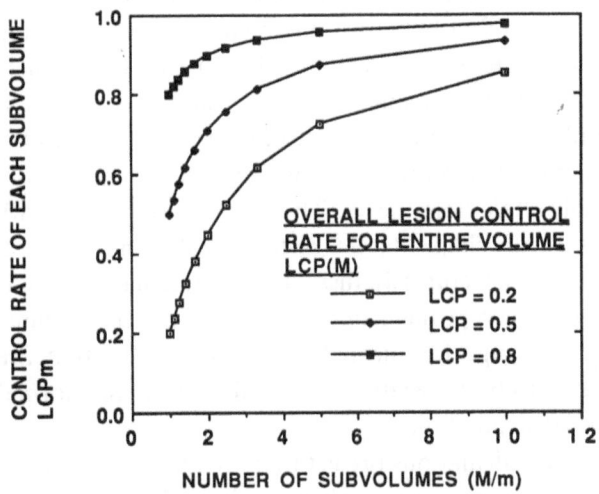

Fig. 4. The subregion control probability (LCP_{m_1}) as a function of the size of the subvolume (m/M) and the overall lesion control rate (LCP_{M_1}). See Eqs. 4 and 8A

Fig. 3. Calculated results of the model are graphically shown. The absolute control rate with heterogeneity is shown for the three clinical situations where $LCP_{M_1} = 20, 50,$ and 80%, respectively, in panels a, b, and c. Eight values of $\Delta D/D_0$ are shown varying from -4 to 4. Negative values are cold spots (underdosage) and positive values are hot spots (overdosage). Values beyond ± 4 show minimal further changes

shown in Fig. 3b). In a relative sense, the new control rate is 80% of the initial rate (40/50 = 0.8), as shown in Fig. 2b. This detrimental effect may be offset by escalating the dose to other regions in the target. In the same example, increasing the dose to ≈ 30% of the lesion by ≈ two D_0's , or to ≈ 40% of the lesion by one D_0, will increase the LCP by ≈ 20% ($LCP_{M_2}/LCP_{M_1} = 1.2$, see Fig. 2b). This type of "hot spot" can offset the above mentioned "cold spot" as $0.8 \times 1.2 \approx 1.0$.

The graphical results shown are explained by reviewing Eq. 8. The relative LCP (LCP_{M_2}/LCP_{M_1}) depends on both the initial control rate of the subvolume of interest (LCP_{m_1}) and the magnitude of the dose change

relative to $D_0 (\Delta D/D_0)$. As the absolute value of $\Delta D/D_0$ increases, LCP_{M_2}/LCP_{M_1} deviates farther from 1.0. The initial value of LCP_m depends on both the overall LCP_M and the size of the subvolume (m/M), as shown in Eq. 4 and Fig. 4. LCP_m increases rapidly as the size of the involved regions decreases (as m/M decreases and the number of subvolumes increases). The initial value of LCP_m and its location on a "typical" dose-response curve determines how sensitive the subvolume is to changes in its dose. For example, if a subregion has an LCP_{m_1} that is very high, higher doses in that region are not likely to have any impact upon the overall lesion control probability, since the lesion control rate in this volume is already very high. However, in this same instance, a reduction in dose to this region can cause a reduction in the LCP_{m_1}. In other words, when LCP_{m_1} is high, there is not much room for it to go up, but there is ample room for it to go down. Alternatively, if LCP_{m_1} is of intermediate value or low, there can be room for it go either up or down with changes in dose. When LCP_{m_1} approaches 100% (for example when m/M is extremely small) even large changes in dose have only a small impact since LCP_{m_1} is on the flat asymptotic portion of the dose-response curve. This is shown in Figs. 2 and 3, where when m/M is very small, the relative lesion control rate is very close to 1 at all values of $\Delta D/D_0$.

Discussion

The calculations presented suggest that dose uniformity within the target volume is not always necessary.

The detrimental effects of small, underdosed regions may be offset by overdosing regions elsewhere within the lesion. There are some clinical situations where the delivery of a uniform dose to the target volume is only possible if the dose of radiation delivered to the surrounding normal brain is increased beyond a clinically "tolerable" level. This is often the case with unusually shaped targets or targets adjacent to critical normal structures. In these situations, it may be preferable to accept the heterogeneity within target volume in exchange for the reduced toxicity risks that are likely to be associated with a reduction in the normal tissue irradiation.

The calculations predict that even in the absence of a cold spot, one can often significantly increase the LCP by escalating the dose to only part of lesion. This approach may be very useful, especially in situations where the expected LCP is not high. For example, when the LCP with a homogeneous dose is 20%, marked increases in LCP are predicted with modest dose escalations to part of the lesion (see Fig. 3).

The impact of dose heterogeneity on the overall lesion control rate (LCP_{M_1}) depends principally on the location of the subregion control rate (LCP_{m_1}) on the typical sigmoidal dose response curve. As shown in Fig. 4 and Eq. 4, LCP_{m_1} depends on both the size of the subvolume involved (m/M) and the overall lesion control probability (LCP_{M_1}). When very small subvolumes are considered (m/M < 0.1), the subregion control rate (LCP_{m_1}) is very high and lies on the "flat" asymptotic portion of the dose-response curve. In these instances, changes in dose, either up or down, to the subregion have minimal effect on the subregion and total lesion control rates. Thus, very small hot and cold spots within the lesion maybe can be ignore when reviewing treatment plans.

The calculations presented are clearly idealized[3,8,12,14]. While the assumption that the target cells are uniformly distributed within the lesion is reasonable for small tumors, it may not be reasonable for larger tumors or arteriovenous malformations. For larger tumors, areas of hypoxia and/or necrosis may not contain viable tumor cells[2,4,9] and, therefore, irradiation of that portion of the lesion may not really be necessary. For arteriovenous malformations, the target cells appear to be the endothelial cells of the feeding arteries and their distribution within the overall lesion is probably not uniform[10]. These calculations also do not consider variations in radiation sensitivity within the target cells[4,14]. If these variations are considered, the overall control rate is determined primarily by the radiation response of the most resistant population of target cells. If these "resistant" cells are uniformly distributed throughout the target volume, then the model is still useful as it applies to this sub-population of target cells. Changes in these assumptions would have quantitatively, but not qualitatively, altered the results.

The variations in dose considered are clinically relevant. Typical values for D_0 are in the $\approx 1-3$ Gy range[12]. Thus, a value of $\Delta D/D_0$ of 1–4 represents a 1–12 Gy dose fluctuation. As typical prescriptions during radiosurgery are 15 to 30 Gy at the 50–90% isodose line, fluctuations of this magnitude are commonly seen.

The various assumptions in the model prevent strict interpretation of the equations. Nonetheless, the model and calculations presented may be useful in that they provide some quantitative estimate as to the effect on the lesion control probability to be expected from dose heterogeneities. This type of information may be useful when comparing competing treatment plans and this mathematical formulation can be integrated into treatment planning programs.

Acknowledgement

Thanks to Jane Hoppenworth for her skillful assistance in the preparation of this manuscript. Dr. Marks is the recipient of an American Cancer Society Career Development Award, #92-53.

References

1. Fletcher GH (1980) Textbook of radiotherapy, 3rd Ed. Lea and Febiger, Philadelphia
2. Koutcher JA, Okunieff P, Neuringer L, Suit H, Phil D, Brady T (1987) Size dependent changes in tumor phosphate metabolism after radiation therapy as detected by ^{31}P NMR spectroscopy. Int J Radiat Oncol Biol Phys 13: 1851–1855
3. Malaise EP, Firtil B, Chavaudra N, Guichard M (1986) Distribution of radiation sensitivities for human tumor cells of specific histologic types: Comparison of in vitro and in vivo data. Int J Radiat Oncol Biol Phys 12: 617–624
4. Moulder JE (1984) Hypoxic fractions of solid tumors experimental techniques, methods of analysis, and a survey of existing data. Int J Radiat Oncol Biol Phys 10: 695–712
5. Nedzi LA, Kooky H, Alexander E, III, et al (1991) Variables associated with the development of complications from radiosurgery of intracranial tumors. Int J Radiat Oncol Biol Phys 21: 591–599
6. Podgorsak EB (1982) Physics for radiosurgery with linear accelerators. Neurosurg Clin N Am 3: 9–34
7. Podgorsak Ev, Pike GB, Olivier A, Pla M, Souhami L (1989) Radiosurgery with high energy photon beams: a comparison among techniques. Int J Radiat Oncol Biol Phys 16: 857–865
8. Quiet CA, Weichselbaum RR, Grdina DJ (1991) Variation in radiation sensitivity during the cell cycle of two human squamous cell carcinomas. Int J Radiat Oncol Biol Phys 20: 733–738

9. Rasey JS, Koh WJ, Grierson JR, Grunbaum Z, Krohn KA (1989) Radiolabeled fluoromisonidazole as an imaging agent for tumor hypoxia. Int J Radiat Oncol Biol Phys 17: 985–991

10. Steiner L, Leksell L, Greitz T, Forster DMC, Backlund EO (1972) Sterotactic radiosurgery for cerebral arteriovenous malformations. Acta Chir Scand 138: 459–464

11. Suit HD, Urano M (1988) Radiation biology for radiation therapy. In: Wang CC (ed) Clinical radiation oncology. PSG, Littleton, pp 17–55

12. Thames HD, Hendry JH (1987) Fraction in radiotherapy. Taylor and Francis, London

13. Wu A (1982) Physics and dosimetry of the gamma knife. Neurosurg Clin N Am 3: 35–50

14. Yaes RJ (1989) Tumor heterogeneity, tumor size, and radioresistance. Int J Radiat Oncol Biol Phys 17: 993–1005

Correspondence: Lawrence B. Marks, M.D., Department of Radiation Oncology, Box 3085, Duke University Medical Center, Durham, NC 27710, U.S.A.

Acta Neurochir (1994) [Suppl] 62: 18–27
© Springer-Verlag 1994

Intrinsic and Extrinsic Characteristics of Human Tumors Relevant to Radiosurgery: Comparative Cellular Radiosensitivity and Hypoxic Percentages*

J. T. Leith[1], **S. Cook**[1], **P. Chougule**[2], **P. Calabresi**[3], **L. Wahlberg**[4], **C. Lindquist**[4], and **M. Epstein**[4]

[1]Radiation Research Laboratories, Department of Radiation Medicine, Brown University, Providence, RI, Departments of [2]Radiation Therapy, [3]Medicine and [4]Neurosurgery, Rhode Island Hospital, Providence, RI, U.S.A.

Summary

We have collected the in vitro x-ray radiation survival characteristics of 181 lines from 12 different classes of exponentially growing human tumor cells (sarcomas, lung cancers, colo-rectal cancers, medulloblastomas, melanoma, breast cancers, prostate cancers, renal cell cancers, grades III and IV brain tumors, ovarian, and head and neck cancers). This information was used to intercompare survival after single high doses of 20–40 Gy for each tumor line. Radiosensitivities could roughly be divided into two groups. The more radiosensitive group included: sarcoma, small-cell lung cancer, non-small cell lung cancer, colorectal cancer, medulloblastoma and melanoma. The more radioresistant group included breast, prostate, renal cell, primary brain tumors, ovarian tumors, and head and neck cancers. Using a model of a 3 cm diameter brain lesion containing about 1.4×10^9 oxic cells, the single doses calculated to reduce survival to 1 cell were: sarcoma and small cell lung cancers – 22–23 Gy; melanoma – 25 Gy; non-small cell lung and colorectal cancer – 26 Gy; medullo-blastoma – 28 Gy; breast, prostate, renal cell, primary brain tumors, ovarian tumors, and head and neck cancers – 30–36 Gy. If, however, tumors contained on average 20 percent hypoxic cells, the dose needed for equivalent cell killing increased by about a factor of 2.6–2.8. Also, there was no correlation between the ranking of relative radiosensitivities of the various classes of tumor cells at high doses (as in radiosurgery) to the sensitivity at low doses (as in conventional fractionated radiotherapy).

Conclusion: available information on the intrinsic radiosensitivity of human tumor cells indicates that meaningful differences exist among different histological classes of neoplasm that are relevant to the single high doses used in radioneurosurgery, and which could constitute a basis for "tailoring" the administered dose to the particular neoplasm. However, if intracerebral lesions contain a large number of hypoxic cells (e.g., 20%), this may constitute a significant problem.

Keywords: Human tumor cell radiosensitivity; lung cancer; medulloblastoma; breast cancer; colorectal cancer; prostate cancer; renal cell cancer; melanoma; central nervous system cancer; ovarian cancer; head and neck cancer; metastases; radiosurgery; hypoxia.

Introduction

About 50% of all intracranial tumors are metastases from systemic disease[19], and the annual number of such cases in the United States is probably greater than 100,000[32]. Mehta et al.[32], and Coia[8] have pointed out that high dose external beam irradiation of metastases can be done using focused multisource isotope units (Gamma knife) or a linear accelerators with multiarc rotation. The most common use of this radiosurgery approach has been for treatment of solitary recurrences in patients who have received previous irradiation for brain metastases, although patients with initial brain metastases have also been treated[8]. Coia[8] notes that increased patient survival would be predicted because of a more effective dose distribution and because administration of high radiation doses should result in increased tumor cell killing. With regard to the success of such a scenario however, two factors deserve analysis. These are, first, the intrinsic radiation sensitivity of a given tumor class, and second, whether significant intratumor hypoxia might exist.

With regard to the first consideration, many publications have compared the radiosensitivities of different classes of human tumor cells at dose levels given in conventional fractionated regimens (e.g., 2 Gy per fraction)[12,13]. However, similar attention has not been given to relative radiosensitivity rankings at high dose levels[28], i.e., in radiosurgery. For example, single doses have ranged from 13–50 Gy, with median doses of 20–30 Gy[14,19,32]. Because of this wide range, we gathered radiation response information for human tumor cell lines of different histological classes to assess whether significant differences exist.

With regard to the second consideration, intratumor

*Research supported by a Grant from the National Cancer Institute 1P20 CA60170.

hypoxia may also play a fundamental role in the success of high dose treatments. Because the chemistry of radiation generated free radicals is different in oxic and hypoxic conditions, hypoxic cells are markedly less sensitive to ionizing radiation than are oxic cells. Therefore high dose radiosurgery might preferentially spare hypoxic cells which will undergo reoxygenation as the oxic, radiation inactivated, cells are cleared, with risk of subsequent regrowth. Therefore, we have gathered existing information on the extent of hypoxia within xenografted human tumors to relate this factor to tumor radiocurability.

We have summarized as much information on the relative radiosensitivity of various classes of human cancer cell lines as possible. Data were available on lung (both small cell and non-small cell lung cancers), sarcoma, colorectal, prostate, renal cell, breast, melanoma, ovarian, head and neck, and primary brain tumors. In this regard, as enumerated by Coia[8] and Egawa *et al.*[11], lung cancer was typically the most frequent primary malignancy (54%), followed by breast (15%), and colo-rectal (6%) cancer. Melanoma or head and neck metastases contributed about 5% or less. In a study by Kihlström *et al.*[19], the percentages of brain metastases were: melanoma-36%, lung-21%, kidney and gastrointestinal-12% each, gynecological 9%, breast-6%, and sarcoma-3%. It should be noted that the radiobiological information that exists on these classes of neoplasms varies greatly in extent. Some classes (e.g., colo-rectal, melanoma, primary brain tumors) are well characterized, while others (breast, renal, prostate cancers) are poorly defined. Radiosensitivity characteristics of primary brain tumor cell lines are included for comparison purposes, and because such cells typically exhibit a high degree of radioresistance.

For purposes of comparison among tumor classes, we have chosen doses of 20–40 Gy, which are in the range of the doses used in radioneurooncology[14,19,32]. A previous publication on the high dose radiation responses of human tumor cells has been published[25] which has addressed many biological concerns involved in proper interpretation of results. However, the current paper includes significant new survival information, and also addresses for the first time, the problem of intratumor hypoxia in high dose radiosurgery.

Methods and Materials

1. Selection of Survival Data

While most data were taken from published information, some unpublished data on melanoma and colo-rectal cancer cells are included. We limited analysis to data on responses of exponentially growing human tumor cells, as data on plateau phase cultures and xenograft tumor radiation responses are not sufficiently extensive to allow histological intercomparisons. For lung cancer, results have been separated into small cell and non-small cell cancers, as there appear to be significant differences in radiosensitivity between the two classes[33].

2. Estimation of Survival at 20–40 Gy

There exist problems in the analysis of high dose radiation responses of human tumor cells. Because in vitro data extend typically only to about 3 logs of cell killing, data must be extrapolated to obtain survival estimates relevant to radiosurgery. A related problem concerns the survival curve formalism chosen for extrapolations. The most frequently used models are the single-hit, multitarget (SHMT) and linear-quadratic (LQ) equations. Because the LQ equation is generally not considered valid below about 1% survival[1], we have used the SHMT formalism, within which three parameters of response are defined: n (extrapolation number) – classically thought to represent the number of "targets" in the cell; D_q(Gy) or quasi-threshold dose – interpreted as representing the ability of the cell to accumulate radiation injury; and D_o(Gy) or the mean lethal dose – interpreted as that amount of dose which produces, on average, one lethal lesion per cell. An equation was generated using SHMT values given by various investigators which was used to determine extrapolated survival at a single doses of 20–40 Gy. From each set of survival data for each class of neoplasm, the mean survival values and SEMs were determined[16]. This calculation represents the putative survival of completely (100%) oxic cells within a neoplasm.

3. Levels of Intratumor Hypoxia

Levels of intratumor hypoxia were taken from published experimental studies. Two types of information are availabe. The first is data from experiments in which irradiated tumors are excised and disaggregated into single cells with subsequent determination of cell survival in vitro by comparing paired survival curves of anoxic and mixed anoxic/oxic cells[23,24,36]. The second type of information is obtained from microelectrode readings of actual intratumor oxygen tensions within patient solid tumors[45]. Although such information

Table 1. *Radiation Survival Parameters of Human Sarcoma cell Lines in vitro*[a]

No.	Cell line	n	D_q^b(Gy)	D_o(Gy)	S_{20}(%)
1.	STSAR-7	11.8	1.60	0.65	5.09×10^{-11}
2.	STSAR-23	10.4	1.57	0.67	1.13×10^{-10}
3.	STSAR-33	5.6	1.29	0.75	1.47×10^{-9}
4.	STSAR-35	15.0	2.00	0.74	2.75×10^{-9}
5.	STSAR-21	9.5	1.80	0.80	1.32×10^{-8}
6.	STSAR-22	3.6	1.14	0.89	6.26×10^{-8}
7.	STSAR-10	4.5	1.44	0.96	4.04×10^{-7}
8.	STSAR-11	3.7	1.28	0.98	5.06×10^{-7}
9.	STSAR-20	2.5	0.92	1.00	5.12×10^{-7}
10.	STSAR-2	4.6	1.50	0.98	6.34×10^{-7}
11.	STSAR-64	3.6	1.32	1.03	1.32×10^{-6}
12.	STSAR-34	3.4	1.40	1.14	8.16×10^{-6}
13.	STSAR-6	1.5	0.50	1.22	1.15×10^{-5}
14.	STSAR-43	1.3	0.41	1.56	3.48×10^{-4}

[a]All data taken from[47].
[b]D_1 values obtained from the relationship $D_q = \ln n \times D_o$.

is scanty, there are enough data to make the evaluation of the impact of intratumor hypoxia on radiosurgical response important. To estimate the effect of hypoxic cells upon survival, we assumed that the effect of hypoxia within the SHMT fromalism was strictly dose-modifying. That is, that although cells become more resistant in the hypoxic state, the extrapolation number of any given survival curve will remain the same in the oxic and hypoxic conditions. Second, we assumed that ratio of enhancement of cell killing in the oxic versus the hypoxic state was 3 (i.e., an oxygen enhancement ratio of 3), which increases the oxic D_o dose by 3. Third, we assumed an average intratumor level of hypoxia of 20%.

Results

Data for the radiation sensitivities of individual cell lines from 12 different histological classes of human tumors, from the most sensitive to the most resistant, are summarized in Tables 1–12. Survival at a dose of 20 Gy (S_{20}) was used to rank cell lines within these tables. In Table 13, we summarize the group mean values found for n, D_q, D_o, and S_{20}. In Table 13, we have indicated the single doses needed to reduce survival to one surviving cell for the various classes of tumor, for both completely oxic and partially (20%) hypoxic neoplasms. The ratio of doses needed for equivalent cell killing the oxic versus the hypoxic conditions varies by a factor of 2.6–2.8.

In Fig. 1, we plot the mean survival values found for these 12 classes of human tumor cell lines for doses of 20–40 Gy. It is clear that there exist clear differences

Table 2. *Radiation Survival Parameters of Human Small Cell Lung Cancer Cell Lines in vitro*

No.	Cell line	n	D_q[a](Gy)	D_o(Gy)	S_{20}(%)[b]	Ref.
1.	NCI H449	1.1	0.05	0.52	3.05×10^{-15}	33
2.	NCI H249	1.49	0.32	0.80	2.23×10^{-9}	33
3.	HC39	2.19	0.70	0.89	3.85×10^{-8}	10
4.	OH-1[c]	12,738$^{\pm}$	2.97	0.42	3.16×10^{-7}	17
5.	NCI H69	1.32	0.28[d]	1.00	3.22×10^{-7}	7
6.	NCI H187	1.00	0.00	1.10	1.28×10^{-6}	7
7.	HC38	1.82	0.70	1.17	6.75×10^{-6}	10
8.	HX149	1.51	0.49	1.19	7.48×10^{-6}	10
9.	HC12	2.75	1.24	1.23	2.38×10^{-5}	10
10.	NCI H209	1.43	0.49	1.37	6.53×10^{-5}	10
11.	NCI H146	1.08	0.11	1.40	9.04×10^{-5}	10
12.	HC41	1.46	0.60	1.59	5.04×10^{-4}	10
13.	HX149M[e]	2.79	1.83	1.78	3.67×10^{-3}	10

[a] D_q for the data of[7,10,33] determined from the relationship $D_q = \ln n \times D_o$.
[b] Survival at a dose of 20 Gy. Data have been rank ordered from lowest to the highest survival.
[c] Data refer to late-passage OH-1 cells[17].
[d] n determined from the relationship $\ln n = D_q/D_o$.
[e] Described as a variant small-cell carcinoma[10].

Table 3. *Radiation Survival Parameters of Human Non-Small Cell Lung Cancer Cell Lines in vitro*

No.	Cell line	Class[a]	n	D_q(Gy)	D_o(Gy)	S_{20}(%)	Ref.
1.	NCI N417	LC	11.1	1.93	0.80	1.63×10^{-8}	7
2.	NCI H82	LC	5.60	1.57	0.91	1.65×10^{-7}	7
3.	NCI H23	car	2.0	0.67	0.97	2.22×10^{-7}	33
4.	NCI H157	LC	14.0	2.38	0.90	3.13×10^{-7}	33
5.	LX1	car	1.20	0.19	1.14	5.55×10^{-7}	21
6.	NCI H324	car	1.3	0.27	1.04	5.78×10^{-7}	33
7.	NCI H125	car	2.0	0.78	1.13	4.12×10^{-6}	33
8.	Calu-6	LC	1.5	0.53	1.30	3.40×10^{-5}	33
9.	HX148M	M	6.44	2.59	1.39	3.65×10^{-4}	10
10.	HX1417	LC	3.77	1.96	1.48	4.96×10^{-4}	10
11.	HX144	car	1.34	0.53	1.81	2.14×10^{-3}	10
12.	HX148	car	1.99	1.25	1.82	3.29×10^{-3}	10
13.	A549	car	3.0	2.09	1.90	8.05×10^{-3}	33

[a] Histology of individual tumor line: *LC* large cell carcinoma; *car* carcinoma; *M* mixed adenocarcinoma/large-cell carcinoma.

Table 4. *Radiation Survival Parameters of Human Melanoma Cell Lines in vitro*

No.	Cell line	n	D_q(Gy)	D_o(Gy)	S_{20}(%)	Ref.
			Radiation survival parameters			
1.	Mel Tang	4.61	0.88	0.57	3.80×10^{-13}	a
2.	MeWo	7.2	1.32	0.67	7.37×10^{-11}	12
3.	Mel5	2.73	0.73	0.73	3.07×10^{-10}	a
4.	SK-MEL 26	6.28	1.59	0.86	5.76×10^{-8}	44
5.	CAL 1	8.1	2.15	1.03	2.86×10^{-6}	9
6.	CAL 7	6.6	2.02	1.07	5.08×10^{-6}	9
7.	KINOSHITA	2.01	0.80	1.14	5.29×10^{-6}	44
8.	9/19/26-4	40	3.69	1.00	8.28×10^{-6}	3
9.	CAL 4	9.2	2.40	1.08	8.55×10^{-6}	9
10.	19-4	35	3.62	1.02	1.03×10^{-5}	3
11.	Le Ca 39.4	14	2.90	1.10	1.75×10^{-5}	37,42
12.	A375	1.56	0.56	1.25	1.98×10^{-5}	53
13.	HMV	7.0	2.28	1.17	2.70×10^{-5}	18
14.	A875	1.58	0.59	1.29	2.91×10^{-5}	53
15.	Ma 111	7.8	2.46	1.20	4.37×10^{-5}	52
16.	IHARA	2.42	1.26	1.43	1.99×10^{-4}	44
17.	Mel H	4.3	2.04	1.40	2.65×10^{-4}	50
18.	C-143	1.2	0.28	1.51	2.65×10^{-4}	44,47
19.	RPMI-7951	1.6	0.71	1.50	2.84×10^{-4}	29
20.	G361	5.54	2.38	1.39	3.09×10^{-4}	44
21.	Be 211	2.7	1.48	1.49	3.99×10^{-4}	50
22.	Na 11	2.7	1.48	1.49	4.00×10^{-4}	50
23.	SK-MEL 28	4.8	2.90	1.85	9.62×10^{-3}	29
24.	C-32	1.7	1.12	2.11	1.31×10^{-2}	47

[a]J. Leith, unpublished data, September 1993.

Table 5. *Radiation Survival Parameters of Human Colo-Rectal Cancer Cell Lines in vitro*

No.	Cell line	No.[a]	n[b]	D_q(Gy)	D_o(Gy)	S_{20}(%)
			Radiation survival parameter			
1.	SKCO-1	36	1.00(0.51–1.34)	0.00	0.90(0.10)	2.76×10^{-8}
2.	COLO320HSR	28	5.76(2.03–16.3)	1.52	0.87(0.16)	5.41×10^{-8}
3.	SW48	23	2.56(1.42–4.62)	0.90	0.95(0.12)	1.91×10^{-7}
4.	SW480	36	8.98(4.90–16.5)	2.04	0.93(0.11)	3.94×10^{-7}
5.	HCT116	20	4.86(2.91–8.12)	1.54	0.97(0.10)	5.59×10^{-7}
6.	HCT-8	23	5.66(3.44–9.33)	1.72	0.99(0.11)	9.74×10^{-7}
7.	SW620	32	5.02(2.84–8.88)	1.62	0.98(0.12)	1.13×10^{-6}
8.	HCT-15	28	3.25(1.73–6.09)	1.24	1.06(0.15)	1.59×10^{-6}
9.	clone A	28	5.58(3.04–10.2)	1.82	1.06(0.15)	3.39×10^{-6}
10.	LoVo	24	4.31(2.45–7.58)	1.58	1.08(0.14)	4.05×10^{-6}
11.	LS174T	18	2.29(0.67–7.86)	0.93	1.12(0.33)	4.16×10^{-6}
12.	SW948	28	2.49(0.78–7.92)	1.06	1.16(0.33)	7.77×10^{-6}
13.	clone D	28	3.58(2.43–5.26)	1.48	1.16(0.11)	1.20×10^{-5}
14.	DLD-2[b]	19	5.10(2.41–10.2)	1.86	1.14(0.19)	1.25×10^{-5}
15.	GEO	12	2.99(1.93–4.63)	1.29	1.18(0.21)	1.26×10^{-5}
16.	CCL237	16	3.54(1.07–11.3)	1.50	1.19(0.35)	1.71×10^{-5}
17.	CBS	12	3.38(1.84–6.21)	1.46	1.20(0.19)	1.92×10^{-5}
18.	T-84[b]	16	3.62(2.04–6.42)	1.59	1.24(0.26)	3.44×10^{-5}
19.	FET	29	4.12(2.85–5.96)	1.77	1.25(0.11)	4.50×10^{-5}
20.	MOSER	10	3.62(2.03–6.46)	1.82	1.42(0.25)	2.62×10^{-4}
21.	SW403	18	1.27(0.76–2.14)	0.40	1.67(0.32)	7.71×10^{-4}
22.	CACO-2	23	2.46(1.28–4.75)	1.47	1.63(0.38)	1.12×10^{-3}
23.	HT-29	26	1.99(1.11–3.55)	1.21	1.76(0.39)	2.36×10^{-3}
24.	WiDR	42	2.23(1.67–2.99)	1.44	1.16(0.13)	3.31×10^{-3}
25.	SW1116	18	1.13(0.26–4.43)	0.28	2.27(0.64)	1.72×10^{-2}

Data taken from published information on colon tumor cells[22], reanalyzed using single-hit, multitarget equation (DLD-2, GEO, CBS, T-84, and MOSER data have not been previously published).

[a]Indicates the number of determinations used to estimate n, D_o, and D_q.

[b]95% confidence limits on the range of the extrapolation number and on D_o.

Table 6. *Radiation Survival Parameters of Human Medulloblastoma Cell Lines in vitro*

No.	Cell line	n	D_q(Gy)	D_o(Gy)	S_{20}(%)	Ref.
1.	D283MED	3.14	1.01	0.88	4.54×10^{-8}	31
2.	TX-14	1.62	0.63	1.31	3.70×10^{-5}	46
3.	TX-7	1.49	0.54	1.35	5.55×10^{-5}	46
4.	DAOY	3.43	2.33	1.89	8.72×10^{-3}	31

Table 8. *Radiation Survival Parameters of Human Prostate Cancer Cell Lines in vitro*

No.	Cell line	n	D_q(Gy)	D_o(Gy)	S_{20}(%)	Ref.
1.	PC-3	2.84	1.02	1.06	3.67×10^{-7}	24
2.	LNCaP	1.26	0.41	1.80	1.60×10^{-3}	26
3.	DU-145	1.92	1.25	1.91	5.63×10^{-3}	24

Table 7. *Radiation Survival Parameters of Human Breast Cancer Cell Lines in vitro*

No.	Cell line	n	D_q(Gy)	D_o(Gy)	S_{20}(%)	Ref.
1.	B370	13.6	2.53	0.97	1.49×10^{-6}	4
2.	3558	30.0	3.29	0.97	3.15×10^{-6}	4
3.	MCF7	1.3	0.35	1.34	4.01×10^{-5}	46
4.	MDA-231	1.2	0.25	1.35	4.38×10^{-5}	46
5.	B313	2.6	1.52	1.59	9.01×10^{-4}	4
6.	B364	2.7	3.41	3.43	7.97×10^{-1}	4

Table 9. *Radiation Survival Parameters of Human Renal Cell Cancer cell Lines in vitro*

No.	Cell line	n	D_q(Gy)	D_o(Gy)	S_{20}(%)	Ref.
7.	PAS	1.20	0.24	1.31	3.02×10^{-5}	47
6.	RS	1.15	0.20	1.42	9.79×10^{-5}	27
1.	ACHN	4.33	1.92	1.31	1.01×10^{-4}	39
2.	Caki-1	2.14	1.12	1.48	2.69×10^{-4}	39
3.	A-704	1.64	1.76	1.53	3.64×10^{-4}	39
8.	T1	4.20	2.11	1.46	5.20×10.4	5
4.	A498	1.42	0.72	2.08	8.36×10^{-3}	39
5.	RR	1.91	1.51	2.35	3.62×10^{-2}	27

Table 10. *Radiation Survival Parameters of Human Brain Tumor Cell Lines in vitro*

No.	Cell line	Class[a]	n	D_q(Gy)	D_o(Gy)	S_{20}(%)	Ref.
1.	D54MG	GBM	10.5	2.47	1.05	5.66×10^{-6}	41
2.	HGL16	GBM	5.5	1.88	1.10	7.32×10^{-6}	41
3.	A2	GBM	5.28	1.85	1.11	8.14×10^{-6}	15
4.	IN 1265	AST3	31.5	3.76	1.09	3.38×10^{-5}	51
5.	G1	AST3	2.7	1.26	1.27	3.83×10^{-5}	41
6.	MMC2	GBM	4.5	1.94	1.29	8.30×10^{-5}	41
7.	TX-13	GBM	1.36	0.44	1.43	1.16×10^{-4}	46
8.	G9	GBM	5.6	2.24	1.30	1.17×10^{-4}	41
9.	U251MG	GBM	2.8	1.43	1.39	1.56×10^{-4}	41
10.	IN 859	AST3	6.25	2.42	1.32	1.65×10^{-4}	54
11.	KNS-42	GBM	1.7	0.77	1.45	1.76×10^{-4}	30
12.	KNS-60	GBM	1.30	0.39	1.50	1.86×10^{-4}	30
13.	HGL9	GBM	6.01	2.49	1.39	3.33×10^{-4}	41
14.	HGL4	GBM	1.2	0.29	1.58	4.16×10^{-4}	41
15.	G25	AST3	1.9	0.99	1.55	4.43×10^{-4}	41
16.	A2	AST3	6.70	2.68	1.41	4.59×10^{-4}	15
17.	A3	AST4	11.7	3.39	1.38	5.83×10^{-4}	15
18.	A7	GBM	14.9	3.78	1.56	9.23×10^{-4}	15
19.	U-87MG	GBM	6.8	2.84	1.48	9.33×10^{-4}	35
20.	MMC1	GBM	3.1	1.78	1.57	9.36×10^{-4}	41
21.	A7	GBM	5.9	2.77	1.56	1.60×10^{-3}	15
22.	T98G	GBM	8.3	3.41	1.61	3.38×10^{-3}	41
23.	HGL5	GBM	2.72	1.60	1.60	1.01×10^{-3}	41
24.	HGL13	GBM	8.3	3.15	1.49	1.21×10^{-3}	41
25.	HGL12	GBM	3.7	2.20	1.68	2.53×10^{-3}	41
26.	HGL11	GBM	4.1	2.40	1.70	3.21×10^{-3}	41
27.	U-118-MG	GBM	4.7	2.63	1.70	3.63×10^{-3}	34
28.	WF	GBM	2.3	1.60	1.92	6.92×10^{-3}	41
29.	EO1	olig	2.73	1.95	1.94	9.17×10^{-3}	41
30.	U-87MG	olig	1.4	0.76	2.25	1.99×10^{-2}	41
31.	SB	AST3	1.46	0.82	2.18	1.43×10^{-2}	54
32.	U251MG	GBM	4.0	3.12	2.25	5.53×10^{-2}	41
33.	G19	GBM	1.77	1.63	2.86	1.61×10^{-1}	41

[a]*GBM* glioblastoma multiforme; *AST3* astrocytoma grade 3/4; *olig* oligodendroglioma grade 3[41].

Table 11. *Radiation Survival Parameters of Human Ovarian Cancer Cell Lines in vitro*[a]

No.	Cell line	n	D_b[b](Gy)	D_o(Gy)	S_{20}(%)
1.	OVC-102	1.3	0.28	1.05	9.44×10^{-7}
2.	OVC-52	1.3	0.29	1.10	1.80×10^{-6}
3.	DOVC-1	2.0	0.83	1.20	1.12×10^{-5}
4.	OVC-106	1.5	0.57	1.40	9.94×10^{-5}
5.	OVC-1	1.6	0.74	1.57	4.87×10^{-4}
6.	OVC-105	1.4	0.54	1.60	5.42×10^{-4}
7.	OVC-73	1.5	0.65	1.60	5.73×10^{-4}
8.	OVC-100	1.5	0.70	1.65	1.40×10^{-3}
9.	OVC-50	1.4	0.62	1.85	2.71×10^{-3}
10.	OVC-77	1.4	0.71	2.10	1.07×10^{-2}
11.	OVC-2	1.1	0.21	2.20	1.26×10^{-2}
12.	OVC-62	1.6	1.03	2.20	1.74×10^{-2}
13.	OVC-23	1.8	1.37	2.33	3.38×10^{-2}
14.	OVC-44	1.7	1.27	2.40	3.99×10^{-2}

[a]All data taken from[51].
[b]D_q values determined from $D_q = (\ln n)(D_o)$.

in radiosensitivity among the various classes, and that this differential is preserved as doses increase from 20 to 40 Gy (i.e., as survival decreases).

In Fig. 2, we plot the calculated doses needed to reduce survival to one cell assuming a lesion of 3 cm diameter containing 1.4×10^9 cells. The closed triangles

Table 12. *Radiation Survival Parameters of Human Head and Neck Cell Lines in vitro*[a]

No.	Cell line	n	D_q[b](Gy)	D_o(Gy)	S_{20}(%)
1.	SCC-73	1.2	0.20	1.08	1.10×10^{-6}
2.	SCC-61	1.8	0.63	1.07	1.38×10^{-6}
3.	SCC-13	2.1	0.95	1.28	3.46×10^{-5}
4.	SCC-66	2.1	0.96	1.29	3.88×10^{-5}
5.	SCC-9	1.4	0.45	1.34	4.63×10^{-5}
6.	SCC-25	1.5	0.58	1.42	1.15×10^{-4}
7.	SQ-9G	1.4	0.49	1.46	1.56×10^{-4}
8.	SQ-38	1.8	0.85	1.46	2.02×10^{-4}
9.	SQ-43	2.0	1.01	1.46	2.25×10^{-4}
10.	SCC-71	1.5	0.65	1.60	5.62×10^{-4}
11.	SCC-4	1.5	0.68	1.69	1.08×10^{-3}
12.	SCC-4	1.6	0.80	1.70	1.24×10^{-3}
13.	SQ-29	1.6	0.81	1.73	1.52×10^{-3}
14.	SCC-50	1.3	0.47	1.79	1.84×10^{-3}
15.	SCC-35	1.6	0.86	1.84	3.05×10^{-3}
16.	HN-SCC-28	1.0	0.00	1.96	3.71×10^{-3}
17.	HN-SCC-68	2.8	1.87	1.82	4.62×10^{-3}
18.	SCC-76	1.5	0.80	1.97	5.86×10^{-3}
19.	SQ-39	1.0	0.00	2.13	8.38×10^{-3}
20.	SQ-31	1.4	0.76	2.26	1.98×10^{-2}
21.	SQ-20B	1.4	0.80	2.39	3.24×10^{-2}
22.	HN-SCC-131	1.3	0.66	2.50	4.36×10^{-2}
23.	HN-SCC-29	2.4	2.04	2.33	4.49×10^{-2}
24.	JSQ-3	1.7	1.40	2.63	8.48×10^{-2}

[a]All data taken from[51]
[b]D_q values not given by authors: determined from $D_q = (\ln n)(D_o)$.

Table 13. *Summary of Single-Hit, Multitarget Survival parameters for Various Class of Human Tumor Cells*

Tumor class	N[a]	n[b]	D_q (Gy)	D_o (Gy)	S_{20}(%) (Oxic)	D_{3cm}[d] (oxic, Gy)	D_{3cm} (hypoxic, Gy)
Sarcomas	14	4.55(3.74–5.53)	1.30(0.12)	0.96(0.07)	$1.1 \times 10^{-7}(3.4 \times 10^{-8}–3.8 \times 10^{-7})$	20.4	52.4
Small cell lung cancer	12[c]	1.57(1.43–1.73)	0.57(0.15)	1.22(0.08)	$1.0 \times 10^{-6}(1.3 \times 10^{-7}–7.9 \times 10^{-6})$	22.8	64.8
Melanoma	24	4.64(3.83–5.61)	1.74(0.20)	1.22(0.07)	$8.2 \times 10^{-6}(2.6 \times 10^{-6}–2.6 \times 10^{-5})$	25.3	66.9
Non-small cell lung cancer	13	3.00(2.38–3.77)	1.29(0.23)	1.28(0.10)	$1.2 \times 10^{-5}(3.3 \times 10^{-6}–4.0 \times 10^{-5})$	26.0	67.3
Colo-rectal	25	3.20(2.78–3.56)	1.34(0.10)	1.21(0.06)	$1.2 \times 10^{-5}(6.2 \times 10^{-6}–2.5 \times 10^{-5})$	26.1	68.5
Medullo-blastoma	4	2.26(1.82–2.81)	1.13(0.41)	1.36(0.21)	$3.0 \times 10^{-5}(2.5 \times 10^{-6}–3.7 \times 10^{-4})$	27.6	73.2
Breast	6	4.06(2.38–6.93)	1.89(0.57)	1.61(0.38)	$1.4 \times 10^{-4}(2.0 \times 10^{-5}–1.0 \times 10^{-3})$	30.2	77.8
Prostate	3	1.90(1.50–2.40)	0.89(0.25)	1.59(0.27)	$1.5 \times 10^{-4}(7.2 \times 10^{-6}–3.1 \times 10^{-3})$	30.9	86.0
Renal	8	1.98(1.65–2.38)	2.07(2.06)	1.62(0.14)	$5.1 \times 10^{-4}(2.2 \times 10^{-4}–1.2 \times 10^{-3})$	33.4	87.0
Primary brain tumors	33	4.01(3.51–4.60)	2.03(0.17)	1.57(0.07)	$6.2 \times 10^{-4}(4.1 \times 10^{-4}–1.0 \times 10^{-3})$	33.8	90.0
Ovarian	14	1.49(1.43–1.55)	0.70(0.09)	1.73(0.12)	$6.7 \times 10^{-4}(2.6 \times 10^{-4}–1.7 \times 10^{-3})$	34.9	93.6
Head and neck	24	1.57(1.50–1.65)	0.78(0.10)	1.76(0.09)	$8.8 \times 10^{-4}(4.7 \times 10^{-4}–1.6 \times 10^{-3})$	35.6	95.9

[a]Indicates the number of survival curves analyzed (see Tables 1–12).
[b]Values in parentheses are SEMs.
[c]The data on the OH-1 line (Table 2) have been omitted in the calculation of n, D_o, and S_{20} (percent survival at a dose of 20 Gy).
[d]Dose needed to reduce survival to one cell in either completely oxic or partially hypoxic tumors based on the average radiosensitivity parameters of a 3 cm neoplasm containing 1.4×10^9 cells.

The value of 20% was calculated as the mean of the experimental values of hypoxia established by either clonogenic assay or by oxygen tension measurements by microelectrode[10,23,36,45]. The value of 20% was obtained as the unweighted mean hypoxic percentage of the logs of values reported for SCLC (23.4%)[10], NSCLC (46.4%)[10], colon cancer (10.4%)[23], prostate cancer (19.4%)[23], melanoma (28.9%)[36], ovarian cancer (14.1%)[36], and breast cancer (18%)[45].

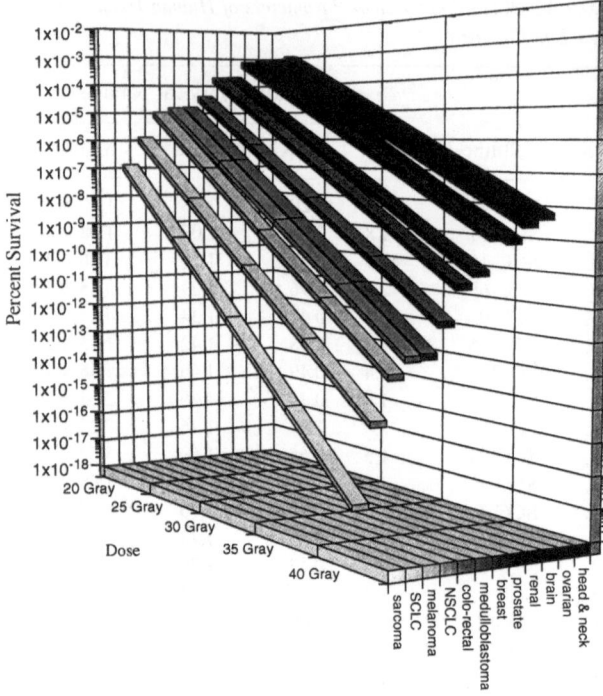

Fig. 1. Plot of the mean survival of exponentially growing human tumor cells at single doses of 20–40 Gy for various neoplastic classes

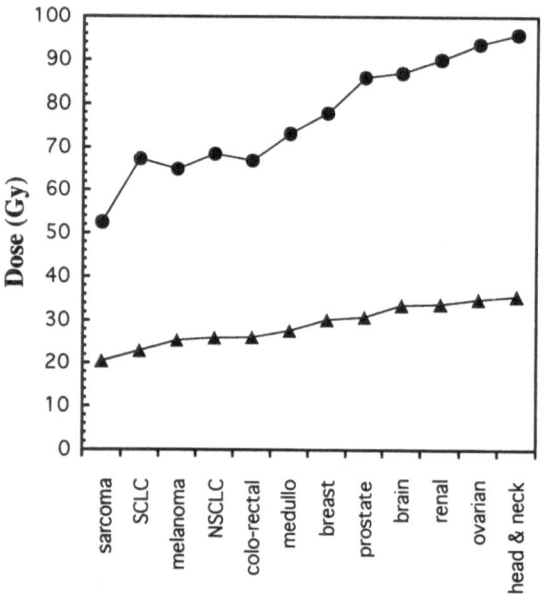

Fig. 2. Estimated single doses needed to reduce survival to one cell for model neoplasms of 3 cm diameter containing 1.4×10^9 clonogenic cells. The closed triangles represent doses for completely oxic neoplasms of various histological classes, while the closed circles represent doses required if the tumors contained 20% hypoxic cells

represent responses assuming that all cells within the neoplasm are oxic, while the closed circles represent equivalent doses that are needed if, on average, 20% of the tumor cells are hypoxic at the time of irradiation.

Discussion

The primary findings of this work are illustrated in Fig. 1, where, using doses of 20–40 Gy for comparison, we show that there are marked differences in the radiosensitivity of the 12 different classes of human cancer cells. In Table 13, we have listed the relative survival of the various tumor classes. In order, using the mean survival at 20 Gy, the qualitative ranking of neoplastic classes from radiosensitive to radioresistant is: *sarcoma > small cell lung cancer > melanoma ≥ non-small cell carcinomas ≥ colorectal > medulloblastoma > breast ≥ prostate > renal ≥ primary brain tumors ≥ ovarian ≥ head & neck*. From the most sensitive tumor class (sarcomas), there is a difference of 3–4 log units to the most resistant tumor class (head and neck cancers).

The large variation in radiosensitivity within a given class of tumor occurs for two resons. First, because limited data exist on the radiosensitivity of certain tumor classes (e.g., small cell lung cancer, breast cancer) and second, because even in situations where there is extensive experimental information (e.g., colon cancer and primary brain tumors), significant heterogeneity in response within tumor classes exists (i.e., there is a large variation in intrinsic radiosensitivity). More experimental data are needed for rigorous definition of the variability in tumor cell radiosensitivity as a function of histological class (e.g., breast cancers). Regardless, it is clear that class specific differences in radiosensitivity exist at the high dose levels reported herein, although the biological reasons for these differences in radiation sensitivity are unknown. For these high dose data, the parameter predicting relative radioresistance is the D_o value (Table 13), which shows a statistically significant correlation with S_{20} (cc = 0.945, p < 0.05)[16]. It is also important to point out that there is no correlation *between the radiosensitivity of tumor classes at low doses and radiosensitivity at high doses*. The estimated survival at 20 Gy may be used to rank order the relative sensitivities of tumor classes. This ranking may then be compared using the non-parametric signed-rank test[41], to the relative low dose sensitivity of these tumor classes obtained using the mean quasi-threshold dose (D_q) listed in Table 13. The result indicates a non-significant correlation between the two rankings ($p > 0.20$). To restate, there is no correlation between high and low dose radiosensitivity, or *relative radiation resistance seen at low doses, as in conventional fractionated radiotherapy, can not necessarily be used to predict the high dose responses of tumor cells in radiosurgery.*

The overall rationale for this work was to determine first, if any significant differences in high dose radiation sensitivity existed among various tumor classes, and second, if there were, how might these estimates be used as guides in stereotactic neuroradiosurgery? The first part of this question has been answered above. In regard to the second part of this question, consider the results of Egawa *et al.*[11], which indicate that the incidence of types of brain metastases as a percent of the total number of metastases were: lung (small cell) = 7.6%, sarcomas = 1.9%, lung (non-small cell) = 45.8%, colo-rectal = 4.2%, breast = 10.6%, melanoma = 1.1%, and head and neck = 1.5% (the remaining 27.3% of metastases were of other varied histologies). In the work of Kilström *et al.*[18], the most frequent type of metastases to brain was melanoma. It is interesting that the lung cancers (both SC and NSCLC) and melanoma, lie on the more radiosensitive side of the spectrum as illustrated by the data presented in Fig. 1. These results raise the issue of whether dose should be "tailored" to the metastasis. In this regard, doses given to brain metastases vary considerably, i.e., from 13 to 50 Gy, with median doses of about 20–30 Gy[14,19,32]. From review of the literature, it appears that the choice of the doses was based primarily on considerations of tumor volume, although the logic of how doses were chosen, is not discussed in detail. To emphasize the importance of the relationship between dose, intrinsic radiosensitivity, and tumor volume, Coia[8] notes that "dimensions of brain metastases are rarely reported in the literature", and cites data taken from Smalley *et al.*[38] who indicated that, in patients with single metastases, 41% were less than or equal to 3 cm diameter, while 53% were greater than 3 cm diameter (6% were of unknown size). In patients studied by Kihlström *et al*[19], volumes varied from 0.3 to 15 cm^3, with mean and median volumes of 5.8 and 3.5 cm^3 (diameters of 2.2 and 1.9 cm respectively). In a study by Mehta *et al.*[32], the mean tumor volumes and diameters were 5.2 cm^3 and 2.15 cm.

Consider for modeling purposes, a spherical brain lesion of 3 cm diameter (volume approximately 14 cm^3). Data from many studies of disaggregated solid tumors yield typical values of about 10^8 clonogenic cells/gram (e.g.[20,23,24]). Therefore, for such a lesion, there would be about 1.4×10^9 clonogenic cells. To cure, sufficient dose must be given to reduce the percentage of surviving cells to 7.14×10^{-8} or less-*given that neoplasms contain no hypoxic cells. If hypoxia exists, the required doses will be higher.* The SHMT values summarized in Table 13 may be used to generate the level of dose used in single fraction to produce sufficient cell killing, and these doses are listed in Table 13 (D_{3cm}, Gy). Only for sarcomas and small cell lung cancers would a dose of 20 Gy provide roughly sufficient cell killing for an oxic tumor of 3 cm diameter. Needed doses range from about 20 Gy for sarcomas to 33–36 Gy for more resistant tumors such as renal, ovarian, head and neck metastases, or primary brain tumors. If however, tumors contained on average 20% hypoxic cells, then the required doses increase to 52.4 Gy for sarcomas, and 87.0–95.9 Gy for the more resistant tumor types. Several comments can be made with respect to this potential problem of intratumor hypoxia in the radioneurosurgical setting. First, with the exception of work done on the 9L gliosarcoma rat brain tumor model[20], there exist no data on the hypoxic status of intracerebral neoplasms, a lack of information that has forced us to use information on peripherally located solid human tumors. More baseline information is needed in this regard. Second, clinical responses after single high dose radioneurosurgery appear to be more positive than results that would be predicted from an assumption of 20% tumor hypoxia (Wahlberg, unpublished data, 1993) which suggests that intratumor hypoxia may not be as bad a problem as postulated. Clinical information indicates for example, that intracerebral melanoma appears to be responding well to doses used in radiosurgery (Kihlström, unpublished data presented at the 1st International Conference on Stereotactic Neurosurgery, Stockholm, Sweden, June, 1993). Given that peripherally located melanoma typically exhibits high average levels of hypoxia, on the order of 30%[37], such good responses would not have been predicted. These results raise an intriguing possibility. Perhaps intratumor levels of hypoxia are less for lesions growing intracerebrally then for lesions growing peripherally. The local micro-environment (e.g., levels of angiogenic growth factors) might be significantly different for intracerebral versus peripheral neoplasms, leading to a differential expression of intratumor hypoxia. This is an experimentally testable hypothesis, relevant to optimal use of radiosurgery. Related to the overall considerations of the problems of differential intrinsic radiosensitivity and intratumor hypoxia, combined modality therapy could be considered for all situations in which the more resistant metastases are to be treated (e.g., prostate, renal, ovarian, head and neck – Table 13). In this regard, agents that modify the slope (D_o) of the survival curve should be of particular interest (e.g., bleomycin, 5-fluorouracil, taxol)[2,43]. Conversely, rather than sensitizing tumor cells to ionizing radiation, it might be possible to administer an agent such as WR-2721, which could protect normal tissue. Lastly, if intratumor hypoxia proves to be a significant clinical problem, then radiosensitizing agents[6] could be administered.

References

1. Alper T (1980) Survival curve models. In: Meyn RE, Withers HR (eds) Radiation biology in cancer research. Raven, New York, pp 3–18
2. Bellamy AS, Hill BT (1984) Interactions between clinically effective antitumor drugs and radiation in experimental systems. Biochim Biophys Acta 738: 125–166
3. Barranco SC, Romsdahl MM, Humphrey RM (1971) The radiation response of human malignant melanoma cells grown in vitro. Cancer Res 31: 830–833
4. Besch GJ, Tanner MA, Sattler CA, Wolberg WH, Howard SP, Gould MN (1986) Radiation survival of human mammary carcinoma cells: criteria for an agar-based clonogenic assay. Int J Radiat Oncol Biol Phys 12: 75–81
5. Blakely EA, Tobias CA, Yang TCH, Smith KC, Lyman JT (1979) Inactivation of human kidney cells by high-energy monoenergetic heavy-ion beams. Radiat Res 80: 122–160
6. Brown JM, Lemmon MJ (1991) SR 4233 – a tumour specific radiosensitizer active in fractionated radiation regimes. Radiother Oncol 20: 151–156
7. Carney DN, Mitchell JB, Kinsella TJ (1983) In vitro radiation and chemotherapy sensitivity of established cell lines of human small cell lung cancer and its large cell morphological variants. Cancer Res 43: 2806–2811
8. Coia LR (1992) The role of radiation therapy in the treatment of brain metastases. Int J Radiat Oncol Biol Phys 23: 229–238
9. Courdi A, Gioanni J, Lalanne CM, Fischel JL, Schneider M, Ettore F, Lambert JC (1983) Establishment, characterization, and response to cytotoxic and radiation treatment of three human melanoma cell lines. In Vitro 19: 453–461
10. Duchesne GM, Peacock JH, Steel GG (1986) The acute in vitro and in vivo radiosensitivity of human lung tumour lines. Radiother Oncol 7: 353–361
11. Egawa S, Tukiyama I, Akine Y, Kajiura Y, Yanagawa S, Watai K, Nomura K (1986) Radiotherapy of brain metastases. Int J Radiat Oncol Biol Phys 12: 1621–1625
12. Fertil B, Deschavanne PJ, Lachet B, Malaise EP (1980) In vitro radiosensitivity of six human cell lines. A comparative study with different statistical models. Radiat Res 82: 297–309
13. Fertil B, Dertinger H, Courdi A, Malaise EP (1984) Mean inactivation dose: a useful concept for intercomparison of human cell survival curves. Radiat Res 99: 73–84
14. Fuller BG, Kaplan ID, Adler J, Cox RS, Bagshaw MA (1992) Stereotaxic radiosurgery for brain metastases: the importance of adjuvant whole brain irradiation. Int J Radiat Oncol Biol Phys 23: 413–418
15. Gerweck L, Kornblith P, Burlett P, Wang J, Sweigert S (1977) Radiation sensitivity of cultured human glioblastoma cells. Radiology 125: 231–234
16. Goldstein A (1965) Biostatistics. Academic Press, New York, pp 140–150
17. Goodwin G, Baylin SB (1982) Relationships between neuroendocrine differentiation and sensitivity to γ-radiation in culture line OH-1 of human small cell lung carcinoma. Cancer Res 42: 1361–1367
18. Inada T, Kasuga T, Nojiri I, Hiraoka T, Furuse T (1977) Comparative study on radiosensitivities of cultured cell lines derived from several human tumors under hypoxic conditions. Gann 68: 357–362
19. Kihlstrom L, Karlsson B, Lindquist C (1992) Gamma knife surgery in brain metastases. In: Lundsford LD (ed) Stereotactic radiosurgery update. Elsevier, New York, pp 429–434
20. Leith JT, Schilling WA, Wheeler KT (1975) Cellular radiosensitivity of a rat brain tumor. Cancer 35: 1545–1550
21. Leith JT, Dexter DL, De Wyngaert JK, Zeman EM, Chu MY, Calabresi P, Glicksman AS (1982) Differential responses to X-irradiation of subpopulations of two heterogeneous human carcinomas in vitro. Cancer Res 42: 2556–2561
22. Leith JT, Padfield G, Faulkner LE, Quinn P, Michelson S (1991) Effects of feeder cells on the X-ray sensitivity of human colon cancer cells. Radiother Oncol 21: 53–59
23. Leith JT, Padfield G, Faulkner L, Michelson S (1991) Hypoxic fractions in xenografted human colon tumors. Cancer Res 51: 5139–5142
24. Leith JT, Quaranto L, Padfield G, Michelson S, Hercbergs A (1993) Radiobiological studies of PC-3 and DU-145 human prostate cancer cells: x-ray sensitivity in vitro and hypoxic fractions of xenografted tumors in vivo. Int J Radiat Oncol Biol Phys 25: 283–287
25. Leith JT, Cook S, Chougule P, Calabresi P, Lindquist C, Epstein M (1993) Responses of various classes of human tumor cells to high X-ray doses: implications for stereotactic external beam irradiation. Cancer Res Therapy and Control 3: 153–166
26. Leith JT (1993) In vitro Radiation Sensitivity of the LNCaP Prostatic Tumor Cell Line. The Prostate 24: 119–124
27. Leung SW, Mitchell JB, Al-Nabulsi I, Friedman N, Newsome J, Belldegrun A, Kasid U (1993) Effect of L-buthionine sulfoximine on the radiation response of human renal carcinoma cell lines. Cancer 71: 2276–2285
28. Loeffler JS, Larson DA (1992) Subspecialization in radiation oncology: impact of stereotactic radiosurgery. Int J Radiat Oncol Biol Phys 24: 885–887
29. Marchese MJ, Minarik L, Hall EJ, Zaider M (1985) Potentially lethal damage repair in cell lines of radioresistant human tumours and normal skin fibroblasts. Int J Radiat Biol 48: 431–434
30. Masuda K, Aramaki R, Takaki T, Wakisaka S (1993) Possible explanation of radioresistance of glioblastoma in situ. Int J Radiat Oncol Biol Phys 9: 255–258
31. McMillan TJ (1993) In vitro radiosensitivity of human medulloblastoma cell lines. J Neurooncol 15: 91–92
32. Mehta MP, Rozental JM, Levin AB, Mackie TR, Kubsad SS, Gehring MA, Kinsella TJ (1992) Defining the role of radiosurgery in the management of brain metastates. Int J Radiat Oncol Biol Phys 24: 619–626
33. Morstyn G, Mitchell J, Carney D, Gazdar A, Glatstein E (1983) Radiation biology of human lung cancer (HLC) cell lines (CL) of different histologies. Proc Am Assoc Cancer Res 24: 33
34. Nilsson S, Carlsson J, Larsson B, Ponten J (1980) Survival of

irradiated glia and glioma cells studied with a new cloning technique. Int J Radiat Bio 37: 267–279

35. Raaphorst GP, Feeley M, Da Silva V, Danjoux C, Gerig L (1989) A comparison of heat and radiation sensitivity of three human glioma cell lines. Int J Radiat Oncol Biol Phys 17: 615–622

36. Rockwell S, Moulder JE (1990) Hypoxic fractions of human tumors xenografted into mice. A review. Int J Radiat Oncol Biol Phys 19: 197–202

37. Rofstad EK (1986) Radiation biology of malignant melanoma. Acta Radiol 25: 1–10

38. Smalley S, Schray M, Lans E, O'Fallon J (1987) Adjuvent radiation therapy after surgical resection of solitary brain metastasis: association with pattern of failure and survival. Int J Radiat Oncol Biol Phys 13: 1611–1616

39. Strachan LR, Hercbergs A, Leith JT (1994) Radiation sensitivity of human renal carcinoma cells in vitro. Int J Radiat Biol: in press

40. Taghian A, Suit H, Pardo F, Gioiso D, Tomkinson K, duBois W, Gerweck L (1992) In vitro intrinsic radiation sensitivity of glioblastoma multiforme. Int J Radiat Oncol Biol Phys 23: 55–62

41. Tate MW, Clelland RC (1957) Nonparametric and shortcut statistics. Interstate, Danville, IL, pp 101–104

42. Thompson LF, Smith RA, Humphrey RM (1975) The response of a human malignant melanoma cell line to high LET radiation. Radiology 117: 155–158

43. Tisler RB, Geard CR, Hall EJ, Schiff PB (1992) Taxol sensitizes human astrocytoma cells to radiation. Cancer Res 52: 3495–3497

44. Utsumi H, Elkind MM (1993) Human melanoma cells: relationship between their radiosensitivity and the repair of potentially lethal damage. Radiat Oncol Inves 1: 29–33

45. Vaupel P, Schlenger K, Knoop C, Höckel M (1991) Oxygenation of human tumors: evaluation of tissue oxygen distribution in breast cancers by computerized O_2 tension measurements. Cancer Res 51: 3316–3322

46. Weichselbaum RR, Epstein J, Little JB (1976) In vitro cellular radiosensitivity of human malignant tumors. Eur J Cancer 12: 47–51

47. Weichselbaum RR, Nove J, Little JB (1980) X-ray sensitivity of human tumor cells in vitro. Int J Radiat Oncol Biol Phys 6: 437–440

48. Weichselbaum RR, Schmit A, Little JB (1982a) Cellular repair factors influencing radiocurability of human malignant tumours. Br J Cancer 45: 10–15

49. Weichselbaum RR, Malcom AW, Little JB (1982b) Fraction size and the repair of potentially lethal radiation damage in a human melanoma cell line. Radiol 142: 225–229

50. Weichselbaum RR, Little JB (1983) The heterogeneity in response of human tumor cells to x irradiation in vitro. In: Nygaard OF, Simic MG (eds) Radioprotectors and anticarcinogens. Academic Press, New York, pp 607–613

51. Weichselbaum RR, Rotmensch J, Ahmed-Swan S, Beckett MA (1989) Radiobiological characterization of 53 human tumour cell lines. Int J Radiat Biol 56: 553–560

52. Weininger J, Guichard M, Joly AM, Malaise EP, Lachet B (1978) Radiosensitity and growth parameters in vitro of three human melanoma cell strains. Int J Radiat Biol 34: 285–290

53. Wollin M, FitzGerald TJ, Santucci MA, Menon M, Longcope C, Reale R, Carson J, Sakakeeny MA, Greenberger JS (1989) Radiosensitivity of human prostate cancer and malignant melanoma cell lines. Radiother Oncol 15: 285–293

54. Yang X, Darling JL, McMillan TJ, Peacock JH, Steel GG (1990) Radiosensitivity, recovery and dose-rate effect in three human glioma cell lines. Radiother Oncol 19: 49–56

Correspondence: John T. Leith, Ph.D. Division of Biology and Medicine, Brown University, Box G, Room B-004, Providence, RI 02912, U.S.A.

Acta Neurochir (1994) [Suppl] 62: 28–32

A Universal, Multi-Modality Localization System for Animal Radiosurgery

T. D. Solberg[1,2], A. A. F. De Salles[2], D. Hovda[2], and F. E. Holly[1]

[1]Radiation Oncology, and [2]Neurosurgery, Jonsson Comprehensive Cancer Center and UCLA School of Medicine, Los Angeles, CA, U.S.A.

Summary

We have developed a stereotactic localization system allowing a radiosurgical approach in a number of animal models. The system utilizes fixation adapters specially designed for a particular animal, which in turn are attached to a common Brown–Roberts–Wells (BRW) compatible Delrin head ring. Each fixation adapter is constructed using materials compatible with CT, MRI, PET, and angiographic imaging studies. With such a system, radiographic localization, computerized treatment planning, and stereotactic radiation delivery can subsequently be performed in a manner identical to the procedures used for humans.

Keywords: Animal experiments; stereotactic radiosurgery; fixation systems; stereolactic localization system.

Introduction

With the increasing role of stereotactic radiosurgery in the treatment of both malignant and benign disease, the need for animal models to evaluate the effects of high dose irradiation in tumor, vasculature, and normal brain has become more important. In many respects, the modality has found popular use despite lack of a firm understanding of the basic biological mechanisms involved, as the number of good radiosurgery animal models which exist are limited[3,6-14].

We are developing a porcine AVM model, tumor models in rats, and normal tissue models in cats, pigs, and primates. For each of these models, specialized stereotactic radiosurgery adapters have been constructed.

For any model to be successful, one needs to simulate the problem, in this case, radiosurgery in humans, as closely as possible. High dose Cobalt-60 irradiation with a single field, for example, is obviously an inadequate representation of a radiosurgical procedure, and inferences drawn from such a model would be of limited use. Thus in designing our animal models, the importance of closely mimicking clinical procedures, from imaging to treatment planning to radiation delivery, is highly stressed. By doing so, we are able to obtain the same high level of mechanical and dosimetric precision in animals as in humans.

Methods and Materials

UCLA uses the SRS200 clinical radiosurgery system developed at the University of Florida[2] and manufactured by Philips, in combination with a Varian Clinac 18 linear accelerator[1]. The system consists of a BRW fixation system mounted to an isocentric floor stand. With the isocentric subsystem, an average mechanical accuracy of less than 0.3 mm has been obtained[4]. Accuracy of coordinate transformation from CT to the BRW headstand is slightly more than one-half of the slice thickness used, while that for angiographic localization is just less than 0.5 mm on average[5].

At the heart of our system for animal radiosurgery is a Delrin (plastic) ring, identical to the commercial BRW ring in most respects, which allows stereotactic localization and treatment procedures to be performed in a manner consistent with that in humans (see Fig. 1). Individual adapters are attached to the ring to secure animals for imaging or radiosurgery procedures. Bodies of the larger animals are supported by the treatment couch, while smaller animals can be supported entirely by the frame and floor stand.

Fixation for the pig is accomplished using the device shown in Fig. 2 (left). The device consists of a plastic cylinder, with a portion cut away to allow the radiation arcs to impinge on the animal unobstructed, while the lower portion acts to support the animal's head and neck. Two pins are affixed to dorsal portion of the animal's skull, with an additional pin in either corner of the lower mandible. the pins are mounted to a sliding attachment allowing adjustment of their position within the plane of the ring. A future version of this adapter will allow for an additional degree of movement in the direction perpendicular to the ring.

The primate stereotactic device is most similar to the human frame (Fig. 2, right), and unlike those for our other animal models, the primate adapter attaches to the underside of the Delrin ring. As in humans, fixation is accomplished at four points in the skull. Posts holding the pins may be raised, lowered and rotated about the animal independent of one another. In Fig. 3, attachment of the CT and MR localization devices to the porcine and primate frames is demonstrated.

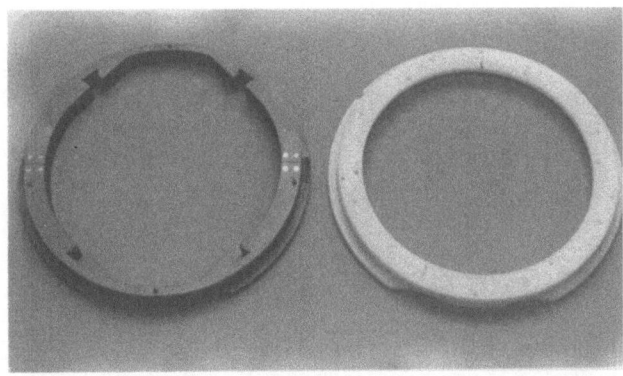

Fig. 1. Delrin base ring (right) and the BRW base ring upon which it is modeled. All animal fixation devices attach to the Delrin ring, which in turn is compatible with commercially available localization devices

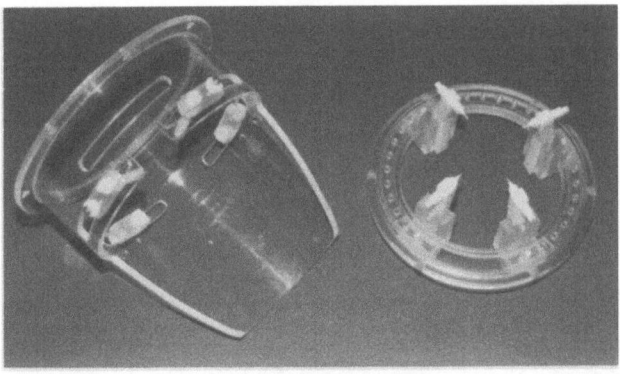

Fig. 2. Left: The four-point porcine fixation adapter. The upper part of the plastic cylinder is cut away where the radiation arcs are incident on the skin while the animal's jaw and neck rest on the bottom portion for increased stability. Bony fixation is accomplished through two aluminum-tipped plastic screws in the skull and one either corner of the mandible. Right: The four-point primate fixation adapter. Though similar to the human frame in most respects, the primate frame has an additional degree of movement allowing the posts to rotate about the animal's head in the axial plane

Fixation device for feline and rat models (Fig. 4) have been modeled after commercial devices used for surgical studies (David Kopf Instruments, Tujunga, CA). Fixation for the rat is accomplished using opposed ear bars and a bite block. With its body fully supported underneath, this three-point fixation is more than sufficient for an anesthetized rat. An additional advantage is that the frame geometry is identical to a similar device used for stereotactic tumor implantation. Additional support for feline models is added through bars positioned at the inferior rim of the orbits.

Prior to radiosurgery, a CT or MRI scan is performed to provide image data for computerized treatment planning and dose calculation. With the exception of the primate and porcine angiogram, all animals are imaged and treatment in the prone position. For vasculature studies, target coordinates must be obtained from angiogram.

Results

Pre-radiosurgery exams and radiosurgery planning was performed in the porcine, primate, feline, and murine models. Figure 5 shows a PA contrast enhanced angiogram of the intracranial target of our porcine AVM model prior to radiosurgery, with the fiducial markers on the angio box, labeled A-H, clearly visible. Figure 6 shows a axial CT cut of the animal with the calculated isodose distributions superimposed. In this case, each of the bilateral AVM-mimicking structures was treated. Though these structures are separated by only 2 cm, the flexibility of the linear accelerator-based system allows us to tailor the dose distributions to each side very precisely. While results of this model will be discussed in a later publication, pathologic and radiographic studies in four animals treated with various doses to date have verified our ability to cover the intended target, each of which measures approximately 1.5 cm in diameter.

Similarly, Fig. 7 shows MRI studies used for treatment planning in the primate and feline models, with fiducials from the localization box visible at the peri-

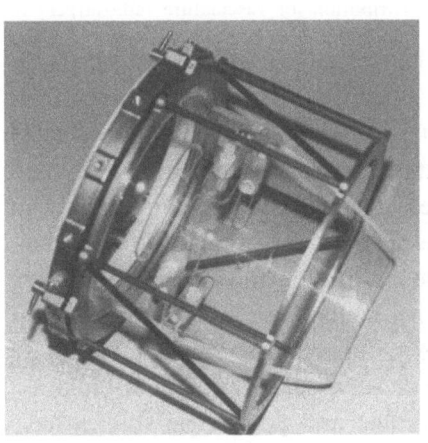

a

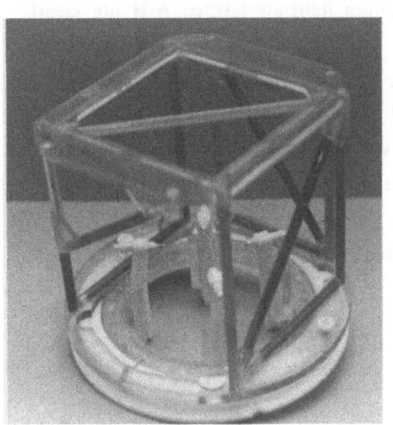

b

Fig. 3. (a,b) The porcine and primate frames of Fig. 3 shown attached to the Delrin ring with CT and MRI localization devices in place

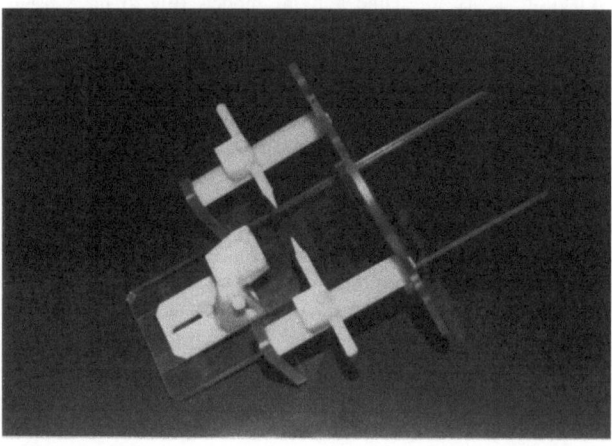

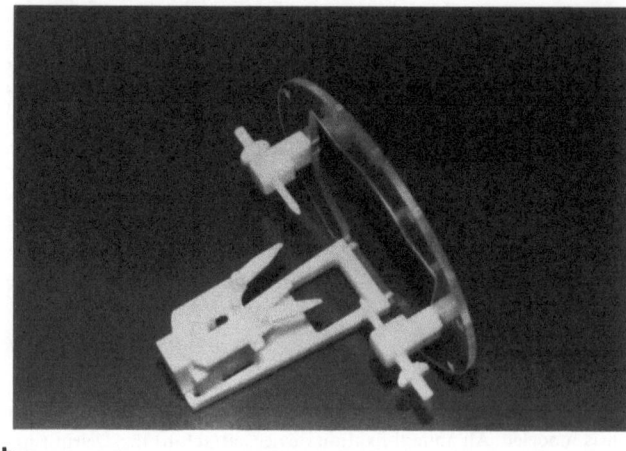

a

b

Fig. 4. Fixation device for rat (a) and cat (b) are modeled after commercially available stereotactic surgery devices. Fixation for the rat is accomplished via the ears and a bar for the upper fangs, while the cat frame has additional support on the inferior rim of the orbits

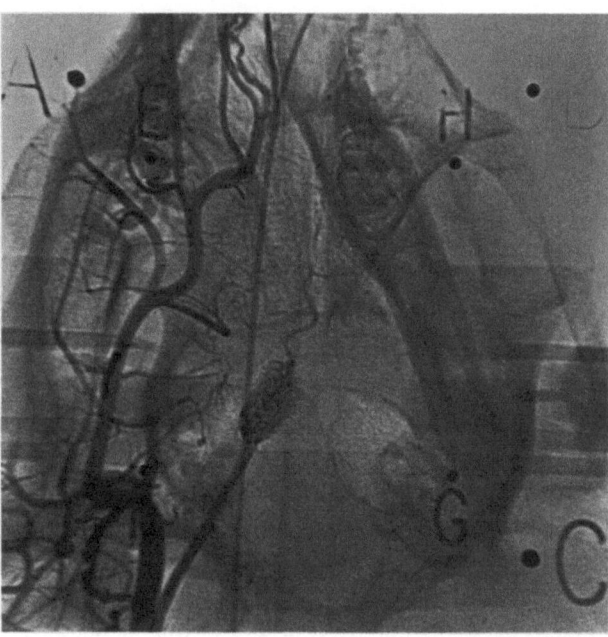

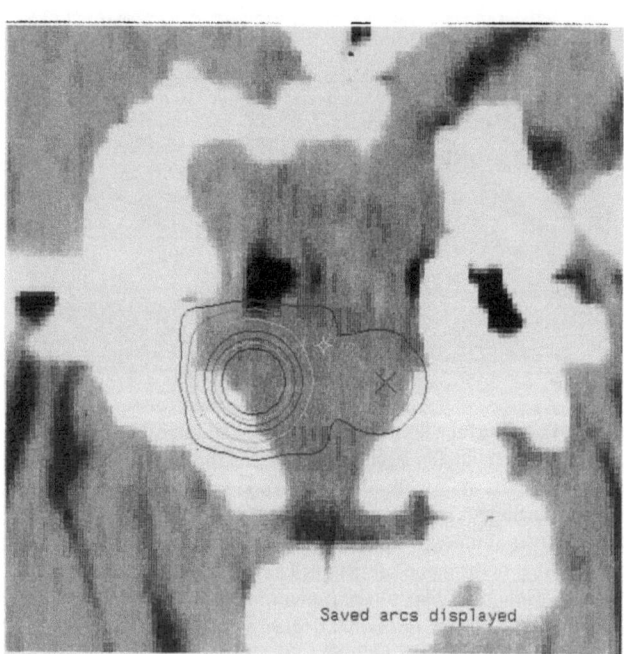

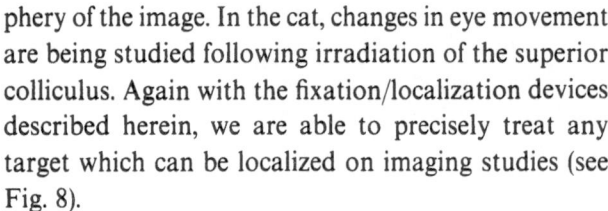

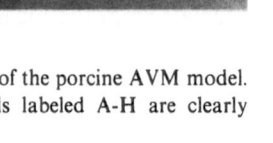

Fig. 5. Constrast enhanced angiogram of the porcine AVM model. The angiographic localization fiducials labeled A-H are clearly visible

Fig. 6. Axial isodose distribution for vasculature radiosurgery in the pig. The left and right sides were treated to doses of 80 and 30 Gy respectively, using a 12 mm collimator

phery of the image. In the cat, changes in eye movement are being studied following irradiation of the superior colliculus. Again with the fixation/localization devices described herein, we are able to precisely treat any target which can be localized on imaging studies (see Fig. 8).

Discussion

In order to properly extrapolate results in animal models to humans, the procedures applied to each must be as consistent as possible. We have constructed a number of fixation devices for animal surgery and radiosurgery. These devices, through their attachment to a common Delrin ring, are compatible with commercially available localization and treatment planning systems. While other methods have been employed for animal radiosurgery, our systems provides for accurate and reproducible fixation, localization, and radiation delivery. Radiographic and pathologic studies have demonstrated the ability to pinpoint a surgical or radiosurgical target localized in such a manner.

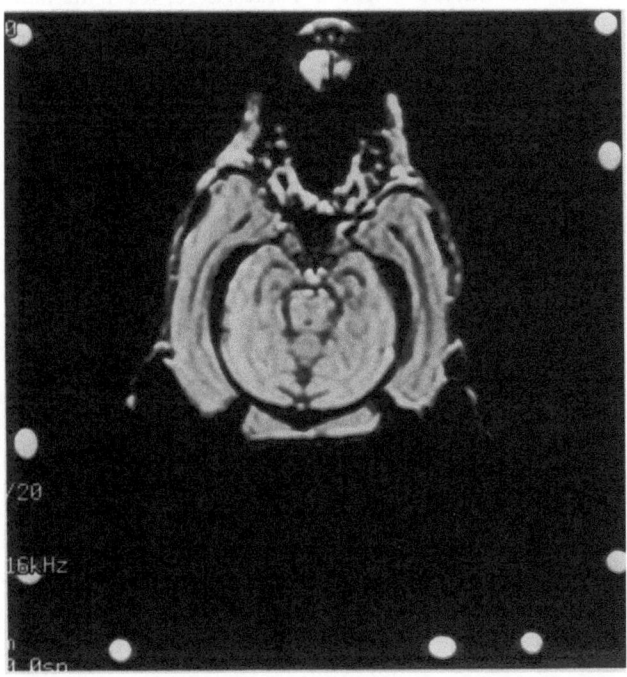

a

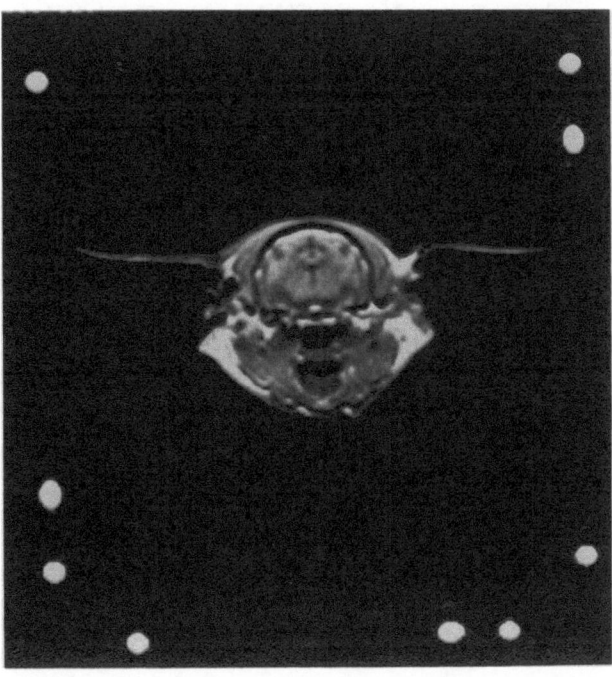

b

Fig. 7. In the primate (a) and feline (b) models, MRI is used for both target localization and treatment planning

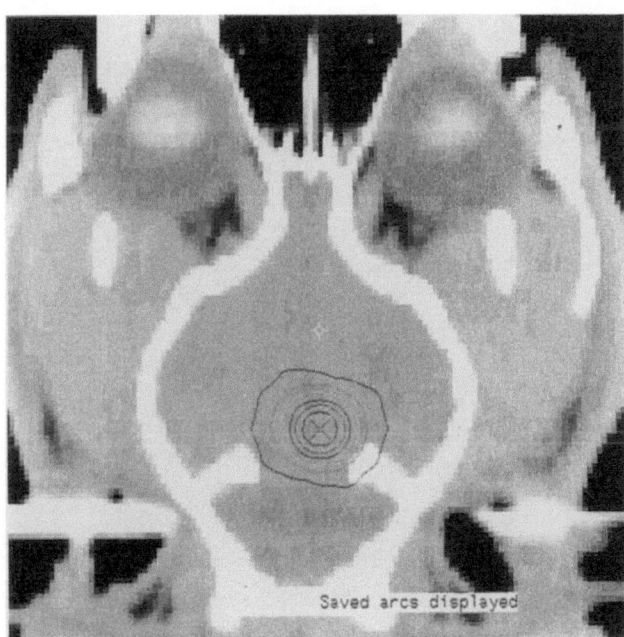

Fig. 8. Axial isodose distribution in the feline brain. Using a 5 mm collimator, doses to 150 Gy have been delivered

Each animal model developed for radiosurgery studies addresses a variety of radiosurgery applications, including AVMs (porcine model), tumor (rat model), functional radiosurgery (primate), and cranial nerves and other normal tissue (porcine and feline models). Each of these animals have perculiarities that make them excellent models for the particular applications described. Work is underway to further characterize each of these models.

The system is not limited to the animal models presented here. Additional fixation devices can be constructed for a number of animals, provided that the design be compatible with the BRW system, and that materials compatible with various imaging studies.

References

1. De Salles AAF, Bajada CL, Goetsch SJ, Selch MT, Holly FE, Solberg TD, Becker DP (1993) Radiosurgery of cavernous sinus tumors. Acta Neurochir (Wien) [Suppl] 58: 101–103
2. Friedman WA, Bova FJ (1989) The University of Florida radiosurgery system. Surg Neurol 32: 334–342
3. Friedman WA, Blatt DR, Bova FJ (1993) Experimental radiosurgery. In: De Salles AAF, Goetsch SJ (eds) Stereotactic surgery and radiosurgery. Medical Physics Publishing, Madison, pp 267–275
4. Holly FE, Miller GE, Solberg TD, Goetsch SJ, Smathers JB, Selch MT, De Salles A, Sutton C (1992) Assessment of a quality control program for the Philips SRS 200 stereotactic radiotherapy system medical physics 19: 791
5. Holly FE, Solberg TD, De Salles AAF, Goetsch SJ, Smathers JB, Selch MT (1993) Inherent accuracies of subsystems of the Philips/BRW SRS 200 radiosurgery system. Proceedings of the

International Conference and Course on Stereotactic Radiotherapy/Surgery, May 6–8, 1993 Amsterdam, The Netherlands

6. Kondziolka D, Linskey ME, Lunsford LD (1993) Animal models in radiosurgery. In: Alexander E *et al* (eds) Stereotactic radiosurgery. McGraw-Hill, New York, pp 51–64
7. Kondziolka D, Lunsford LD, Claassen D, Maitz AH, Flickenger JC (1992) Radiobiology of radiosurgery: Part I. The normal rat brain model. Neurosurgery 31: 271–279
8. Kondziolka D, Lunsford LD, Claassen D, Pandalai S, Maitz AH, Flickenger JC (1992) Radiobiology of radiosurgery: Part II. The rat C6 glioma model Neurosurgery 31: 280–288
9. Larsson B (1960) Blood vessel changes following local irradiation of the brain with high-energy protons. Acta Societatis Medicorum Upsaliensis 65: 61–71
10. Leksell L, Larsson B, Anderson B, Rexed B, Sourander P, Mair W (1960) Lesions in the depth of the brain produced by a beam of high energy protons. Acta Rad 54: 251–264

11. Lunsford LD, Altschuler EM, Flickenger JC, Wu A, Martinez AJ (1990) In vivo biological effects of stereotactic radiosurgery: a primate model. Neurosurgery 27: 373–382
12. Nilsson A, Wennerstrand D, Leksell D, Backlund EO (1978) Stereotactic gamma irradiation of basilar artery in cat. Acta Radiol Oncol 17: 150–160
13. Siegfried J, Ervin FR, Koehler A, Kjellberg RN (1962) Effects d'une radiation localisée de protons sur lrs potentiels électrophysiologiques évoqués dans le genglion geniculatum laterale du chat. Helv Physiol Acta 20: C83–84
14. Spiegelmann R, Friedman WA, Bova FJ, Theele DP, Mickle JP (1993) LINAC radiosurgery: an animal model. J Neurosurg 78: 638–644

Correspondence: Timothy D. Solberg, M.S., Department of Radiation Oncology, 200 UCLA Medical Plaza, Suite B265, Los Angeles, CA 90024-6951, U.S.A.

Acta Neurochir (1994) [Suppl] 62: 33–38
© Springer-Verlag 1994

Stereotactic Radiosurgery for Pituitary Adenomas: Imaging, Visual and Endocrine Results

B. E. Pollock[1], **D. Kondziolka**[1,3], **L. D. Lunsford**[1,2,3], and **J. C. Flickinger**[1,3]

Departments of [1]Neurological Surgery, [2]Radiology, and [3]Radiation Oncology, University of Pittsburgh School of Medicine and the Specialized Neurosurgical Center, Presbyterian University Hospital, Pittsburgh, Pennsylvania, U.S.A.

Summary

To determine the endocrine, ophthalmologic, and tumor growth control responses after stereotactic radiosurgery using the gamma unit, we reviewed our experience in 35 patients with pituitary adenomas. Twenty-four females and 11 males (mean age 47 years, range 9–81 years) had radiosurgery with average follow-up of 26 months (range 6–60 months). Most patients were refractory to surgical removal.

Fifteen patients had Cushing's disease. Prior transsphenoidal resection was performed in 14 patients (6 had two prior operations), fractionated radiotherapy in 3, and adrenalectomy in 2. In 11 evaluable patients, the hormone response was normalized in 8, decreased in 2 and increased in 1. Five patients remained on cortisol suppression. Of 12 patients with imaging follow-up, 4 had decreased tumor size, 6 had no change, and 2 had an increase; these 2 patients underwent subsequent surgery.

Ten patients had acromegaly, and 6 had undergone prior surgery. Of 8 evaluable patients, growth hormone secretion has normalized in 3, decreased in 3, and increased in 2. Six tumors decreased in size, and 2 were unchanged. One patient had repeat resection 21 months after radiosurgery and one patient underwent repeat radiosurgery.

Ten patients had non-secreting adenomas; all 10 had prior operations (1–4 operations, 6 underwent frontal craniotomy) and 5 had undergone fractionated radiotherapy. Eight patients had panhypopituitarism prior to radiosurgery. Four tumors decreased in size and 6 were without change. One patient had worsening of vision and had optic nerve decompression without improvement; 2 had improvement in visual function after radiosurgery. One patient died 16 months later from hypothalamic insufficiency (after 4 prior operations and fractionated radiotherapy).

Radiosurgery is a potentially effective management option for recurrent small pituitary adenomas or for primary management of tumors unsuitable for microsurgery. Radiosurgical dose planning with selective beam blocking and shifting is necessary to preserve visual function. Dose escalation or repeat irradiation may be necessary to improve endocrine control in secreting tumors.

Keywords: Pituitary adenoma; radiosurgery; brain tumor; Cushing's disease; acromegaly.

Introduction

Pituitary adenomas are histologically benign tumors that can behave aggressively if they compress adjacent neurovascular structures or if they are hormonally active. Transsphenoidal resection of hormone secreting pituitary adenomas producing acromegaly or Cushing's disease is the accepted initial treatment for small, non-invasive tumors; cure rates range from 52–85%[1,4,10,23,24]. Prolactinomas, even when large and invasive, are generally treated with bromocriptine[25]. Dopamine agonist therapy has been less effective for acromegaly[3]. Octreotide, a long-acting somatostatin analog, normalized growth hormone levels in 45% of patients with acromegaly but requires subcutaneous injection every 8 hours and is very expensive[26]. Fractionated radiotherapy has been reported to achieve clinical remission in between 55–100% of patients with pituitary adenomas[7,11,12,18,19]. However, conventional fractionated external beam irradiation of the pituitary gland requires several years to control tumor growth and reduce hormone secretion, and almost all of patients develop hypopituitarism within 5 to 7 years after treatment[16].

Stereotactic radiosurgery has been used to manage patients with pituitary adenomas[2,13,15,21,22,29], especially those who have failed surgical resection. Charged-particle radiosurgery has a long history and has proven to be an effective treatment modality[13,15], with 70–90% of patients in remission 1–4 years after irradiation. Experience with the cobalt-60 gamma unit has been reported[2,20–22]; in these early efforts the majority of patients had tumor localization using pneumoencephalopathy alone. Stephanian et al.[21] previously reported our initial experience with pituitary adenomas in 18 patients where computed tomography (CT) or magnetic resonance imaging (MRI) was used for stereotactic localization. Tumor growth control was obtained in 17 of 18 patients, however follow-up was short and

Table 1. *Clinical Characteristics of 35 Patients with Pituitary Adenomas*

Characteristic	No. patients
Endocrinological function	
ACTH secreting tumors	15
GH secreting tumors	10
Non-secreting tumors	10
Panhypopituitarism	8
Normal pituitary function	4
Ophthalmological function	
Blind	1
Visual field loss	4
Normal visual function	30
Prior surgery	
Transsphenoidal operation (1–3 resections)	30
Frontal craniotomy (1–3 resections)	6
Adrenalectomy	2
Prior fractionated radiation therapy[a]	8

[a]Average dose, 46 Gy (range 39.5–50 Gy).
ACTH adrenocorticotrophic hormone; *GH* growth hormone.

only 3 to 10 patients had normalization of hormone secretion.

To better define the endocrine, ophthalmologic and tumor growth control responses of pituitary adenomas after stereotactic radiosurgery, we retrospectively reviewed our five year experience.

Methods and Materials

Thirty-five patients (24 females and 11 males) with imaging, endocrinological, or surgical evidence of a pituitary adenoma underwent radiosurgery with the 201-source cobalt-60 gamma unit (Elekta Instruments, Atlanta, GA). The mean age of the patients was 47 years (range 9–81 years). Thirty patients previously underwent attempted microsurgical removal (one to four resections). The clinical characteristics of the patients are shown in Table 1.

Stereotactic localization of the tumor volume was performed with either CT or MRI (MRI only over the past three years). Selective beam blocking, small beam diameters, and multiple isocenters were used to reduce the dose delivered to the optic apparatus to ≤ 8 Gy[8,9] (Fig. 1). Selection of the radiosurgery dose was based on published results[5,14,17,21], the prediction of radiation related complications as determined by the integrated logistic formula[6], and the determined isodose containing the optic nerve or chiasm.

Follow-up consisted of clinical and neuroimaging examinations performed at 6-month intervals. Endocrinological follow-up was performed by the patients' internist or endocrinologist.

Results

Radiation Dosimetry

The radiation planning and dose parameters used in these patients are presented in Table 2. A single isocenter was used in 18 cases (51%); multiple isocenters (range 2–8 isocenters; mean, 3.4 isocenters) were used in 17

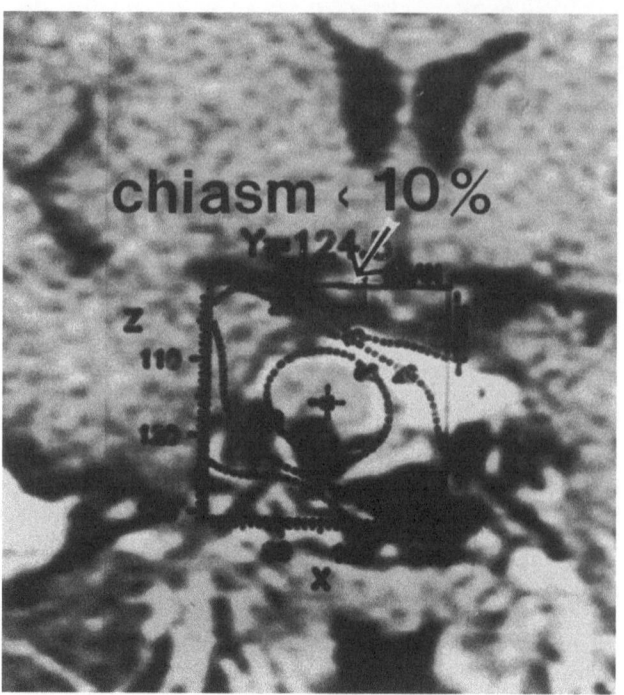

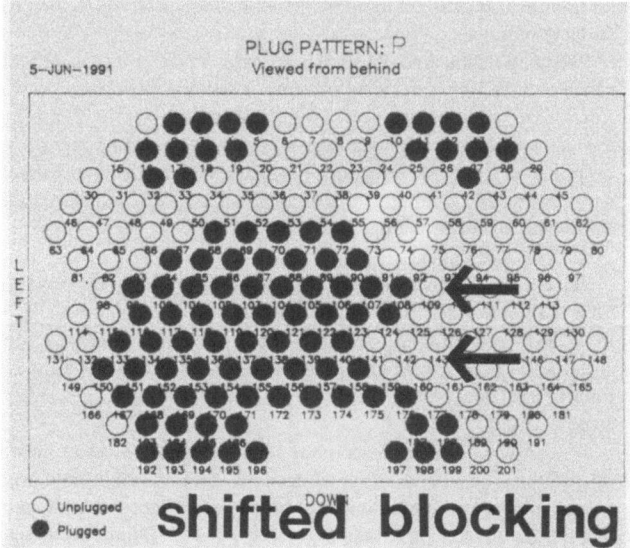

Fig. 1. Stereotactic MRI dose plan for growth-hormone producing macroadenoma. Top: Coronal T_1 spin-echo MRI showing optic chiasm (arrow) receiving $< 10\%$ (< 4.2 Gy) of maximum radiation dose. Bottom: Cobalt source blocking pattern with shift to limit radiation delivery to the optic chiasm and nerves

cases (49%). Thirty-two of 35 patients were treated at the 50% or greater isodose line to take advantage of the sharp fall-off of the radiation field outside the target volume[27].

Clinical and Neuroimaging Evaluation

Thirty of 35 patients had clinical and neuroimaging follow-up at least 6 months after radiosurgery (mean

Table 2. *Radiosurgical Dosimetry in 35 Patients with Pituitary Adenomas*

Characteristic	No. patients
Tumor size	
No mass identified[a]	3
Microadenoma[b]	14
Macroadenoma[c]	18
Marginal treatement isodose (%)	
30	1
40	2
50	25
60	5
70	2
Radiation dose to tumor margin (Gy)[d]	
10–17	8
18–24	15
24–30	12

[a]Focal gland irradiation in residual ACTH producing pituitary neoplasms despite prior surgical resection.
[b]Microadenoma – mass <1 cm in greatest dimension.
[c]Macroadenoma – mass >1 cm in greatest dimension.
[d]Maximum tumor dose ranged from 20 to 60 Gy (mean = 40 Gy).

Table 3. *Postradiosurgical Neuroimaging in 30 Patients with Pituitary Adenomas*

Tumor	Decreased	Unchanged	Increased
ACTH secreting	4	6	2
GH secreting			
Microadenoma	2	2	0
Macroadenoma	4	0	0
Non-secreting			
Microadenoma	1	0	0
Macroadenoma	3	6	0

follow-up 26 months). Two patients had improvement of their visual function after radiosurgery. One patient with a non-secreting adenoma was blind preoperatively after 4 prior resections (3 transsphenoidal operations and 1 frontal craniotomy) and conventional fractionated radiotherapy. He regained functional vision in his right eye 6 months after radiosurgery. This patients died 16 months after radiosurgery because of hypothalamic insufficiency despite improved visual function and decreased tumor size. The second patient had improvement of a bi-temporal hemianopsia. One patient with a left homonymous hemianopsia after 2 prior resections (1 transphenoidal operation and 1 frontal craniotomy) and conventional fractionated radiotherapy, had visual acuity deterioration in the left eye 7 months after radiosurgery. Although a repeat MRI showed a slight reduction in tumor size, the patient underwent repeat transsphenoidal tumor resection without improvement in visual function. Visual function in 27 patients remained normal after radiosurgery.

Two Cushing's disease patients underwent repeat transsphenoidal operation at 15 and 26 months after radiosurgery because imaging studies showed that their tumors had increased in size. One patient with acromegaly and a pre-operative growth hormone level of 150 ng/ml, refused resection of a macroadenoma before radiosurgery. Operative removal of tumor was performed 27 months after radiosurgery when the growth hormone level remained elevated and she was unable to tolerate octreotide therapy. One patient who

originally received 17 Gy to the margin of a growth hormone producing macroadenoma, underwent repeat radiosurgery 24 months later because of persistently elevated growth hormone levels.

Neuroimaging results are shown in Table 3. Twenty-eight of 30 patients had either a decrease or no change in the size of their tumor after radiosurgery (tumor growth control of 93%) (Fig. 2).

Endocrine Evaluation

Endocrine results in 11 evaluable patients with Cushing's disease and 8 evaluable patients with acromegaly after radiosurgery are presented in Table 4. Function of the hypothalamic-pituitary-adrenal axis was considered normal if either the 24 hour urinary free cortisol level <90 mg/day, or the a.m. plasma adrenocorticotrophic hormone level <80 pg/ml. Normal growth hormone secretion was considered a fasting plasma a.m. growth hormone level <5 ng/ml. Eight of 11 (73%) of patients with ACTH secreting tumors had normalization of the hypothalamic-pituitary-adrenal axis, although 5 patients remained on cortisol suppression. Three of 8 patients (38%) with growth hormone secreting tumors had normal growth hormone secretion after radiosurgery. No patient in this series developed post-operative pituitary insufficiency.

Discussion

The goals of pituitary adenoma therapy are to control tumor growth, to decrease abnormal hormone hypersecretion when observed, and avoid hypopituitarism whenever possible. Current management strategies for symptomatic pituitary adenomas include pharmacologic suppression, surgical resection, fractionated radiation therapy, and more recently, stereotactic radiosurgery. In this retrospective analysis, tumor

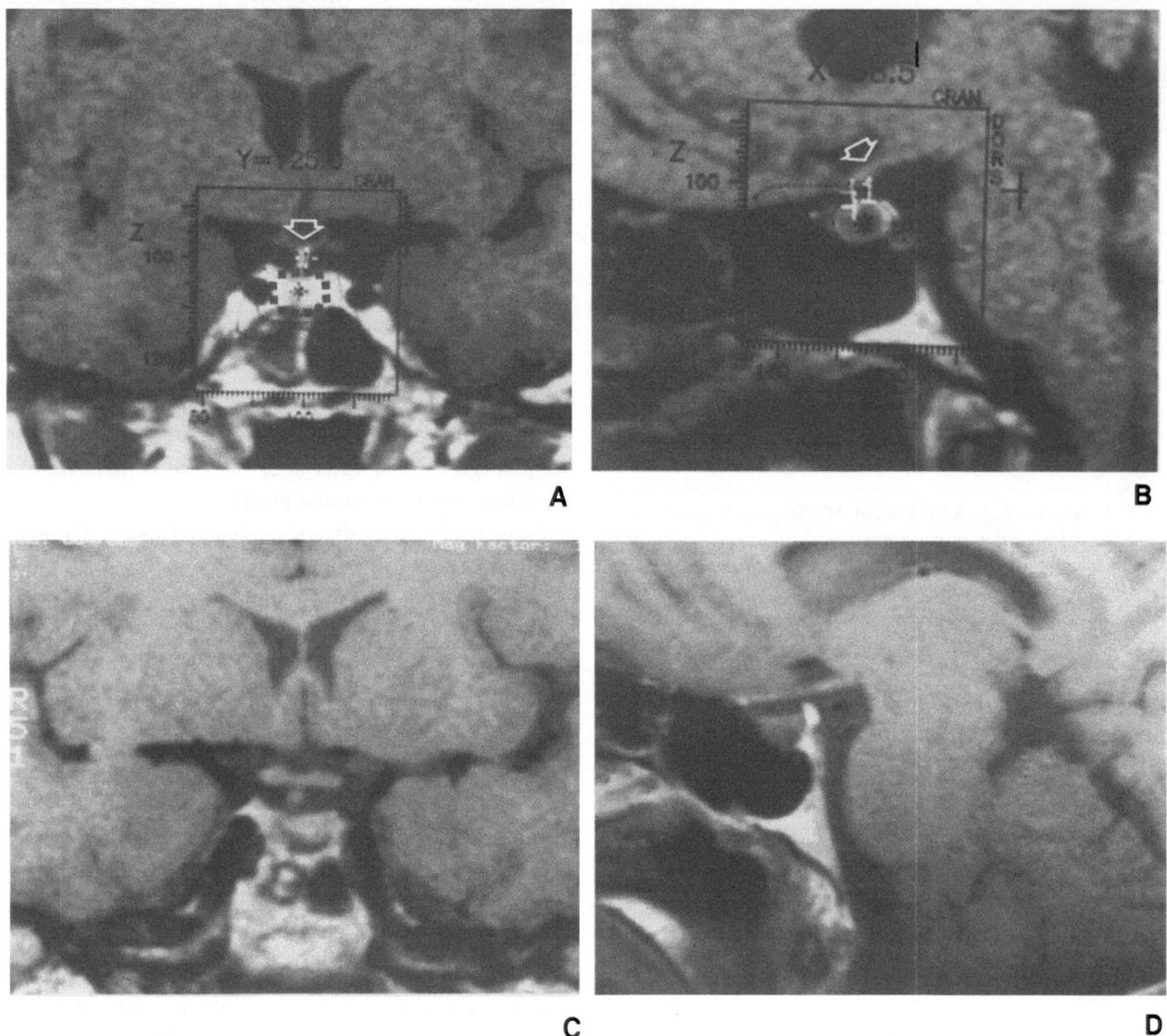

Fig. 2. Stereotactic MRI dose plan for ACTH-hormone producing microadenoma. Coronal (A) and sagittal (B) T_1 spin-echo MRI showing optic chiasm (arrow) receiving < 10% (< 4.5 Gy) of maximum radiation dose. Coronal (C) and sagittal (D) 1 year follow-up T_1 spin-echo MRI showing decrease in size of tumor

Table 4. *Endocrine Results After Radiosurgery of ACTH and GH Producing Pituitary Adenomas*

Tumor	Normal	Decreased	Increased
ACTH secreting	8[a]	2	1
GH secreting	3[b]	3	2

[a] Function of the hypothalamic-pituitary-adrenal axis was normal if either the 24 hour urinary free cortisol level < 90 mg/day or the a.m. plasma adrenocorticotrophic hormone level < 80 pg/ml. (Five patients remained on cortisol suppression).

[b] Normal growth hormone secretion was a fasting plasma a.m. growth hormone level < 5 ng/ml.

growth control was obtained in 93% of patients with pituitary adenomas after radiosurgery; most of these patients had failed either operative resection (86%) or fractionated radiotherapy (23%), or both. No patient developed pituitary insufficiency after radiosurgery, and only one patient had a decline in visual function after radiosurgery. Normalization of hormone secretion was realized in 8 of 11 patients with Cushing's disease and 3 of 8 patients with acromegaly.

The radiosurgical approach to management of patients with pituitary adenomas has evolved with improvements in tumor localization[2,20,22,26]. In Stockholm, patients undergoing radiosurgery before 1985 had stereotactic localization by pneumoencephalography. Results in patients with ACTH-secreting tumors (who first received between 70–100 Gy maximum dose to the medial-posterior part of the anterior lobe) revealed that 82% ultimately were cured after radiosurgery[20]. Most patients required multiple radiosurgical procedures in adjacent parts of the sella; 22% developed some degree of hormonal insufficiency. In 19 patients treated after 1986, target localization was performed with stereotactic CT or MRI. Complete remission was achieved in 13 of 19 patients (68%), though almost one-third require hormonal replacement therapy[20]. Thoren *et al.*[22] reported the Stockholm experience with GH-secreting tumors and found 10 to 21 (48%) of patients had GH levels < 5 ng/ml after radiosurgery. Two of 13 (15%) of patients not treated with previous conventional radiotherapy developed delayed pituitary insufficiency. The higher remission rate noted in Cushing's disease compared to acromegaly can be attributed to two features: (1) the higher radiation dose received by the ACTH-producing tumors (70 to 100 Gy compared to 40–70 Gy), and (2) ACTH-producing tumors were generally microadenomas.

Stereotactic radiosurgery effectively controls tumor growth in most small pituitary adenomas, either as a primary management strategy or after failed microsurgical resection. Normalization of hormonal hypersecretion have been less impressive. Several techniques may improve the endocrine results after radiosurgery. First, stereotactic MRI for tumor localization and sophisticated computer work station volumetric dose planning may allow us to increase the radiation dose to the target volume and yet continue to restrict the dose to adjacent optic apparatus. Second, repeat stereotactic radiosurgery can be utilized if the patient does not show a decrease in hormonal secretion within 24 months. Third, ongoing research investigating the radiation tolerance of the optic nerves and the possible use of neural protective agents or tumor sensitizers during radiosurgery may enable a more effective radiation dose to be delivered.

Acknowledgement

The authors would like to Trish DiGiannurio for preparation of the manuscript.

References

1. Arnott RD, Pestell RG, McKelvie PA, Henderson JK, McNeill PM, Alford FP (1990) A critical evaluation of transsphenoidal pituitary surgery in the treatment of Cushing's disease: Prediction of outcome. Acta Endocrinol (Copenh) 123: 423–430
2. Backlund EO, Ganz JC (1993) Pituitary adenomas: Gamma Knife. In: Alexander E, Loeffler JS, Lunsford LD (eds) Stereotactic radiosurgery. McGraw-Hill, New York, 167–173
3. Bell P, Atkinson AB, Hadden DR, Kennedy L, Leslie H, Merrett D, Sheridan B (1986) Bromocriptine reduces growth hormone in acromegaly. Arch Intern Med 146: 1145–1149
4. Davis DH, Laws ER, Ilstrup DM, Speed JK, Caruso M, Shaw EG, Abboud CF, Scheithauer BW, Root LM, Schleck C (1993) Results of surgical treatment for growth-hormone secreting pituitary adenomas. J Neurosurg 79: 70–75
5. Duma CM, Lunsford LD, Kondziolka D, Harsh GR, Flickinger JC (1993) Stereotactic radiosurgery of cavernous sinus meningiomas as an addition or alternative to microsurgery. Neurosurgery 32: 699–705
6. Flickinger JC (1989) An integrated logistic formula for the prediction of complications from radiosurgery. Int J Radiat Oncol Biol Phys 17: 879–885
7. Flickinger JC, Nelson DB, Martinez AJ, Deutsch M, Taylor F (1989) Radiotherapy of nonfunctional adenomas of the pituitary gland: results with long-term follow-up. Cancer 63: 2409–2414
8. Flickinger JC, Lunsford LD, Wu A, Maitz A, Kalend A (1990) Treatment planning for gamma knife radiosurgery with multiple isocenters. Int J Radiat Onc Biol Phys 18: 1495–1501
9. Flickinger JC, Maitz A, Kalend A, Lunsford LD, Wu A (1990) Treatment volume shaping with selective beam blocking using the Leksell gamma unit. Int J Radiat Oncol Biol Phys 19: 783–789
10. Friedman RB, Oldfield EH, Nieman LK, Chrousos GP, Doppman JL, Cutler GF, Loriaux DL (1989) Repeat transsphenoidal surgery for Cushing's disease. J Neurosurg 71: 520–527
11. Goffman TE, Dewan R, Arakaki R, Gorden P, Oldfield EH, Glatstein E (1992) Persistent or recurrent acromegaly: long-term endocrinologic efficacy and neurologic safety of postsurgical radiation therapy. Cancer 69: 271–275
12. Howlett TA, Plowman PN, Wass JR, Rees LH, Jones AE, Bessner GM (1989) Megavoltage pituitary irradiation in the management of Cushing's disease and Nelson's syndrome: long-term follow-up. Clin Endocrinol 31: 309–323
13. Kjellberg RN, Klimen B (1979) Lifetime effectiveness – a system of therapy for pituitary adenomas, emphasizing Bragg peak photon hypophysectomy. In: Linfoot JA (ed) Recent advances in the diagnosis and treatment of pituitary tumors. Raven, New York, pp 269–288
14. Kondziolka D, Lunsford LD, Coffey RJ, Flickinger JC (1991) Stereotactic radiosurgery of meningiomas. J Neurosurg 74: 552–559
15. Levy RP, Fabrikant JI, Frankel KA (1993) Particle-beam irradiation of the pituitary gland. In: Alexander E, Loeffler JS, Lunsford LD (eds) Stereotactic radiosurgery. McGraw-Hill, New York, pp 157–165
16. Littley MD, Shalet SM, Beardwell CG, Ahmed SR, Applegate G, Sutton ML (1989) Hypopituitarism following external radiotherapy for pituitary tumors in adults. Q J Med 70: 145–160
17. Lunsford LD, Flickinger JC, Lidner G, Maitz A (1989) Stereotactic radiosurgery of the brain using the first United States 201 cobalt-60 source gamma knife. Neurosurgery 24: 151–159
18. McCollough WM, Marcus RB, Rhoton AL, Ballinger WE, Million RR (1991) Long-term follow-up of radiotherapy for pituitary adenoma: the absence of late recurrence after > 4500 Gy. Int J Radiation Oncol Biol Phys 21: 607–614
19. Moberg E, Trampe E, Wersall J, Werner S (1991) Long-term effects of radiotherapy and bromocriptine treatment in patients with previous surgery for macroprolactinomas. Neurosurgery 29: 200–205
20. Rahn T (1993) Gamma knife surgery in pituitary adenomas. Presented at the International Stereotactic Radiosurgery Society Meeting, Stockholm, Sweden

21. Stephanian E, Lunsford LD, Coffey RJ, Bissonette DJ, Flickinger JC (1992) Gamma knife surgery for sellar and suprasellar tumors. Neurosurg Clin North Am 3: 207–218

22. Thoren M, Rahn T, Guo WY, Werner S (1991) Stereotactic radiosurgery with cobalt-60 gamma unit in the treatment of growth hormone-producing pituitary tumors. Neurosurgery 29: 663–668.

23. Tindall GT, Herring CJ, Clark RV, Adams DA, Watts NB (1990) Cushing's disease: results of transsphenoidal microsurgery with emphasis on surgical failures. J Neurosurg 72: 363–369

24. Tindall GT, Oyesiku NM, Watts NB, Clark RV, Christy JH, Adams DA (1993) Transsphenoidal adenomectomy for growth hormone-secreting pituitary adenomas in acromegaly: outcome analysis and determinants of failure. J Neurosurg 78: 205–215

25. Vance ML, Evans WS, Thorner MO (1984) Bromocriptine. Ann Intern Med 100: 78–91

26. Vance ML, Harris AG (1991) Long-term treatment of 189 acromegalic patients with the somatostatin analog octreotide. Arch Intern Med 151: 1573–1578

27. Wu A, Lindner G, Maitz A, Kalend AM, Lunsford LD, Flickinger JC, Bloomer WD (1990) Physics of gamma knife approach on converent beams and stereotactic radiosurgery. Int J Radiat Oncol Biol Phys 18: 941–949

Correspondence: Bruce E. Pollock, M. D., Department of Neurological Surgery, Presbyterian University Hospital, Suite B-400, 200 Lothrop Street, Pittsburgh, PA 15213, U.S.A.

Acta Neurochir (1994) [Suppl] 62: 39–42

Tumour Volume Reduction Following Gamma Knife Radiosurgery: The Relationship Between X-ray and Histological Findings

J. C. Ganz[1], S. Aanderud[2], S. J. Mork[3], and A.-I. Smievoll[4]

Departments of [1] Neurosurgery, [2] Endocrinology, [3] Pathology, and [4] Radiology, Haukeland Hospital, University of Bergen, Norway

Summary

The case histories of two young ladies with Cushing's disease are described. Both patients were treated first with Gamma Knife radiosurgery and subsequently by microsurgery. The radiosurgery caused a marked reduction in tumour volume but only a partial relief of the endocrinopathy.

Comparison of the histological findings with the radiological findings following radiosurgery indicates that confluent necrosis is not a prerequisite for a reduction in tumour volume. It seems more likely that the reduction in tumour volume is related to changes in cellular dynamics.

Keywords: Cushing's disease; Gamma Knife radiosurgery; microsurgery; histological findings; tumour necrosis.

Introduction

The primary application of conventional fractionated radiotherapy has been for the treatment of malignant disease. This means that the aim of treatment is radiation induced destruction of the entire tumour cell population. It could be assumed that a similar aim also applies to radiosurgery. However, in the case of benign tumours this may not necessarily be true. This question has recently been raised by Professor Börje Larsson[4]. Nonetheless, it seems to be widely assumed that when radiosurgery produces a radiologically demonstrable reduction in tumour volume, a histologically visible confluent necrosis has occurred. This notion gains support from published reports[6].

The aim of the present study is to examine the question whether confluent necrosis will necessarily be found when tumour volume reduction can be demonstrated radiologically.

Material and Methods

The effects on the pituitary adenomas in two young women with Cushing's disease are reported. They were assessed for primary treatment with the Gamma Knife on the basis of endocrinological and CT and/or MRI findings. Follow up was by 6 monthly endocrinological and CT/MRI examinations. Both patients received a radiation dose of 50 Gy to the centre of the tumour and 25 Gy to the edge and less than 10 Gy to the visual pathways. Both patients had an unsatisfactory improvement of their endocrinopathy, and were therefore treated about 18 months after radiosurgery by microsurgery. Tumour tissue obtained at operation was examined histologically. A comparison of the radiological and histological findings form the basis of this report.

Results

Case 1. This 18 year old young lady suffering from Cushings disease was treated with the Gamma Knife for a pituitary microadenoma, 11 by 7 mm in diameter (Fig. 1a) on 4.1.89. Prior to treatment the 8 a.m. plasma cortisol was 473 nmol/l and the 8 p.m. was 423 nmol/l. Four months later in May 1989, the tumour was 6 by 4 mm in diameter (Fig. 1b). However, the Cushing endocrinopathy did not improve adequately and in November 1990 the 8 a.m. serum cortisol was 358 nmol/l and the 8 p.m. serum cortisol was 1256 nmol/l. During the period since Gamma Knife treatment, she had received metapyrone and while clinically improved was by no means well. Thus, she was operated on 26.03.91 and there were no operative findings that could have been definitely attributed to the previous radiosurgery. The histological picture showed no sign of clear cut necrosis, though there were some tissue changes which could have been the result of the prior radiosurgery (Fig. 2). As a result of the operation the patient achieved an isolated deficit of ACTH production producing a secondary adrenal insufficiency and requiring cortisone substitution therapy.

Case 2. This 19 year old young lady was treated with the Gamma Knife for a pituitary microadenoma (Fig. 3a) on 1.8.90. Prior to treatment the 8 a.m. plasma cortisol was 568 nmol/l and the 8 p.m. was 484 nmol/l. After the Gamma Knife treatment she had a total clinical improvement while on metapyrone and there was an obvious, radiologically demonstrated reduction in tumour volume (Fig. 3b). However, after stopping the medication the 8 p.m. serum cortisol rose to 450 nmol/l. Thus she was operated on 13.01.92. There was no particular special change at operation that could definitely have been related to the previous radiosurgery. The histological examination again showed no sign of clear cut necrosis (Fig. 2a and b). There may have been some more diffuse fibrosis than usual, but it was not marked. As a result of the operation the patient achieved an endocrinological cure without any pituitary insufficiency, requiring hormone substitution therapy.

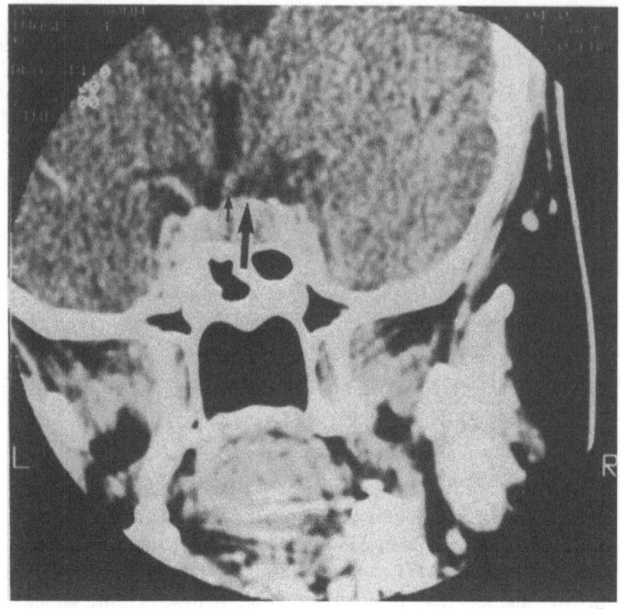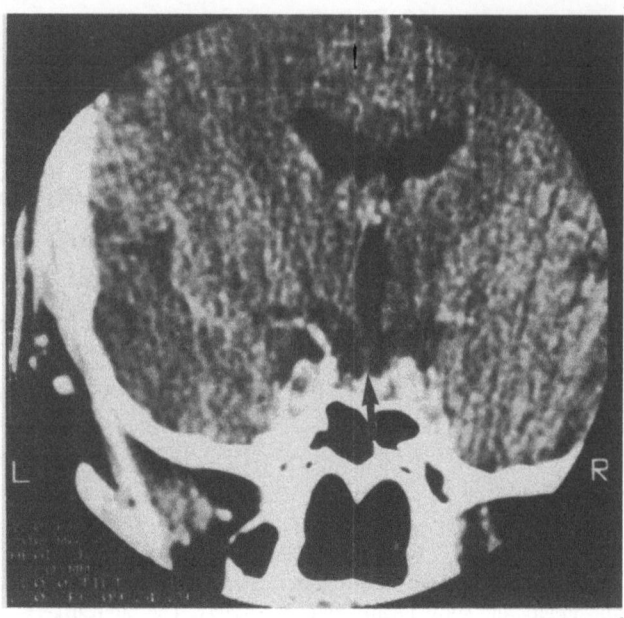

a   b

Fig. 1. (a) Pre-treatment coronal CT with iv contrast (Omnipaque). Note the convex upper margin of the tumour (arrow) and the dislocated pituitary stalk (thin arrow). (b) Post-Gamma Knife treatment coronal CT with iv contrast (Omnipaque). Note the volume reduction of the tumour and the straight mid-line pituitary stalk (arrow)

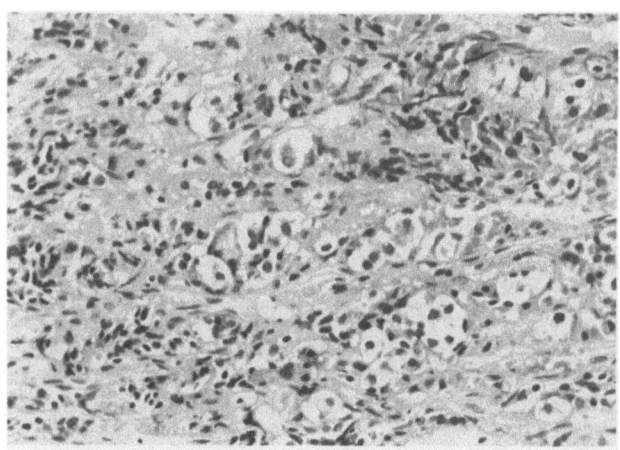

Fig. 2. Pituitary adenoma with a slight but distinct focal increase in connective tissue (HE, × 250)

Discussion

These two patients received only 25 Gy to the edge of the tumour. This is rather lower than the 35 Gy which Rähn and co-workers have found necessary to achieve an endocrinological cure[2,7]. However, there was no choice in these patients as the size of the tumour precluded a higher target edge dose, because the visual pathways would then have received over 10 Gy, which is the generally accepted highest tolerable dose[2,7].

Thus, the failure to achieve an endocrinological cure over the duration of the follow-up was not surprising. Nonetheless, the effect of the radiosurgery in achieving a reduction in tumour volume was impressive. This is in keeping with our findings in a larger series of patients, in that a lower dose is required for control of pituitary tumour growth than is required for endocrinological control[1,3].

The histological material is striking because of the lack of any clear-cut, irrefutable evidence of radiation changes. There is no vascular hyperplasia, no hyaline change and no obvious necrosis. However, it could be argued that the material was not representative of the tumour as a whole, or that some material was lost at surgery. These tumours are small and soft and it can be difficult to harvest them in their entirety. As far as the surgeon (JCG) could judge all available material was removed in case 2.

Thus, the findings indicate that these tumours can reduce in volume without the development of confluent necrosis: a process which would be expected to be followed by scarring and shrinkage. This is in keeping with Larsson's hypothesis that tumour "sterilisation" is not necessary for the radiosurgical control of benign tumours[4]. It is also in keeping with conventional radiobiological concepts. The definition of radiation induced cell death is that the cell loses the capacity to

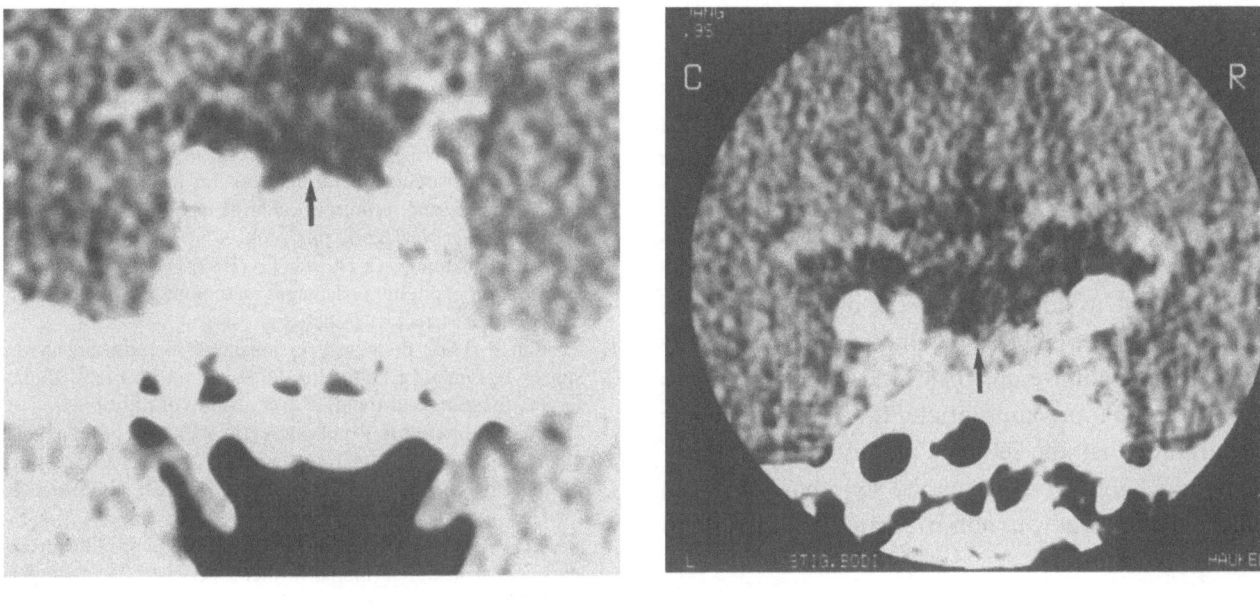

a   b

Fig. 3. (a) Pre-treatment coronal CT with iv contrast (Omnipaque). Note the convex upper margin of the tumour (arrow). (b) Post-Gamma Knife treatment coronal CT with iv contrast (Omnipaque). Note the volume reduction of the tumour and the concave upper margin (arrow)

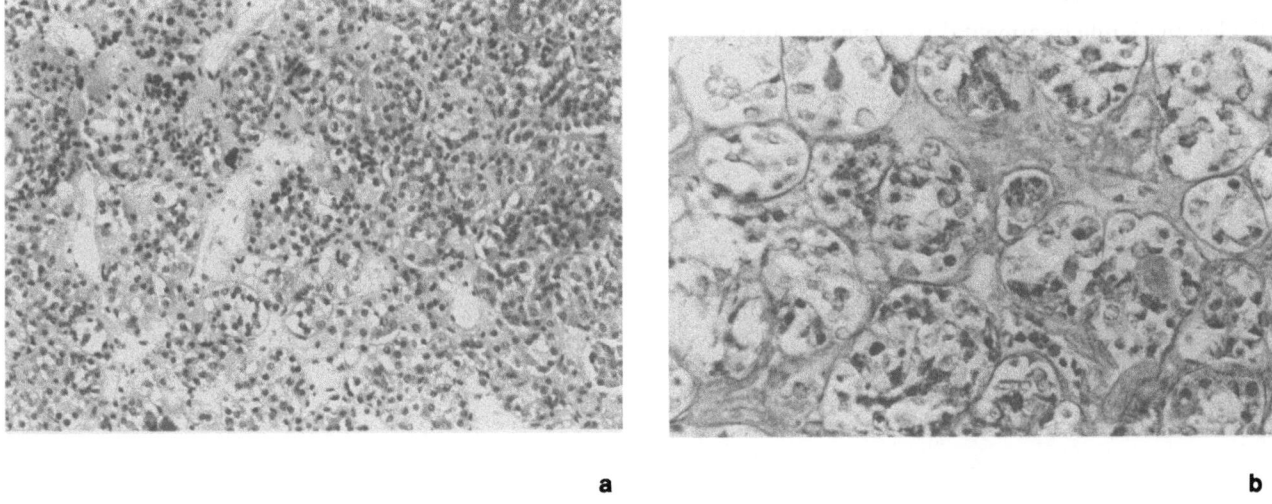

a   b

Fig. 4. (a) Representative area of the pituitary adenoma of patient 2. Note the lack of necrosis and the lack of any of the typical features of radiation damage (HE, × 140). (b) The same tumour showing some focal increase in connective tissue (Reticulin, × 450)

divide indefinitely[8]. Thus cell damage at the time of radiation may still be followed by a number of subsequent cell divisions before a given cell dies. Since cell death in this material cannot be related to a confluent necrosis it seems reasonable to suggest that the reduction in volume is the result of a disturbance of the dynamic balance between cell birth and cell death, present in all tissues. It is known that the tumour

volume doubling time of even malignant tumours is much slower than would be accounted for by the cell division rate[8]. This is explained by the continuing cell death concurrent with the cell division. It is suggested that the radiosurgical lesion has shifted the dynamic balance in the direction of cell death so that over time the total number of cells in the tumour is reduced and thus the volume is reduced. Moreover, apoptosis-, programmed cell death – might also play a part in this scenario.

The endocrinological improvement without cure is consistent with the results of others using different radiosurgical techniques[5], where it has been a consistent observation that endocrinological improvement is a continuing process spread over many years. It could be argued that one should have waited for the improvement to continue. On the other hand, since Cushing's disease is such a debilitating and potentially dangerous condition, microsurgical intervention was deemed to be more appropriate. It is a point of some importance that the findings at surgery were in no way remarkable, when compared with those observed during operations on non-irradiated patients with Cushing's disease.

Conclusions

1. Evidence of confluent necrosis is not a necessary concomitant of a reduction in volume following Gamma Knife Radiosurgery.
2. Volume reduction must be related to changes in tumour cell dynamics favouring a net loss in the number of cells.
3. Gamma Knife treatment does not necessarily make subsequent surgery more difficult.

References

1. Backlund E-O, Ganz JC (1993) Pituitary adenomas: Gamma Knife. In: Alexander E, Loeffler JS, Lunsford LD (eds) Stereotactic radiosurgery. McGraw Hill, New York, pp 167–173
2. Backlund E-O (1979) Stereotactic radiosurgery in intracranial tumours and vascular malformations. In: Krayenbühl H *et al* (eds) Advances and technical standards in neurosurgery, Vol 6. Springer, Wien New York, pp 1–37
3. Ganz JC, Backlund E-O, Thorsen FA (1993) The effects of gamma knife surgery of pituitary adenomas on tumour growth and endocrinopathies. Stereotact Funct Neurosurg:
4. Larsson B (1992) Biological fundamentals of radiosurgery. In: Steiner L, Lindquist C, Forster D, Backlund E-O (eds) Radiosurgery: baseline and trends. Raven, New York, pp 7–8
5. Levy RP, Fabrikant JI, Frankel KA (1993) Particle beam irradiation of the pituitary gland. In: Alexander E, Loeffler JS, Lunsford LD (eds) Stereotactic radiosurgery. McGraw Hill, New York, pp 157–165
6. Norén G, Arndt J, Hindmarsh T (1983) Stereotactic radiosurgery in cases of acoustic neurinoma: further experiences. Neurosurgery 13: 12–22
7. Rähn T, Thorén M, Hall K, Backlund E-O (1980) Stereotactic radiosurgery in cushing's disease: acute radiation effects. Surg Neurol 14: 85–92
8. Withers H, Peters LJ (1978) Biologic aspects of radiation therapy. In: Fletcher G (ed) Textbook of radiotherapy. Lea and Febiger, Philadelphia, pp 103–180

Correspondence: J. C. Ganz, M.A., Ph.D., FRCS, Department of Neurosurgery, Hankeland Hospital, University of Bergen, N-5027 Bergen, Norway.

Acta Neurochir (1994) [Suppl] 62: 43–46

Radiosensitive Craniopharyngiomas: The Role of Radiosurgery

H. K. Inoue[1], H. Kohga[1], T. Kakegawa[1], N. Ono[1], M. Hirato[1], M. Nakamura[1], C. Ohye[1], T. Shibazaki[2], Y. Andou[2], J. Tamada[3], and I. Handa[3]

[1] Department of Neurosurgery, Gunma University School of Medicine, Maebashi, [2] Gamma Unit Center, Hidaka Hospital, and [3] National Takasaki Hospital, Takasaki, Japan

Summary

Clinical characteristics of radiosensitive craniopharyngiomas and histologically identical tumours were re-evaluated from among 53 patients. There were 9 squamous cell type and 3 mixed type tumours. Early effects of radiosurgery for two recent cases are reported. Radiosurgery may have an important role to play in the treatment of craniopharyngiomas, especially of the squamous cell type.

Keywords: Craniopharyngioma; squamous cell type; radiosensitivity; gamma knife surgery; non-radical open surgery.

Introduction

Craniopharyngioma is an histologically benign extramedullary tumour. In spite of advances in modern microsurgical techniques, location of the tumour in the hypothalamic-pituitary axis makes treatment controversial[1]. Total surgical resection is often complicated by endocrinological deficits and the tumour may recur after a long period due to finger-like tumour invasion into the surrounding brain tissue. To decrease the surgical risk, conservative surgery coupled with radiation therapy has been utilized. Long-term follow-up of patients treated with this combined therapy has demonstrated the efficacy of radiation therapy[7,10].

We have treated these tumours with conventional irradiation after partial or subtotal resection and found that some tumours, that were histologically the squamous cell type of craniopharyngioma, responded completely to radiation therapy. We called this "radiosensitive craniopharyngioma"[12].

In 1989, Backlund *et al.* reported their long-term results with a stereotactic approach to craniopharyngiomas[6]. As conventional irradiation may damage the surrounding brain, especially in children[11,15], intracavitary irradiation of cystic tumours and radiosurgery of solid tumours seems to be the ideal mode of radiation for craniopharyngiomas.

This article discusses the clinical characteristics of radiosensitive craniopharyngiomas and the role of radiosurgery. We include preliminary results with gamma knife surgery.

Materials and Methods

Craniopharyngiomas which disappeared after conventional irradiation and histologically identical tumours that were not irradiated from 53 patients treated between 1956 and 1992 were studied. Our therapeutic policy was non-radical open surgery combined with radiation therapy. After partial or subtotal resection, the residual tumour was usually treated with 50 to 60 Gy of fractionated irradiation. The histological characteristics of each tumour were determined by routine light microscopic observation of haematoxylin and eosin-stained surgical specimens. Two recent patients were treated with radiosurgery using a gamma unit.

Results

Clinical Characteristics

Our study was comprised of 27 males and 26 females, from 2 to 66 years of age (mean 26). The age and sex distribution is shown in Fig. 1. Histological re-evaluation was available in 46 cases. There were 35 cases of the adamantinomatous type of craniopharyngioma (76%), 9 cases of the squamous cell type of craniopharyngioma, and 3 cases of mixed type.

In the adamantinomatous type, 21 cases were under 20 years of age and 14 cases were adults (Fig. 1). The main symptoms and signs were headache, visual disturbances, and those related to endocrine dysfunction. Visual disturbances were recognized in 78% of cases. Endocrinological symptoms and signs were polyuria

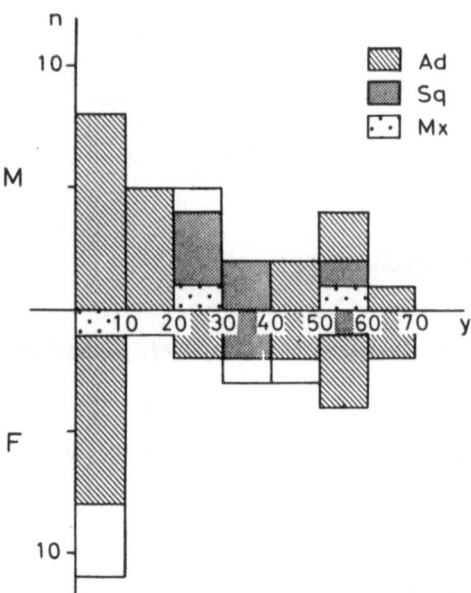

Fig. 1. Age and sex distribution of 53 craniopharyngiomas. *M* male. *F* female. *Ad* adamantinomatous type. *Sq* squamous cell type. *Mx* mixed type

and/or polydypsia, obesity and/or dwarfism, loss of axillary and pubic hair, decreased libido, amenorrhoea, and severe fatigue. These symptoms were observed in 53% of the cases. Polyuria and obesity were dominant in children and hypogonadal functions dominated adults. Neuroradiological examination with CT scan was performed in 14 patients. Calcification was detected in 12 cases (86%) and the tumour mass was low density in 11 cases, high density in 2 cases, and isodense in one case. Tumour cysts were recognized in 13 cases (93%) and the contents were typical "motor oil" in 9 cases and yellowish in 4 cases.

All of the patients with the squamous cell type and mixed type were adults (20 to 57 years of age) except for one 4 year old with a mixed type of tumour (Fig. 1). The main symptoms were headache and visual disturbances (67% of the patients). Symptoms and signs due to endocrine dysfunction were observed in only 3 cases (25%) and these were polyuria and amenorrhoea. CT scans were available in 6 cases and no calcification was seen. Tumours were low density in 4 cases and isodense in 2 cases. Tumour cysts were seen in 3 cases (50%) with yellowish fluid content in all 3. Three squamous cell craniopharyngiomas disappeared after conventional irradiation, as reported previously.

In adults (over 20 years of age), squamous and mixed tumours were found in 11 out of 24 cases (46%). In children, adamantinomatous tumours were found in 21 out of 22 cases (96%).

Early Results of Radiosurgery

Case 1. A 32-year-old female complained of amenorrhoea and progressive decrease in vision. A CT scan demonstrated a large intra- and suprasellar, uncalcified low density mass which extended to near the foramen of Monro. A cystic tumour was partially resected and an Ommaya's reservoir was placed with a catheter in the cystic cavity. Histology showed a squamous cell craniopharyngioma. Postoperative imaging studies (CT scan and MR imaging) showed a marked decrease in the size of the mass and a gadolinium-enhanced solid part in the suprasellar region. The solid part was treated with a gamma unit with marginal dose 9.9 Gy (Fig. 2A). One year after radiosurgery, the solid part decreased markedly. However, the cystic part had expanded again (Fig. 2B) requiring aspiration of cyst fluid.

Case 2. A 56-year-old male presented with progressive deterioration of vision and headache 6 years after the first treatment for craniopharyngioma (subtotal resection and 60 Gy irradiation). MR imaging showed a recurrent tumour in the suprasellar region. A 2-cm solid mass was subtotally resected. Histological diagnosis was that of a mixed type of craniopharyngioma. His visual acuity improved after surgery. However, follow-up MR imaging revealed a regrowth of tumour 2 years later (Fig. 3A). The tumour was then treated with a gamma unit with marginal dose 12 Gy (Fig. 3B). MR imaging 5 months after radiosurgery showed a marked decrease in the size of the tumour (Fig. 3C).

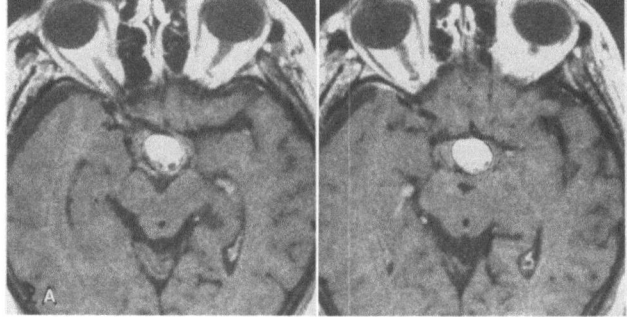

A

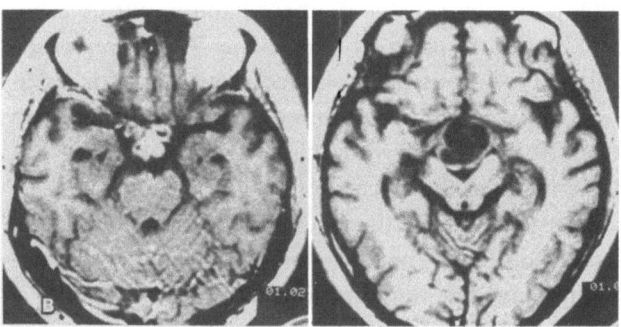

B

Fig. 2. (A) Stereotactic MR imaging (gadolinium-enhanced Tl-weighted) of a 32-year-old female (case 1, squamous cell type of craniopharyngioma) during radiosurgery using a gamma unit. A solid part of the tumour was treated with a 30% isodose, 9.9 Gy. (B) MR imaging (Tl-weighted) one year after radiosurgery showing marked decrease of solid part of the tumour but re-expansion of the cystic part

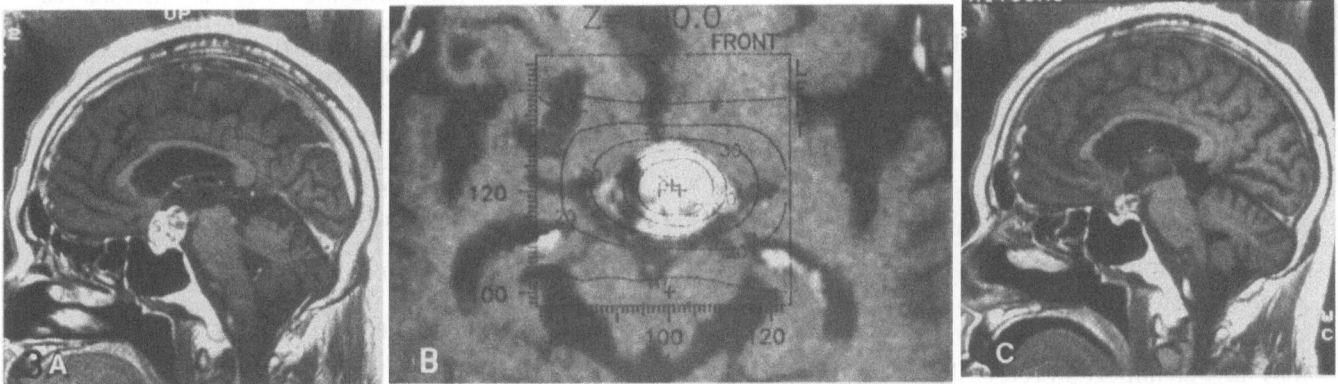

Fig. 3. (A) Sagittal MR imaging (gadolinium-enhanced Tl-weighted) of a 56-year-old male (case 2, mixed type) showing a recurrent tumour before radiosurgery. (B) Stereotactic MR imaging during radiosurgery. The tumour was treated with a 50% isodose, 12 Gy. (C) Five months after treatment, the enhanced mass decreased markedly

Discussion

Long-term follow-up studies of conservative surgery coupled with radiation therapy have demonstrated the efficacy of radiation therapy in the treatment of craniopharyngiomas[7,10]. However, there were no reports describing the relationship between radiosensitivity and the histology of craniopharyngioma until our recent report which demonstrated that squamous cell craniopharyngiomas are radiosensitive tumours[12]. Clinical and histological comparisons of adamantinomatous and squamous cell craniopharyngiomas have been described and the findings suggest that squamous cell craniopharyngiomas represent a distinct clinical entity[8,13].

In this article we have demonstrated clinical differences between adamatinomatous and squamous cell craniopharyngiomas based on re-evaluation of 46 cases. Most adamantinomatous tumours were cystic and occured in children. In adults, about half the patients revealed squamous cell or mixed type histology. These tumours were solid or partly solid and lacked calcification. Depending on the site and extension of tumours, patients with squamous cell craniopharyngiomas had less frequent endocrine symptoms than those with the adamatinomatous type. In some cases prediction of histological type may be possible from these clinical and radiological findings. If the tumour is diagnosed as of the squamous cell type from an intraoperative frozen section, extensive resections may be avoided and postoperative radiation therapy may provide safe and successful treatment. Radiosensitive squamous cell craniopharyngiomas may be curable with conventional irradiation and radiosurgery may

be useful for minimizing the adverse effects of radiation therapy[9,14,16,17].

Although long-term follow-up is necessary, early results of radiosurgery for squamous cell type and mixed type of craniopharyngiomas are encouraging and further trials are warranted. The second case had received full dose conventional irradiation but recurred after treatment. In cases such a these, further conventional irradiation is dangerous because of potential radiation injury to the surrounding brain. Complete resection of the recurrent tumour is desirable. However, radiosurgery will be an alternative treatment modality as reported here because radical excision of recurrent craniopharyngiomas is difficult and very risky.

Backlund has reported stereotactic treatment for craniopharyngiomas[2,3] with intracystic yttrium-90[4] and gamma unit radiosurgery[5]. In 1989, he and his colleagues reported the long-term follow-up of their treatment[6]. Their results with 10 to 23 year follow-up are good, even in comparison with recent microsurgical operations in experienced hands. Stereotactic approaches have also progressed with the advancement of imaging techniques, MR imaging is now able to demonstrate a multicystic tumour very nicely and to distinguish between the solid and cystic parts. Furthermore, lineation of the optic pathway, pituitary stalk, and hypothalamus is available during stereotactic procedures for intracystic treatment and gamma unit radiosurgery. It is expected that the results of recent stereotactic treatment for craniopharyngiomas will improve even more. Radiosurgery may have an important role for treatment of craniopharyngiomas, especially in the radiosensitive squamous cell type.

Conclusion

Radiosensitive squamous cell craniopharyngiomas and mixed type craniopharyngiomas represented 26% of all craniopharyngiomas and 46% of adult craniopharyngiomas in this series. These tumours were solid or partially solid and without calcification. Endocrinological symptoms were less frequent in those cases than the adamatinomatous type. Early results of radiosurgery for these tumours are encouraging and further trials are warranted. It is concluded that radiosurgery may have an important role in the treatment of craniopharyngiomas, especially of the squamous cell type.

References

1. Adamson TE, Wiestler OD, Kleihues P, *et al* (1990) Correlation of clinical and pathological features in surgically treated craniopharyngiomas. J Neurosurg 73: 12–17
2. Backlund E-O (1969) Stereotaxic treatment of craniopharyngiomas. In: Hamberger CA, Wersall J (eds) Nobel Symposium 10: disorders of the skull base region. Almqvist and Wiksell, Stockholm, pp 237–244
3. Backlund E-O (1970) Stereotaxic treatment of craniopharyngiomas. Acta Neurol Scand 46: 623
4. Backlund E-O (1973) Studies on craniopharyngiomas III. Stereotaxic treatment with intracystic yttrium-90. Acta Chir Scand 139: 237–247
5. Backlund E-O (1979) Solid craniopharyngiomas treated by stereotactic radiosurgery. In: Szikla G (ed) Stereotactic cerebral irradiation. INSERM Symposium No 12. Elsevier North-Holland Biomedical Press, Amsterdam, pp 271–281
6. Backlund E-O, Axelsson B, Bergstrand C-G, *et al* (1989) Treatment of craniopharyngiomas–the stereotactic approach in a ten to twenty-three years' perspective I. Surgical, radiological and ophthalmological aspects. Acta Neurochir (Wien) 99: 11–19
7. Fischer EG, Welch K, Belli JA, *et al* (1985) Treatment of craniopharyngiomas in children. J Neurosurg 62: 496–501
8. Giangaspero F, Osborne DR, Bunger Pc, *et al* (1984) Suprasellar papillary squamous epithelioma ("papillary craniopharyngioma"). Am J Surg Pathol 8: 57–64
9. Guy J, Mancuso A, Beck R, *et al* (1991) Radiation-induced optic neuropathy: A magnetic resonance imaging study. J Neurosurg 74: 426–432
10. Hoogenhout J, Otten BJ, Kazem I, *et al* (1984) Surgery and radiation therapy in the management of craniopharyngiomas. Int J Radiat Oncol Biol Phys 10: 2293–2297
11. Inoue HK, Nakamura M, Ono N, *et al* (1993) Long-term clinical effects of radiation therapy for primitive gliomas and medulloblastomas: a role for radiosurgery. Stereotact Funct Neurosurg 61: 51–58
12. Inoue HK, Nakamura M, Ono N, *et al* (1993) Radiosensitive squamous cell craniopharyngiomas: Clinical and pathological comparison with the adamantinomatous type. Brain Tumor Pathol (Tokyo) 10: 27–31
13. Kahn EA, Gosch HH, Seeger JF, *et al* (1973) Forty-five years experience with the craniopharyngiomas. Surg Neurol 1: 5–12
14. Maat-Schieman ML, Bots GT, Thomeer RT, *et al* (1985) Malignant astrocytoma following radiotherapy for craniopharyngioma. Br J Radiol 58: 480–482
15. Mitchell WG, Fishman LS, Miller JH, *et al* (1991) Stroke as a late sequela of cranial irradiation for childhood brain tumors. J Child Neurol 6: 128–133
16. Satran R, Lapham LW, Kido DR, *et al* (1984) Late cerebral radionecrosis after conventional irradiation of cerebral tumors. Rev Neurol (Paris) 140: 249–255
17. Ushio Y, Arita N, Yoshimine T, *et al* (1987) Glioblastoma after radiotherapy for craniopharyngioma: case report. Neurosurgery 21: 33–38

Correspondence: Hiroshi K. Inoue, M.D., Department of Neurosurgery, Gunma University School of Medicine, Showa-machi 3-39-22, Maebashi 371, Japan.

Acta Neurochir (1994) [Suppl] 62: 47–54

A Comparison of Survival Between Radiosurgery and Stereotactic Implants for Malignant Astrocytomas

B. Stea[1], **K. Rossman**[3], **J. Kittelson**[1], **B. Lulu**[1], **A. Shetter**[3], **J. R. Cassady**[1], and **A. Hamilton**[2]

[1]Department of Radiation Oncology, [2]Division of Neurosurgery University of Arizona Health Sciences Center, Tucson, AZ, and [3]Barrow Neurological Institute, Phoenix, AZ, U.S.A.

Summary

The purpose of this paper is to compare the survial of three groups of patients with high grade supratentorial gliomas who were treated on three sequential protocols with surgical resection, external beam fractionated radiotherapy and a boost to the residual contrasting enhancing mass by either interstitial brachytherapy (IB, n = 33), by interstitial thermoradiotherapy (IT, n = 25) or by stereotactic radiosurgery (SRS, n = 19). The primary aim of this study was to evaluate the role of different boosting techniques in the inital management of primary brain tumors. External beam radiotherapy doses were escalated from one study to the next so that the median doses given to the IB, the IT, and the SRS groups were 41.4 Gy, 48.4 Gy, and 59.4 Gy, respectively. The median dose of interstitial irradiation or stereotactic radiosurgery, were 40 Gy, 32.2 Gy and 10 Gy, respectively, for the same groups.

Follow-up was such that all living patients had been followed for a minimum of 30, 27, 4 months in the IB, IT, and SRS groups, respectively; hence, twelve-month survival was 52% (95% CI: 34%–69%), 80% (95% CI: 64%–96%), and 51% (95% CI: 24%–78%) in the same respective groups. Using a multivariate Cox proportional hazards model, treatment with IT conferred a survival advantage over IB (p = 0.029). Furthermore, survival of patients treated with SRS did not significantly differ from that of patients treated with an implant with or without hyperthermia.

We conclude that within the constraints of the selection factors and different treatment parameters used in these studies, stereotactic radiosurgery offers the same survival advantage as interstitial implant but with reduced morbidity and mortality. However, interstitial brachytherapy can be combined with hyperthermia and this combined modality approach appears to decrease by half the risk of dying from a malignant glioma when compared with interstitial irradiation alone.

Keywords: Gliomas; interstitial irradiation; hyperthermia; radiosurgery.

Introduction

External beam fractionated radiation therapy (EBFRT) is a well established treatment modality in the management of patients with high grade gliomas. The results of randomized clinical trials performed by the Brain Tumor Study Group (BTSG)/Brain Cooperative Group (BTCG) (Walker 1980, Shapiro 1989) and by the Radiation Therapy Oncology Group (RTOG) (Chang 1983) have shown that EBFRT significantly prolongs the median survival of patients with glioblastoma multiforme (GBM) and anaplastic astrocytoma (AA). A dose response relationship with increasing doses of EBFRT of up to 60 Gy has been demonstrated for this neoplasm (Walker 1979). However, the limitations imposed by normal tissue tolerance have prevented a significant escalation of radiation therapy (RT) dose. Furthermore, numerous studies have also shown that despite high doses of EBFRT the vast majority of recurrences occur within two centimeters of the original tumor volume (Hochberg 1980, Wallner 1989).

The prognosis following therapy for adults with supratentorial malignant gliomas remains poor. Therefore, since a RT dose escalation appears to be desirable in order to increase the local control and thereby the survival of these patients, numerous attempts have been made over the past decade to increase the focal dose of radiation to the contrast enhancing part of the tumor. Such attempts have included, among other approaches: both temporary, and permanent implants (Rossman 1985, Leibel 1989, Gutin 1991, Ostertag 1992), three dimensional conformal treatment planning (Thornton 1991), stereotactic radiosurgery, (Loeffler 1992) and fractionated stereotactic radiotherapy (Souhami 1991, Brada 1993).

In an attempt to improve the therapeutic gain, hyperthermia has also been used as an adjuvant to interstitial irradiation by numerous investigators (Roberts 1986, Stea 1990, 1992, Sneed 1992). The rationale for using hyperthermia in conjunction with radiation are the following: a) complementarity of action with RT on cells within different phases of the cell cycle, i.e. hyperthermia is more damaging to cells which are in the S-phase of the mitotic cycle when cells are most resistant to radiation-induced killing; b) effectiveness againt cells growing at low pH and in nutritionally deprived conditions which are believed to exist in the core of the highly malignant GBM; c) thermal radiosensitization by inhibition of sublethal and potential lethal damage repair.

Treatment of malignant brain tumors using interstitial irradiation with Iridium-192 (Ir-192) in conjunction with ferromagnetic seed hyperthermia began at the University of Arizona in March 1988. The first 28 patients were treated in a Phase I study with the primary objective of determining the level of toxicity associated with the treatment. The Phase I study was closed at the end of 1990 and an analysis concluded that treatment could be carried out within acceptable toxicity bounds (Stea 1992) A Phase II study of survival duration was opened in 1991; however, it was closed one year later due to inability to meet the anticipated accrual targets.

Since 1991, we have been using stereotactic radiosurgery to focally escalate the RT dose to the contrast enhancing region of malignant gliomas. Although the technique of SRS goes back 40 years (Leksell 1951), only recently has this technique found application to a wide variety of intracranial neoplasms (Flickinger 1991, Loeffler 1990, Kondziolka 1991) including high grade gliomas (Loeffler 1992).

The purpose of this paper is to compare the survival of patients with high grade supratentorial gliomas, treated in our Phase I/II protocol of interstitial thermoradiotherapy (IT) with that of a similar group of patients treated at the Barrow Neurological Institute (BNI) with interstitial brachytherapy alone (IB), and with the survival of another group of patients treated at the University of Arizona between 1991–1993 with a stereotactic radiosurgery (SRS) boost at the completion of their course of EBFRT.

Materials and Methods

Patient Selection

The three studies under evaluation in this paper were conducted over a period of ten years in a quasi-sequential manner. The investigators involved in the patient selection in the first phase (IB) also collaborated in the IT studies, and investigators in the IT studies were also involved in the SRS studies. Patients in the IB group were treated at the BNI between May 1982 and November 1990. A total of 55 IB patients met the eligibility criteria defined below, however 22 patients were excluded from analysis so that treatment volumes between the IB and the IT groups would be comparable (see *Data Reduction*, below). The IT study was conducted between March 1988 and March 1992, and the SRS study was initiated in June 1991. The present analysis restricts attention to all patients seen through February 1993, who were treated at the time of initial presentation.

Eligibility criteria common to all three studies included: a) biopsy-proven diagnosis of AA of GBM; b) Karnofsky performance status (KPS) of 50 or better; c) at least 18 years of age; d) life expectancy of at least three months; e) tumor location. Although the last criterion was more stringently applied in the implant series (due to the potential for increased morbidity with an invasive techinque), tumors treated on the SRS protocol were also selected based on their location (e.g. patients with tumors located with 5 mm of the optic chiasm were excluded). Patients with brain stem lesions or multicentric tumors were excluded from all studies. Although other studies (Loeffler, 1990, 1992) have been restricted to small tumors, the IB and SRS studies included all patients that could be technically implanted or adequately covered with single or multiple isocenters. The IT study was restricted to tumors less than 100 cm³.

Treatment Protocol

Patients on all three studies first underwent as much of a complete resection as possible for the dual purpose of establishing a diagnosis

Table 1. *Comparison of Patient Populations and Treatment Parameters*

Factor	Level	Interstitial brachytherapy (n = 33)	Interstitial thermoradiotherapy (n = 25)	Stereotactic radiosurgery (n = 19)
KPS[a]	$\% \geq 80$	82	92	74
Histology	% AA	24	32	37
Age	median	51	44	42
	range	(27, 76)	(21, 79)	(22, 72)
Treated vol. (cm³)	median	55.6	54.1	50.5
	range	(14.0, 108.5)	(20.3, 131.9)	(11.7, 158.7)
IB/RS dose (Gy)	median	40.0	32.2	10.0
	range	(24.0, 60.0)	(26.0, 41.4)	(6.5, 15.0)
EBRT dose (Gy)	median	41.4	48.4	59.4
	range	(40.0, 60.0)	(40.0, 54.0)	(44.0, 62.0)

[a]Percentages based on the subset of patients for which KPS was measured (IB = 18, IT = 24, SRS = 19 patients).

as well as to maximally debulk the tumor. This was followed by a course of EBFRT delivered to partial brain fields by appropriate portal arrangements to spare as much normal brain as possible. Margins of 3 cm around the contrast enhancing region on CT scans or 1.5–2 cm around the area of increased signal intensity on the T2 weighted MRI images were used. Patients were treated at conventional fractionation of 1.8 to 2.0 Gy per fraction five days per week. Generally, IB patients tended to receive lower total EBFRT doses, IT patients received an intermediate EBFRT dose, and SRS patients received the highest EBFRT doses (Table 1). Stereotactic implants or SRS were performed two to fours weeks after completion of EBFRT. Brachytherapy was delivered with Iridium-192 in both the IB and IT studies to median doses of 40 Gy and 32.2 Gy, respectively (Table 1). The dose distribution and seed strength were optimized so that the target boundary would receive the prescribed dose at a rate of 30 to 70 cGy per hours. In contrast to patients in the IB group, patients in the IT group had the advantage of computerized dosimetry with display of the isodose lines in multiple planes to ensure that the chosen isodose line fully encompassed the contrast enhancing volume in every plane (Lulu 1990).

Interstitial Catheter Implantation

Operative techniques for the intracranial implantation of silastic catheters have already been described (Rossman 1985, Stea 1990). Both the IB and IT patients underwent stereotactic catheter implantation with the help of a Brown Roberts Wells (BRW) stereotactic system. The technique of template guided implantation used for the IT group has been previously described (Lulu 1990). Briefly, on the morning of the implant procedure, a CT scan with the BRW frame in place and the localizer assembly attached to the base ring was done. Then the trajectory, approach direction, and depth of catheter placement were all computed with a Hewlett Packard HP41C programmable calculator (IB group) or on a computer graphics display station (Lexidata 3700) for the IT group.

The treatment planning process for the IT group consisted of marking the target volume on transverse CT slices using a track ball at the computer graphics display station. A variale margin of up to 15 mm outside of the contrast enhancing edge of the tumor was used whenever possible. Margins were necessarily smaller for tumors that abutted critical structures such as the brain stem or the motor cortex. Once the digitization of the target was completed, and the necessary coordinate transformation derived, an approach direction for catheter placement was determined. Once an approach direction was chosen, the projection of the target volume along the approach direction was computed and displayed on the Lexidata terminal. This helped in the selection and positioning of an appropriate template. The templates differed primarily in the intercatheter spacing. We commonly used an intercatheter spacing of 1.2 cm. Catheter insertion depth required to adequately cover the distal boundaries of the target volume was then computed, and the information relayed to the surgeon who then positioned the catheters within the tumor.

Interstitial Hyperthermia

Hyperthermia was delivered by means of thermally regulating ferromagnetic implants that were afterloaded into the surgically placed catheters. The ferromagnetic implants consisted of either 1×10 mm seeds strung together in ribbons, or multistranded wire bundles of similar dimension (Stea 1992). The ferromagnetic implants were heated by means of a radiofrequency magnetic field induced by a magnetic induction coil. The composition of the ferromagnetic seeds and the details of the hyperthermic technique have been

described previously (Stea 1990, Haider 1991). Hyperthermia was delivered for sixty minutes with the goal of heating as much of the implant volume as possible to a temperature between 42 °C and 45 °C. Hyperthermia treatments were given just prior to and immediately after interstitial brachytherapy. Temperatures were continuously monitored by means of multisensor thermocouple probes or fiber optic thermometers. The patients were monitored during the hyperthermia sessions with continuous vital signs and frequent neurological examination at five to ten minute intervals.

Stereotactic Radiosurgery

Stereotactic radiosurgery was performed by means of a standard 6 MeV linear accelerator (Varian and Associates Inc., Palo Alto, CA), a custom designed floor stand (Lutz 1988) and in-house derived MacIntosh-based treatment planning program. We used a median of two isocenters per tumor with a range of one to four isocenters. The median collimator diameter used was 37.5 mm (range: 15 mm–40 mm). The median minimum dose was 10 Gy (range: 6.5 Gy–15 Gy) dosed to the 80–113% isodose line. The radiosurgical tumor volume was marked on sequential CT slices together with critical structures which were then digitized into the treatment planning software. Following completion of the treatment plan and quality assurance tests, the patient was brought to the Radiation Oncology Department. The patient's head was fixed to the floor stand by means of two screws attached to the BRW stereotactic frame and treatment delivered via the standard four radiosurgery arcs. Tumor and treatment volumes were available from the treatment planning program for the patients who received SRS boost. The tumor volumes ranged from $1.3–115.5$ cm^3 (median 24.1 cm^3). The median treatment volume for the radiosurgery patients was 50.5 cm^3 with a range of $11.7–158.70$ cm^3.

Data Reduction

Due to restrictions in the IT protocol (Stea 1990), treatment volumes in the IB group were substantially larger than those in the IT group (Fig. 1a). Thus, in order to provide a meaningful comparison, the primary analysis was based on a subset of the IB patients that included only those patients with treatment volumes less than 110 cm^3. Restricting the analysis to this subset provided a better match between treatment volume distributions in the three groups (Fig. 1b). As a result, 22 patients were excluded from the 55 patient IB group: 10 because of excessive treatment volume, and 12 because treatment volume could not be accurately verified.

Statistical Methods

Treatment groups were compared based on patient survival. Survival duration was measured from the time of diagnosis. All living patients had recent follow-up visits at the time the analysis was initiated (March 1993). No patients were lost to follow-up.

Survival comparisons were conducted on two levels, an unadjusted analysis in which the differences between the three treatment groups were compared using the logrank test, and an adjusted analysis in which comparisons were made in a Cox proportional hazards model that adjusted for imbalances in prognostic factors between groups. In the unadjusted analysis, survival was estimated using the method of Kaplan and Meier, and the variance of these estimates was calculated using Greenwood's formula (Miller 1981). The adjusted analysis enabled comparison of treatments after adjusting for the effect of important covariates (treated volume, patient age, histology). Hence, if there were imbalances between the treatment groups (e.g.

(a) Untrimmed Volume Distribution

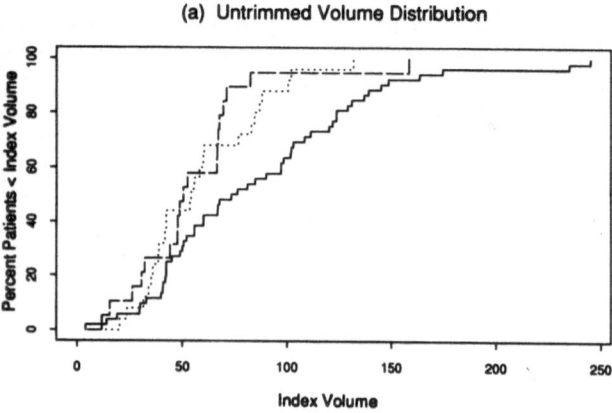

(b) Trimmed Volume Distribution

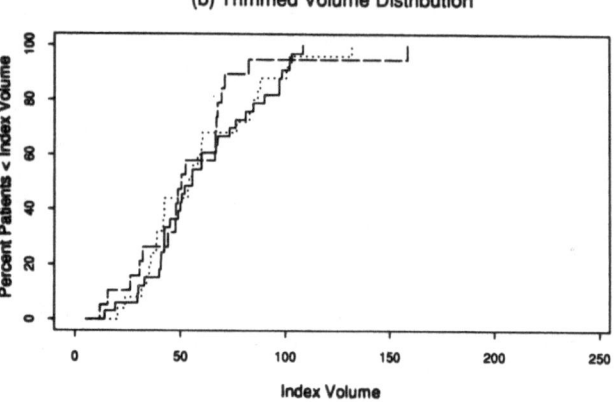

Fig. 1. Distribution of treatment volumes for the three patient populations. Treatment volumes were used as surrogates for tumor volumes as the latter were not available for all patients. Treatment volume was defined as the volume encompassed by the treatment isodose line; (a) the entire population of 55 patients treated with interstitial brachytherapy (solid line) is plotted against the interstitial thermoradiotherapy group (broken line) and the stereotactic radiosurgery group (dotted line); (b) volumes of the interstitial brachytherapy group have been trimmed (n = 33) so that their distribution closely matches that of the other two groups

the interstitial radiation group has somewhat older patients), this type of analysis made appropriate adjustments to the comparison p-values. To select the proportional hazards model that described the data, we used a stepwise elimination process beginning with all treatment groups and covariates. The proportional hazards assumption was checked using a log/log survival plot, residual analysis, and by examining changes in the parameter estimates when they were computed over subintervals of the time range (Fleming and Harrington, 1991).

Results

Patients and Treatment Parameters

The clinical characteristics and the treatment parameters for the three groups of patients analyzed in this study are summarized in Table 1. The three groups consisted of patients who received an interstitial brachy-

therapy boost alone (n = 33); a second group of 25 patients who received a thermoradiotherapy boost, and a third group of 19 patients who received a SRS boost. The median KPS for all the three groups of patients was 90, and the percent of patients with a KPS ≥ 80 was comparable among the three groups. However, an imbalance in the percentage of patients with AA histology was noted; the radiosurgery group having the highest proportion of these patients. These three groups of patients also received different doses of EBFRT and interstitial or SRS boost. These differences reflect changes in treatment philosophy occurring over the decade during which the three studies took place. When considering the two implant studies, the median EBFRT doses were 41.4 Gy and 48.4 Gy for the IB and IT groups, respectively; however, the median interstitial dose of radiation was higher (40 Gy) for the former than the latter (32.2 Gy). Although EBFRT and brachytherapy doses cannot be directly added to one another due to different radiobiological effectiveness, it is notable that the sum of the median doses of EBFRT and brachytherapy was approximately constant for the two implant studies (Table 1). In the thermoradiotherapy study we used a higher proportional dose of EBFRT because early autopsy results had shown that patients treated with brachytherapy alone had marginal recurrences.

Survival

The survival curves for each of the treatment groups are displayed in Fig. 2. Although comparisons based on these curves are not adjusted for the effects of

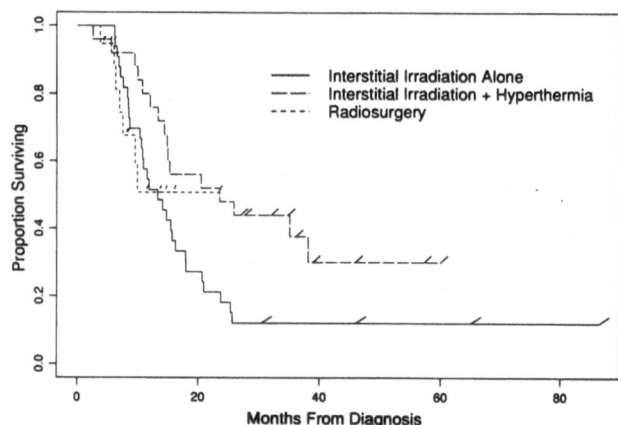

Fig. 2. Kaplan-Meier representation of survival from diagnosis for patients with high grade gliomas treated with a course of external beam fractionated radiotherapy and a "boost" either by interstitial brachytherapy or by interstitial thermoradiotherapy or by stereotactic radiosurgery

imbalances in prognostic factors between treatment groups, they show that the IT group had significantly improved survival when compared to the IB group (p = 0.017, Table 2). There were no significant differences between either IT and SRS (p = 0.22) or IB and SRS (p = 0.98). This analysis was based on the 33 patients remaining in the IB data set after eliminating patients with large treatment volumes. We note that an analysis based on all 55 patients from the IB group demonstrated an even more significant difference between IT and IB (p = 0.0060, analysis not shown), thereby demonstrating that the significant result was not an artifact of the exclusion criteria that we used.

The precision of the study (i.e. the variability of the results) is a function of the number of deaths and pattern of censored observations in the various treatment groups. The unadjusted survival curves (Fig. 2) show that the survival function is most precisely estimated in the IB group (median censored observation = 55.5 months, range = 30.4 to 86.5 months) is least precise in the SRS group (median censored observation = 9.7 months, range = 4.0 to 23.4 months), and is intermediate in the IT (median censored observation = 36.1 months, range = 27.0 to 60.0 months). The precision is formally reflected in the 95% confidence intervals on the estimated survival probabilities at various time points (Table 2), which can be used for comparison to other studies in similar patient populations.

A more complete survival analysis adjusts for imbalances in patient characteristics. The fitted multivariate Cox model (Table 3) shows that patient age and tumor histology (AA vs GBM) are significantly associated with patient survival. Furthermore, the adjustment for these covariates does not really change the conclusions of the unadjusted analysis; that is, of the three possible comparisons, only the IT group differs significantly from the IB group (p = 0.029, Table 3). The multivariate model also estimates the adjusted relative hazard of dying under the different treatment regimens (Table 3). Thus we estimate that patients treated with IT are only half as likely to die (95% CI: 0.36 to 0.69) as patients treated with IB.

Table 2. *Unadjusted Analysis Comparison of Survival Curves*
(a) Comparison of survival curves (logrank test)

Comparison	P-Value
IT vs. IB	0.017
SRS vs. IB	0.98
IT vs. SRS	0.22

(b) Survival estimates (95% Confidence Interval)

Time point (months)	Interstitial brachytherapy	Interstitial thermoradiotherapy	Stereotactic radiosurgery
12	0.52	0.80	0.51
	(0.34, 0.69)	(0.64, 0.96)	(0.24, 0.78)
24	0.18	0.48	—
	(0.050, 0.31)	(0.28, 0.68)	
36	0.12	0.38	—
	(0.0098, 0.23)	(0.18, 0.58)	
48	0.12	0.30	—
	(0.0098, 0.23)	(0.093, 0.51)	
60	0.12	0.30	—
	(0.0098, 0.23)	(0.093, 0.51)	
Median survival (mos.)	13.3	23.5	not reached

Table 3. *Adjusted Model (Cox Proportional Hazards Model)*

Factor	Hazard[a]	95% Conf. interval	p-Value
IB	1.0	—	—
IT	0.50	(0.27, 0.93)	0.029
SRS	1.12	(0.48, 2.64)	0.79
Histology	2.80	(1.26, 6.22)	0.014
Age	1.046	(1.024, 1.069)	0.000049

[a]Estimated instantaneous hazard of dying with IB as reference group. Parameter interpretation: IT group is 0.5 times as likely to die as IB; SRS group is 1.12 times as likely to die as IB, patients with GBM are 2.8 times more likely to die than AA patients; the likelihood of dying increases 1.046 times per year.

Toxicities

Toxicities associated with the implantation of catheters and with the delivery of hyperthermia have been discussed previously (Stea 1990, 1992). There have been three major complications among the IT patients. Briefly, one patient developed an intracranial hemorrhage, a second patient developed hydrocephalus secondary to edema from the trauma of catheter implantation, and a third patient developed pneumoencephalus. All these complications resolved after appropriate surgical intervention. There was also one fatal complication resulting from edema and mass effect secondary to both the implantation of numerous catheters and hyperthermia. Finally, hyperthermia contributed directly to the induction of seizures during the treatment in six patients, and in five patients it contributed to transient worsening of the neurological deficits or brain edema which responded to conservative medical management (Stea 1992). Despite the somewhat large treatment volumes used for stereotactic radiosurgery, none of the 19 patients so treated developed any toxicity or untoward side effects. Three of the 19 patients have undergone re-operation, but in each case, viable tumor was found in the presence of radiation necrosis.

Discussion

Stereotactic interstitial irradiation may play a significant role in the local control and survival of patients with high grade glioma, when used as a focal boost in the initial management of well defined tumor volumes (Loeffler 1990, Prados 1992). Loeffler *et al.* (1990), used a high activity I-125 boost in the initial treatment of 35 patients with GBM. The median survival of this group of patients was 27 months which was significantly higher than the median survival of 11 months for a group of similar patients treated without an implant boost at the same institution. A similar conclusion was reached in a retrospective study from UCSF (Larson 1990) where patients with GBM had a median survival of 95 weeks when treated with an implant boost vs 52 weeks for a group of matched control patients treated with EBFRT only. However, selection biases may significantly contribute to the reported increased in median survival rates for patients receiving implant boosts, since these patients usually represent a subset with favorable prognosis. Indeed a study of patients treated with only EBFRT, but analyzed in terms of the same selection criteria used for stereotactic implants, showed that those patients who would have qualified for a stereotactic implant had a significant longer median survival (16.7 months) than those who were ineligible on the basis of large or diffuse tumor volume (median survival 9.3 months, p = 0.004) (Florell 1992). The value of a stereotactic implant in prolonging survival of patients with high grade supratentorial gliomas is now being tested in a Phase III randomized trial (protocol 8701) by the BTCG. In an attempt to further increase the local control of malignant gliomas, several investigators have used hyperthermia as an adjunct to interstitial irradiation (Roberts 1986, Sneed 1992, Stea 1992). A preliminary survival analysis of patients treated at the University of Arizona with thermoradiotherapy showed a medial survival of 20.6 months from diagnosis for a group of 28 patients with high grade gliomas (Stea 1992). A Phase III randomized trial of implant with or without hyperthermia is being conducted at UCSF to evaluate the effacacy of short duration (60 min) sequential hyperthermia and brachytherapy boost for patients with GBM.

Despite encouraging early results obtained with brachytherapy boosts (with or without hyperthermia),

this approach has significant limitations. Patients of advanced age or with coexisting medical illness may not be suitable candidates for an implant. Furthermore, tumors located in deep supratentorial structures or eloquent parts of the brain or tumors originating in the posterior fossa are usually not considered for an implant due to the potential for serious morbidity and even mortality secondary to surgical trauma. In these situations, stereotactic radiosurgery offers a viable alternative to boosting the RT dose following EBFRT, with significantly reduced risks of complications.

Although stereotactic radiosurgery has been used extensively for brain metastases (Loeffler 1990, Mehta 1992) and benign intracranial neoplasms (Flickinger 1991) very few studies have been published about the efficacy of this technique in the initial management of high grade gliomas. In a recent publication by Loeffler *et al.* (1992), 37 selected patients with malignant gliomas were treated with a median boost dose of 12 Gy delivered by SRS after an EBFRT dose of 59.4 Gy. The median survival for 23 patients with GBM was 26 months. This survival compares well with the median survival of 27 months achieved with an implant boost in a previous study from the same institution (Loeffler 1990).

In this retrospective analysis, we have compared the survival differences of three groups of patients with high grade gliomas who, as part of their initial management, received a boost either by IB, IT, or SRS in three successive studies performed over a span of 10 years. The results show that the IT group survived significantly longer than the IB group, and that there was no difference between survival in the IB and SRS groups or in the IT and SRS groups.

The results of this study must be interpreted with caution since the patient groups differ in factors other than the type of boost received:

IB: Median EBFRT dose of 41.4 Gy, median brachytherapy dose of 40.0 Gy planned without the benefit of 3-D treatment planning software.

IT: Median EBFRT dose of 48.4 Gy, median brachytherapy dose of 32.2 Gy, and a hyperthermia boost. All treatments planned using a 3-D approach.

SRS: Median EBFRT dose of 59.4 Gy, no brachytherapy, and a SRS boost of 10 Gy. All treatments planned using a 3-D approach.

Hence, the observed differences between groups must consider the totality of treatment differences, not simply the type of boost received. In addition, we note that since patients were not randomly assigned to treatment groups, there may be unmeasured imbalances that affect the conclusions (i.e. we cannot rule out the possibility that hyperthermia treatment is a surrogate measure for some unmeasured favorable prognostic factor rather than a causal agent).

In spite of these cautionary notes, we believe that this study provides enough indication to justify further evaluation of a thermoradiotherapy boost in the treatment of malignant gliomas. Furthermore, this study demonstrates reduced morbidity using SRS; hence, combining these results should motivate work on the development of non-invasive hyperthermia devices that can be used to improve the efficacy of SRS treatment (Richards 1993).

References

1. Brada M, Laing RW, Graham J, Warrington AP, Hines F (1993) Fractionated stereotactic radiotherapy in the treatment of recurrent high grade glioma: dose escalation study. Abstract. Acta Neurochir (Wien) 122: 151

2. Chang CH, Horton J, Schoenfeld D, Salazar O, Perez-Tamayo R, Kramer, S, Weinstein A, Nelson J, Tsukada Y (1993) Comparison of postoperative radiotherapy and combined postoperative radiotherapy and chemotherapy in the multidisciplinary management of malignant gliomas. Cancer 52: 997–1007

3. Fleming TR, Harrington DP (1991) Counting processes and survival analysis. Wiley, New York

4. Flickinger JC, Lunsford LD, Coeffey RJ, Linskey ME, Bissonette DJ, Maitz AH, Kondziolka D (1991) Radiosurgery of acoustic neurinomas. Cancer 67: 345–353

5. Florell RC, Macdonald DR, Irich WD, Bernstein M, Leibel SA, Gutin PH, Cairncross JG (1992) Selection bias, survival, and brachytherapy for glioma. J Neurosurg 76: 179–183

6. Gutin PH, Prados MD, Phillips TL, Wara WM, Larson DA, Leibel SA, Sneed PK, Levin VA, Weaver KA, Silver P, Lamborn K, Lamb S, Ham B (1991) External irradiation followed by an interstitial high activity iodine-125 implant "boost" in the initial treatment of malignant gliomas: NCOG study 6G-82-2. Int J Radiat Oncol Biol Phys 21: 601–606

7. Hochberg FH, Pruitt A (1990) Assumptions in the radiotherapy of glioblastoma. Neurology 30: 907–911

8. Kondziolka D, Lunsford LD, Coffey RJ, Flickinger JC (1991) Stereotactic radiosurgery of meningiomas. J Neurosurg 74: 552–559

9. Larson DA, Gutin PH, Leibel SA, Phillips TL, Sneed PK, Wara WM (1990) Stereotaxic irradiation of brain tumors. Cancer 65: 792–799

10. Leksell L (1951) The stereotactic method and radiosurgery of the brain. Acta Chir Scand 102: 316–319

11. Leibel SA, Gutin PH, Wara WM, Silver PS, Larson DA, Edwards MSB, Lamb SA, Ham B, Weaver KA, Barnett C, Phillips TL (1989) Survival and quality of life after interstitial implantation of removable high-activity iodine-125 sources for the treatment of patients with recurrent malignant gliomas. Int J Radiat Oncol Biol Phys 17: 1129–1139

12. Loeffler JS, Alexander E, Wen P, Shea WM, Coleman CN, Kooy H, Fine Howard, Nedzi L, Silver B, Riese N, McL Black P (1990) Results of stereotactic brachytherapy used in the initial management of patients with gliobalstoma. J Nat Cancer Inst 82: 1918–1921

13. Loeffler JS, Alexander E, Shea M, Wen PY, Fine HA, Kooy HM, Black PM (1992) Radiosurgery as part of the initial management of patients with malignant gliomas. J Clin Oncol 10: 1379–1385

14. Loeffler JS, Kooy HM, Wen PY, Fine HA, Cheng C-W, Mannarino EG, Tsai JS, Alexander E (1990) The treatment of recurrent brain metastases with stereotactic radiosurgery. J Clin Oncol 8: 576–582

15. Lulu BA, Lutz W, Stea B, Cetas TC (1990) Treatment planning of template-guided stereotaxic brain implants. Int J Radiat Oncol Biol Phys 18: 951–955

16. Lutz W, Watson KR, Maleki N (1988) A system for stereotactic radiosurgery with linear accelerator. Int J Radiat Oncol Biol Phys 14: 373–381

17. Mehta MP, Rozental JM, Levin AB, Mackie TR, Kubsad SS, Gehring MA, Kinsella TJ (1992) Defining the role of radiosurgery in the management of brain metastases. Int J Radiat Oncol Biol Phys 24: 619–625

18. Miller RG (1981) Survival analysis. Wiley, New York

19. Ostertag CB, Kreth FW (1992) Iodine-125 interstitial irradiation for cerebral gliomas. Acta Neurochir (Wien) 119: 53–61

20. Prados MD, Gutin PH, Phillips TL, Wara WM, Sneed PK, Larson DA, Lamb SA, Ham B, Malec MK, Wilson CB (1992) Interstitial brachytherapy for newly diagnosed patients with malignant gliomas: the UCSF experience. Int J Radiat Oncol Biol Phys 24: 593–597

21. Richards WF (1993) Optimization of power density in microwave hyperthermia. In: Gerner E, Cetas TC (eds) Hyperthermic oncology, Vol 2. University of Arizona, Arizona, pp 223–230

22. Roberts DW, Coughlin CT, Wong TZ, Fratkin JD, Douple EB, Strohbehn JW (1986) Interstitial hyperthermia and iridium brachytherapy in treatment of malignant glioma. J Neurosurg 64: 581–587

23. Rossman KJ, Shetter AG, Speiser BL, Nehls D (1985) Stereotactic afterloading iridium implants in treatment of high-grade astrocytomas. Endocur Hyper Onc 1: 49–57

24. Shapiro WR, Green SB, Burger PC, Mahaley MS, Selker RG, Van Gilder JC, Robertson JT, Ransohoff J, Mealey J, Strike TA, Pistenmaa DA (1989) Randomized trial of three chemotherapy regimens and two radiotherapy regimens in postoperative treatment of malignant glioma. J Neurosurg 71: 1–9

25. Sneed PK, Gutin PH, Stauffer PR, Phillips TL, Prados MD, Weaver KA, Suen S, Lamb SA, Ham B, Ahn DK, Lamborn K, Larson DA, Wara WM (1992) Thermoradiotherapy of recurrent malignant brain tumors. Int J Radiat Oncol Biol Phys 23: 853–861

26. Sneed PK, Stauffer PR, Gutin PH, Phillips TL, Suen S, Weaver KA, Lamb SA, Ham B, Prados MD, Larson DA, Wara WM (1991) Interstitial irradiation and hyperthermia for the treatment of recurrent malignant brain tumors. Neurosurgery 28: 206–215

27. Souhami L, Olivier A, Podgorsak EB, Villemure J-G, Pla M, Sadikot AF (1991) Fractionated stereotactic radiation therapy for intracranial tumors. Cancer 68: 2101–2108

28. Stea B, Cetas TC, Cassady JR, Guthkelch AN, Iacono R, Lulu B, Lutz W, Obbens E, Rossman K, Seeger J, Sheter A, Shimm DS (1990) Interstitial thermoradiotherapy of brain tumors: preliminary results of a phase I clinical trial. Int J Radiat Oncol Biol Phys 19: 1461–1471

29. Stea B, Kittelson J, Cassady JR, Hamilton A, Guthkelch N, Lulu B, Obbens E, Rossman K, Shapiro W, Shetter A, Cetas T (1992) Treatment of malignant gliomas wit interstitial irradiation and hyperthermia. Int J Radiat Oncol Biol Phys 24: 657–667

30. Thornton AF, Hegarty TJ, Ten Haken RK, Yanke BR, LaVigne ML, Fraass BA, McShan DL, Greenberg HS (1991) Three-

dimensional treatment planning of astrocytomas: a dosimetric study of cerebral irradiation. Int J Radiat Oncol Biol Phys 20: 1309–1315

31. Walker MD, Green SB, Byar DP, Alexander E, Batzdorf U, Brooks WH, Hunt WE, MacCarty CS, Mahaley MS, Mealey J, Owens G, Ransohoff J, Robertson JT, Shapiro WR, Smith KR, Wilson CB, Strike TA (1980) Randomized comparisons of radiotherapy and nitrosoureas for the treatment of malignant glioma after surgery. N Engl J Med 303: 1323–1329

32. Walker, MD, Strike TA, Sheline GE (1979) An analysis of dose-effect relationship in the radiotherapy of malignant gliomas. Int J Radiat Oncol Biol Phys 5: 1725–1731

33. Wallner KE, Galicick JH, Krol G, Arbit E, Malkin MG (1989) Patterns of failure following treatment for glioblastoma multiforme and anaplastic astrocytoma. Int J Radiat Oncol Biol Phys 16: 1405–1409

Correspondence: Baldassarre Stea, M.D., PhD, Department of Radiation Oncology, University of Arizona Health Sciences Center, Tucson, AZ 85724, U.S.A.

Acta Neurochir (1994) [Suppl] 62: 55–57

Stereotactic Radiosurgery for Tectal Low-Grade Gliomas

L. Kihlström[1], **C. Lindquist**[1], **M. Lindquist**[2], and **B. Karlsson**[1]

Department of [1]Neurosurgery and [2]Neuroradiology, Karolinska Hospital, Stockholm, Sweden

Summary

We report 7 cases with low-grade gliomas in the tectal region of the midbrain. This series started in 1979 and all tumours were treated by radiosurgery using the Leksell Gamma Knife. All cases were treated by using a single isocenter with the 14 mm collimator. Doses administered ranged from 14 to 35 Gy delivered to the 50–70% isodose line. All tumours but one responded to the treatment and disappeared or ceased growing. In the first two treated cases, the dose was chosen by the early experience from the AVM's, with 30 and 35 Gy as the peripheral dose. These cases developed severe radio-induced oedema with aggravating symptoms and permanent deficits. We conclude that radiosurgery is effective in the treatment of deeply located low-grade gliomas. Cases accepted for treatment should be carefully selected and the peripheral dose should not exceed 14 Gy to avoid uncontrolled radio-induced changes

Keywords: Tectal tumours; radiosurgery; low-grade gliomas; radio-induced changes.

Introduction

The management of brainstem tumours has changed significantly over the last 10 years as a result of improved neuroradiological and neurosurgical techniques. The presence of a small mass in the tectal region of the midbrain causing obstruction of the Sylvian aqueduct and subsequent hydrocephalus is well recognized. Controversy as to management of these tumours still remains, although the historical perception of a uniformly poor prognosis[2,7,15] has been modified with reports of agressive surgical treatment in certain well-defined subgroups[5,9] and conservative treatment with only shunt placement in some[12].

Traditionally, in the management for low-grade gliomas, treatment has been surgery to reduce mass effect and diminish tumour burden for adjuvant therapies, and to reduce the chance of malignant transformation. Previous reports from 5- and 10-year survivals of 13%–38% and 11% respectively suggest that more ex-

tensive resection improves survival following operative intervention without radiation[1,6,11]. Postoperative radiation therapy has commonly been recommended and the 5- and 10-year survivals following subtotal resection and radiation are 40%–68% and 35%–39% respectively[1,6,11,17].

Low-grade brainstem gliomas constitute a small subgroup were total resection is difficult and were conventional radiation is not curative. Stereotactic radiosurgery with the Leksell Gamma Knife affords the possibility to deliver a tumouricidal dose to the lesion and has an established role in the treatment of some brain tumours[3,10,14]. We present our experience with 7 patients who received Gamma Knife surgery for small tectal gliomas between 1979 and 1991.

Methods and Patients

Seven cases with biopsy verified low-grade gliomas were treated by Gamma Knife surgery between 1979 and 1991 (Table 1). In all cases tumour growth was defined by serial CT or MRI investigations and brainstem symptoms (neuro-ophtalmological manifestations) existed even after shunt-operation which were required as an initial treatment in all cases. Six patients were female and 1 male, mean age of 18 years (range 6–40 years) by the time for the treatment. The mean duration of clinical history was 4 years (6-months–17 years). The patients were treated by the Gamma Knife, guided by stereotactic ENC for target localization in the first case, CT for the next 3, and MRI for the last 3 cases. All cases were treated by using a single isocenter with the 14 mm collimator. Doses administered ranged from 14 to 35 Gy delivered to the periphery. The 2 earliest, cases received 30 and 35 Gy respectively to the periphery, reduced to 18–20 Gy in the next 2 cases and to 14 Gy in the last 3 cases in this series. Follow-up was assessed on clinical examination and post-operative CT or MRI investigations.

Results

The patients have been followed 2–15 years (mean 6 years). The results are summarized in Table 2. One

Table 1. *Clinical Summary of Seven Patients with Tectal Tumours Subjected to Gamma Knife Surgery*

Case no.	Age and gender	History before RS	Presentation	Signs referable to tectum	Histology	Tumour size diameter (cm)
1	12 years F	1 year	raised ICP	yes	astrocytoma II	3.0
2	25 years F	17 years	raised ICP	yes	astrocytoma II	2.5
3	13 years F	5 years	raised ICP	yes	astrocytoma II	2.0
4	10 years F	1.5 years	raised ICP	yes	astrocytoma II	1.5
5	21 years M	3 years	raised ICP	yes	astrocytoma II	2.0
6	40 years F	1 year	raised ICP	yes	astrocytoma II	1.5
7	6 years F	6 months	raised ICP	yes	pilocyt. astro.	$6.0 \times 3.0 \times 2.5$

Table 2. *Treatment Parameters and Follow-up in Seven Patients Subjected to Gamma Knife Surgery*

Case no.	Min dose to tumour	Stereotactic technique	Tumour response	Radionecrosis (RN) Radio-induced changes (RIC)	Radiological follow-up	Clinical follow-up	Clinical response
1	30 Gy	ster ENC	disappearence	RN	14 years	15 years	sequelae
2	35 Gy	ster CT	disappearence	RN	7 years	7 years	no change
3	20 Gy	ster CT	regression	RIC	2 years	6 years	improved
4	18 Gy	ster CT	disappearence	RIC	4 years	4 years	improved
5	14 Gy	ster MRI	regression	RIC	3 years	3 years	improved
6	14 Gy	ster MRI	disappearence	RIC	2 years	2 years	improved
7	<14 Gy	ster MRI	progression	–	3 years	4 years	no change

patient with a 6 year follow-up has MR investigation only for up to 2 years after radiosurgery and the tumour was smaller in size at that time (no. 3). In 5 cases, the tumours shrunk progressively after the treatment. In one case (no. 7), a large pilocytic astrocytoma was treated only to its small solid part with 14 Gy to the periphery. The cysts progressed and the patient was operated upon after 3 years with removal of the tumour. Except for this partially treated tumour, no local recurrence or dedifferentiation to malignant glioma has been observed.

The dose selection in the first cases was based on the early results from successful eradication of small arteriovenous malformations (25–30 Gy), and metastases (30–35 Gy). The knowledge of the dose-response effect was at that time not well understood. Except for the large cystic tumour, all tumours had imaging evidence of radiation induced blood-brain barrier breakdown (gadolinium-enhancement on MRI or contrast-enhancement on (CT) in the region surrounding the tumour 4 months–10 months after radiosurgery (mean 5.6 months). The first two treated cases (no. 1, 2) developed severe radio-induced reactions with severe permanent neurological deficit in one. The next two cases (no. 3, 4), treated with 18–20 Gy also presented a progression of aggravating symptoms over a period of months, but these untoward effects were temporary and left no deficits. Even in two cases treated with the reduced dose of 14 Gy and a relative mild radio-induced reaction, a period of diplopia was observed. All seven patients remain alive with a mean follow-up of 6 years after the treatment with clinical improvement in 4, no change in 2 and one with worse symptoms.

Discussion

The diversity and varied biological behaviour of low-grade gliomas can make management decisions difficult. Nevertheless, it is concluded that in cases with verified tumour progression, treatment is indicated. The failure of treatment of low-grade glioma is due to local "recurrence". This phenomenon is due either to continued growth or residual tumour or to transformation to malignant glioma. The most commonly reported figure is about 50% malignant transformation at a median period of 31–56 months postoperatively[13] and there is no firm evidence that tumour resection lessens the incidence of this event but radical resections may achieve prolonged survival. Deeply seated thalamic or brainstem low-grade gliomas constitute a challenge for surgery and radiosurgery may constitute a good alternative to surgery when the tumour volume is small.

Our study shows that low-grade gliomas in the pineal region, can be managed by using Gamma Knife surgery with long term survival and low rate of recurrence. It is an effective technique to treat small distinct tumours but not without complications. Extended series with long term follow-up are needed and will determine the role for radiosurgery in the future.

The dose selection in the first two treated cases was based on the early results from successful eradication of small arteriovenous malformations (25–30 Gy), and metastases (30–35 Gy) and the knowledge of the dose-tissue response effect was by that time not well understood. Volume is clearly an important factor in the risk of complications for radiosurgery and needs to be carefully considered in deciding each dose prescription. Nevertheless, calculating the risks of radiation necrosis from radiosurgery predicted by risk-formulas based on information from other lesions can be dangerous[9]. This retrospective study shows that not only dose-volume effects are important in radiosurgery, also the treated lesion itself plays an important role for the dose-response. This finding is consistent with reported observations of untoward effects after Gamma Knife surgery for cavernous haemangiomas[16] and venous angiomas[4].

We believe that surgery should be considered for all low-grade gliomas as the first treatment choice and Gamma Knife surgery may represent a useful new therapeutic modality in selected cases for small tumours. The doseplanning should be guided by stereotactic MRI and the dose should be carefully selected. Our actual recommendation is 12–14 Gy to the tumour periphery.

References

1. Bouchard J, Pierce PC (1960) Radiation therapy in the management of neoplasmas of the central nervous system with a special note in regard to children: twenty years experience, 1930–1958. AJR 84: 610–628
2. Chapman PH (1989) Indolent gliomas of the midbrain tectum. Concepts in Pediatric Neurosurgery 10: 97–107
3. Lindquist C (1989) Gamma Knife surgery for recurrent solitary metastasis of a cerebral hypernephroma. Neurosurgery 25: 802–804
4. Lindquist C, Guo W, Karlsson B, Steiner L (1993) Radiosurgery for venous angiomas. J Neurosurg 78: 531–536
5. Epstein F, McCleary EL (1986) Intrinsic brain-stem tumours of childhood: surgical indications. J Neurosurg 64: 11–15
6. Fazekas JT (1977) Treatment of grades I and II brain astrocytomas: the role of radiotherapy. Int J Radiat Oncol Biol Phys 2: 661–667
7. Flamm ES, Rovit R, Kricheff II, *et al* (1972) Periaqueductal neoplasms and vascular malformations. NY State J Med 72: 2623–2628
8. Flickinger JC (1989) An integrated logistic formula for prediction of complications from radiosurgery. Int J Radiat Oncol Biol Phys 15: 441–447
9. Hoffman HJ, Becker L, Craven MA (1980) A clinically and pathologically distinct group of benign brainstem gliomas. Neurosurgery 7: 243–248
10. Kihlström L, Karlsson B, Lindquist C (1992) Gamma knife surgery in brain metastases. In: Lunsford LD (ed) Stereotactic radiosurgery update. Elsevier, Amsterdam, pp 4429–4434
11. Liebel SA, Sheline GE, Wara WM, Boldrey EB, Nielsen SL (1975) The role of radiation therapy in the treatment of astrocytoma. Cancer 35: 1551–1557
12. May PL, Blaser SI, Hoffman HJ, Humphreys RP, Harwood-Nash DC (1991) Benign intrinsic tectal "tumours" in children. J Neurosurgery 74: 867–871
13. Müller W, Afra D, Schröder R (1977) Supratentorial recurrences of gliomas: morphological studies in relation to time intervals with astrocytomas. Acta Neurochir (Wien) 37: 75–91
14. Norén G, Arndt J, Hindmarsch J (1983) Stereotactic radiosurgery in cases of acoustic neurinomas: further experiences. Neurosurgery 13: 12–22
15. Sanford RA, Bebin J, Smith RW (1982) Pencil gliomas of the aqueduct of Sylvius. Report of two cases. J Neurosurg 57: 690–696
16. Steiner L, Lindquist C, Steiner M (1992) Radiosurgery. In: Symon L (ed) Advances and technical standards in neurosurgery, Vol 19. Springer, Wien New York, pp 57–59
17. Shaw EG EJ Scheithauer BW, Daumas-Duport K, Laws ER, Gilbertson DT, ÒFallon JR (1987) Postoperative radiation for supratentorial low grade gliomas. Int Radiat Oncol Biol Phys [Suppl 1] 13: 148–156

Correspondence: Lars Kihlström, M.D., Department of Neurosurgery, Karolinska Hospital, S-10401 Stockholm, Sweden.

Acta Neurochir (1994) [Suppl] 62: 58–61

Stereotactic Radiosurgery of Deeply Seated Low Grade Gliomas

J. A. Barcia[1,2], **J. L. Barcia-Salorio**[1,2], **C. Ferrer**[3], **E. Ferrer**[3], **R. Algás**[3], and **G. Hernández**[3]

[1] Servicio de Neurocirugía, Hospital Clínico Universitario, Valencia, [2] Departamento de Cirugía, Universidad de Valencia, Spain, and [3] Servicio de Radioterapia, Hospital Clínico Universitario, Valencia

Summary

The authors report the results of a series of 16 cases of low-grade gliomas in whom radiosurgery was performed. This series started in 1977. All the tumours received a single radiosurgical session (with a mean dose of 21.7 Gy, 5–10 mm. collimator; one patient received two sessions and in another patient two different targets were irradiated in the same session). Prior to radiosurgery, six patients received conventional external fractionated radiotherapy, with two lateral fields of up to 10 × 10 cm. and a mean dose of 55.1 Gy. and another six patients with tumours less than 5 cm. in diameter, received stereotactic radiotherapy using four fields of up to 5 × 5 cm. and a mean dose of 53.1 Gy. In both cases, conventional fractionation was used, giving a dose of 1.8 to 2 Gy/day. The tumour disappeared in 8 cases (50%) and shunk or ceased its growth in 5 additional cases (31%). In 3 cases of brainstem gliomas in which the clinical condition was previously very poor there was no evolutional change and the patients eventually died.

We conclude that radiosurgery is effective in the treatment of deeply seated low-grade gliomas, where it may become the treatment of choice in the absence of other more definitive choices.

Keywords: Stereotactic radiosurgery; stereotactic radiotherapy; low grade gliomas.

Introduction

Deeply seated thalamic or brainstem low-grade gliomas constitute a challenge for neurosurgery, since while surgical access is difficulted due to the functional importance of the structures involved, conventional radiotherapy is not curative, attaining up to a 50% survival at two years in some series[18].

However, the possibility by means of stereotactic radiosurgery of giving higher doses than those given in conventional radiotherapy within the small volume of the tumour, while sparing the surrounding structures, may render these tumours sensitive to treatment.

Since 1977, the authors have performed stereotactic radiosurgery of deeply-seated glial tumours. The initial results were consistent with a good result of the technique in low-grade gliomas (a series of 4 cases), while high grade gliomas (4 additional cases) had a bad outcome[3]. Based on these initial results, we have continued radiosurgery in cases of otherwise intractable deep low grade gliomas. In those cases, not initially suitable for radiosurgery because the volume of the tumour was too large, conventional or stereotactically directed fractionated radiotherapy was performed first.

Other authors have also reported on stereotactic radiosurgery for low-grade gliomas[5,14,17].

Methods and Material

Between July 1978 and October 1991, 16 patients harouring deap seated low-grade gliomas were treated. Criteria for non-operability were location of the tumour in the brain stem or in the thalmus, or any other factor in which surgical resection carried a significant morbidity or mortality risk. Four cases had been subjected to partial resection. Stereotactic biopsy was performed in three cases. In all histologically studied cases, a low-grade (Kernohan's grades I or II) glioma was diagnosed. In the remaining cases, biopsy was not performed because of the potential risk of the procedure. In these cases, the diagnosis of a low grade glioma was stablished by clinical and radiological (CT and MR) criteria. Also included in this group are two cases which were recurrence after radiological cure with surgery and conventional radiotherapy. Tumour size was calculated using the largest diameter as seen on the contrast-enhanced CT or MR slices. In the case of CT slices, the distance between the first and the last plane in 5 mm slices was also taken into account. All cases consisted of rounded tumours, so that this was considered a good correlate to the tumour volume. Clinical features are summarized in Table 1.

Prior to radiosurgery, six patients received conventional external fractionated radiotherapy, with two lateral fields of up to 10 × 10 cm. and a mean dose of 55.1 Gy. and another six patients with tumours less than 5 cm. in diameter, received stereotactic radiotherapy using four fields of up to 5 × 5 cm. and a mean dose of 53.1 Gy. In both cases, conventional fractionation was used, giving a dose of 1.8 to 2 Gy/day.

Nine months (on average) after radiotherapy, all these patients underwent stereotactic radiosurgery, using 10 to 25 fields with a

Table 1

Case	Age	Sex	Localization	Biopsy	Size (mm)	Symptoms and signs
1. AR	6	F	thalamus	yes	$30 \times 30 \times 30$	hemiplegia
2. RG	7	M	brain stem	no	$30 \times 30 \times 30$	hemiparesis
3. JL	23	M	brain stem	no	$30 \times 30 \times 30$	diplopia
4. EM	4	F	thalamus	no	$40 \times 40 \times 45$	hemiparesis
5. IC	10	F	brain stem	yes	$30 \times 30 \times 50$	sleepiness, unilateral weakness
6. JP	39	M	III ventricle	no	$20 \times 20 \times 50$	papillaedema, ataxia
7. TM	66	F	pons	yes	$40 \times 23 \times 20$	hemiparesis
8. HC	57	F	brain stem	yes		headache, unilateral weakness
9. FL	17	M	brain stem	yes	$30 \times 40 \times 55$	causal diagnosis
10. NA	13	F	thalamus	no	$30 \times 30 \times 25$	right arm paresis
11. JP	13	V	mesencephalon	yes	$31 \times 28 \times 26$	hemiparesis
12. NL	42	F	pons	no	$35 \times 32 \times 30$	hemiparesis
13. AR	68	F	IV ventricle	no	$15 \times 15 \times 10$	ataxia, hydrocephalus
14. AM	15	F	cerebellum	yes	$50 \times 50 \times 45$	headache, ocular symptoms
15. FN	55	F	thalamus	no	$27 \times 20 \times 23$	hemiparesis
16. JG	35	M	pons	no	$25 \times 22 \times 21$	hydrocephalus, headache

10 mm. collimator (except in one case in which the 5 mm. collimator was used), and a mean dose of 21.7 Gy. One patient received two sessions and in another patient two different targets were irradiated in the same session to completely cover the target volume. Stereotactic radiosurgery was performed using a conventional gamma source (Theratron 780, Atomic Energy of Canada, Ltd.), optically coupled to a stereoguide. The beam was doubly collimated, a first collimator being attached to the source and the other one (smaller, 5–10 mm. in diameter in this case), attached to the arc of the stereoguide. The stereoguide used is an arc-quadrant target-centered system[2]. One of the cases was initially a cystic tumour. In three additional cases, a cyst developed inside the tumour after irradiation. In these cases, an indwelling catheter was stereotactically placed inside the cyst and connected to a subcutaneous Ommaya reservoir under the scalp. The reservoir was periodically punctured when the patient was symptomic.

Table 2 summarizes the type of therapy and the doses used in all cases.

Table 2

Case	Type of RT	Dose	Dose radiosurgery	Clinical response	Radiological response	Follow up (mo)
1. AR	4 fields (stereotactic)	44 Gy	20 Gy	improved	tumour disappearance	29
2. RG	4 fields (stereotactic)	46 Gy	25 Gy	deterioration	↑ tumor size	9
3. JL	3 fields (stereotactic)	54 Gy	20 Gy	deterioration	↑ tumour size	5
4. EM	2 fields	60 Gy	10 Gy	symptom free	Tumour disappearance	133
5. IC	2 fields	42 Gy	10 Gy	Symptom free	Tumour disappearance	40
6. JP	2 fields	60 Gy	30 Gy	greatly improved	Tumour disappearance	23
7. TM	no	–	35 Gy	symptom free	Tumour disappearance	18
8. HC	4 fields	54 Gy	30 Gy	symptom free	Tumour disappearance	78
9. FL	2 fields	55 Gy	20 Gy	deterioration	↑ tumour size	29
10. NA	4 fields (stereotactic)	60 Gy	11 Gy	Symptom free	Tumour disappearance	53
11. DD	4 fields (stereotactic)	54 Gy	20 Gy	Improved	Tumour disappearance	45
12. NL	no	–	25 Gy	improved	no change	60
13. AR	no	–	25 Gy	symptom free	no change	99
14. AM	2 fields	60 Gy	30 Gy	improved	↓ tumour size	156
15. FN	no	–	30 Gy	no change	no change	76
16. JG	4 fields (stereotactic)	66 Gy	20 Gy	improved	↓ tumour size	48

Patients were followed up both clinically and with CT or MR controls each 3 to 6 months during the first two years after radiosurgery, and then once annually. Radiological criteria for classifying the results were complete response (CR): complete disappearance of the lesion on CT, partial response (PR): reduction of the lesion size with matching imaging methods, stable disease (SD): same size of the lesion than prior to the operation, progression of disease (PD): increase of size. Clinically, results were classified as symptom free, better, equal or worse than prior to the operation.

Data analysis was performed using the survival curves method described by Kaplan and Meier.

Results

Of the 16 low-grade gliomas treated, the tumour disappeared (CR) in 8 cases (50%), diminished in size (PR) in 2 cases (13%) and stopped growing (SD) in 3 additional cases (31%). Clinically, 6 patients are symptom free after treatment, 6 did better and one case remained the same. In 3 cases of brainstem gliomas in which the clinical condition was previously very poor, there was no evolutional change and the patients eventually died. Results are summarized in Table 2. The 10-year actuarial survival rate was 81% ($\pm$10), with a median follow-up of 50 months (5–156 months). Survival curves are plotted in Fig. 1.

Discussion

Prognosis of low-grade brainstem gliomas is still poor (5-year survival rate of 10%), and not very different from the high-grade ones (7%)[1]. Conventional radiotherapy alone achieves initially good results in brainstem gliomas[9–16] but reversal within 3 months occurs in about half of the patients[9,13]. Hyperfractionation radiotherapy is reported to achieve clinical improvement in 70% and radiographic tumour shrinkage in 74% of cases, and has significantly improved

SURVIVAL (%)

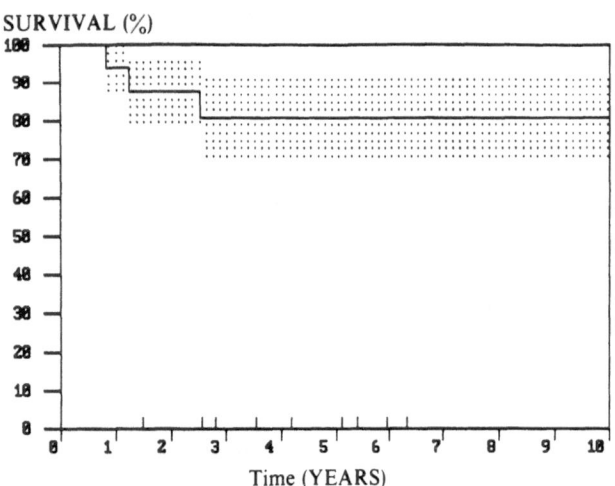

Fig. 1. Low grade gliomas

the prognosis in focal or midbrain lesions, but diffuse lesions at the pons still have a poor prognosis[4,10]. Stereotactic radiosurgery has changed the concept of radiosensitivity. As higher doses can now be delivered to smaller volumes, many earlier radioresistant tumours respond to focal irradiation. This is the case with acoustic neuromas, for example, which are radioresistant tumours, but respond well to stereotactic radiosurgery[12].

Our results are consistent with the published series of stereotactic irradiation of low-grade gliomas by Pozza *et al.*[14], and Souhami *et al.*[17]. In the first series, 14 tumours diagnosed pathologically as low-grade gliomas received stereotactic radiosurgery with a mean dose 23 Gy (16–50 Gy) in either one fraction or two fractions 8 days apart. After a median follow-up of 28 months, 86% of patients had partial or complete response. In the other series, 7 tumours confirmed pathologically as low-grade gliomas received stereotactic irradiation in 6 to 7 fractions of 650–700 cGy. up to a mean dose of 40.7 Gy (37.8–45.5 Gy). There were three radiologically partial responses and one radiological cure, with a 100% clinical improvement, 57% being symptom free.

We have not had any serious complication due to acute post-irradiation toxicity, probably due to the low doses used in the radiosurgical boost. In the other two series cited, only one case in each out of 14 and 7 cases respectively showed transient acute neurological deterioration which could be reversed with corticosteroid therapy. However, the doses used were somewhat higher than in our series. Other studies suggest that previous radiotherapy is not associated with an increased risk of complications after radiosurgery for recurrent tumours[11]. In three cases, a cyst developed inside the tumours and its contents were stereotactically evacuated through an indwelling catheter.

We have included in this group nine true brainstem tumours and seven tumours located outside the brainstem, which may constitute a too heterogeneous group, since thalamic tumours tend to behave more like hemispheric tumours[10]. Our aim when reporting these cases together is to stablish the role of radiosurgery in tumours considered inoperable because of their deep location.

One question can be raised about the radiological diagnosis of brainstem low-grade glioma without biopsy. We agree in that a histological diagnosis must be sought whenever possible. However, our approach to brainstem stereotactic biopsy or open surgery has been very conservative until reports suggesting its safety were published[7]. Kelly[8] has reported good results with computer-assisted resection of intraaxial piloctic astrocytomas. Biopsy is not without risks, and may worsen the clinical condition[15], as well as resection[6]. Our cautions are shared by many surgeons, and the decision to perform surgery or biopsy is biased by certain factors. Surgery is selected more in exophytic lesions, and biopsy in focal lesions located in the medulla or midbrain rather than diffuse lesions located in the pons[4]. Stereotactic radiosurgery may constitute a good alternative for the treatment of these tumours, specially those associated with a higher iatrogenic morbidity.

References

1. Albright AL, Guthkelch AN, Packer RJ, *et al* (1986) Prognostic factors in pediatric brain-stem gliomas. J Neurosurg 65: 751–755
2. Barcia-Salorio JL, Barberá J, Broseta J, *et al* (1977) Tomography in stereotaxis. A new stereoencephalotome disigned for this purpose. Acta Neurochir (Wien) [Suppl] 24: 77–83
3. Barcia-Salorio JL, Hernandez G, Sancho R (1983) Stereotactic radiosurgery in benign gliomas and radiosurgical boost post-cobalt therapy in malignant gliomas. In: Current status of chemotherapy and radiotherapy for cerebral gliomas in adult. VII European Neurosurgical Congress. Brussels
4. Barkovich AJ, Krischer J, Kun L, *et al* (1991) Brain stem gliomas: a classification system based on magnetic resonance imaging. J Pediatr Neurosurg 16: 73–83
5. Colombo F, Benedetti A, Pozza Fea (1986) Radiosurgery using a 4 MeV linear accelerator. Acta Radiol 369 [Suppl]: 303–307
6. Epstein F, Wisoff J (1987) Intra-axial tumors of the cervicomeduallary junction. J Neurosurg 67: 483–487
7. Hood TW, Gebarski S, McKeever PE, *et al* (1986) Stereotaxic biopsy of intrinsic lesions of the brain stem. J Neurosurg 65: 172–176
8. Kelly PJ, Kall BA, Goerss SJ, *et al* (1986) Computer-assisted stereotaxic resection of intra-axial brain neoplasm. J Neurosurg 64: 427–439
9. Kim TH, Chin HW, Pollan S, *et al* (1980) Radiotherapy of primary brain stem tumors. Int J Radiat Oncol Biol Phys 6: 51–57
10. Kovnar EH, Parham DM (1993) Brainstem astrocytomas. In: Black PM, Schoene WC, Lampson LA (ed) Astrocytomas: diagnosis, treatment and biology. Blackwell, Boston, pp 181–201
11. Loeffler JS, Siddon RL, Wen PY, *et al* (1990) Syterotactic radiosurgery of the brain using a standard linear accelerator: a study of early and late effects. Radiother Oncol 17: 311–321
12. Norén G, Arndt J, Hindmarsh T (1983) Stereotactic radiosurgery in cases of acoustic neurinoma: further experiences. Neurosurgery 13: 12–22
13. Panitch HS, Berg BO (1970) Brain stem tumors of childhood and adolescence. Am J Dis Child 119: 465–472
14. Pozza F, Colombo F, Chierego Gea (1989) Low-grade astrocytomas: treatment with unconventionally fractionated external beam stereotactic radiation therapy. Radiology 171: 565–569
15. Reigel DH, Scraff TB, Woodford JE (1979) Biopsy of pediatric brain stem tumors. Childs Brain 5: 329–340
16. Shibamoto Y, Takahashi M, Dokoh S, *et al* (1989) Radiation therapy for brain stem tumor with special reference to CT feature and prognosis correlations. Int J Radiat Oncol Biol Phys 17: 71–76
17. Souhami L, Olivier A, Podgorsak EB, *et al* (1991) Fractionated stereotactic irradiation therapy for intracranial tumors. Cancer 68: 2101–2108
18. Wara WM, Linstadt DE, Larson DA (1991) Management of primary brainstem gliomas and spinal cord gliomas. 1: 50–53

Correspondence: Juan A. Barcia, M.D., Servicio de Neurocirugia, Hospital Clinico Universitario, Av. Blasco Ibáñez 17, 46010 Valencia, Spain.

Acta Neurochir (1994) [Suppl] 62: 62–66

Radiosurgical Treatment of Gliomas of the Diencephalon

J. C. Ganz[1], A.-I. Smievoll[2], and F. Thorsen[3]

Departments of [1]Neurosurgery, [2]Radiology, and [3]Radiophysics, Haukeland Hospital University of Bergen, Norway

Summary

The results of Leksell Gamma Knife treatment of diencephalic gliomas are presented. Eight tumours in seven patients form the basis of this report. 7 patients, 4 males and 3 females. The age range was 7.5 to 33 years with a mean of 18 years. Mean follow-up was 21 ± 12 months. In 4 patients the tumour had been reduced in volume by an open internal decompression procedure. The location of the tumour will determine the risks of treatment. With anterior lesions there is risk of endocrinological and visual pathway damage. With a pineal region lesion there is a risk of diplopia.

In this series no tumour has increased in volume. Four have decreased and one has disappeared. Two patients suffered temporary diplopia. No visual disturbance has been observed to date. No hypothalamic disturbance has been observed yet.

These tumours are dangerous not so much because of their biological nature as because of their location. However, the biological nature of the tumours, with the close concordance between the radiological and actual extent make them appropriate targets for radiosurgery as a primary treatment. The present study gives preliminary support to this line of treatment.

Keywords: Glioma; diencephalon; Gamma Knife; indications; results.

Introduction

The Leksell Gamma Knife now has an established role in the treatment of arteriovenous malformations, acoustic neurinomas, meningiomas and cerebral metastases[4,5,8,9,10–14,17,18]. On the other hand its role in the treatment of glial cell tumours is less well established. Gliomas are a family of disparate neoplasms with differing biological characteristics. The majority are glioblastomas which are highly malignant and differ from metastases in being larger and less well defined radiologically. The Gamma Knife has been used to give a booster dose after surgery and conventional fractionated radiotherapy. This may lead to an increased survival in selected cases[1–3] though the selection criteria and duration of survival remain to be clarified. Of the other commoner gliomas cerebral astrocytomas are often poorly defined radiologically and cerebellar astrocytomas are often large and cystic. This makes both these tumour categories unsuitable for radiosurgery, which is dependent on accurate and reliable radiological definition of a moderate sized preferably solid tumour. In addition to the above, it is widely accepted that the radiologically visible extent of gliomas commonly underestimates the true tumour volume. This is because a significant proportion of these tumour's cells are distributed in a region of apparently normal brain, outside the macroscopically visible extent of the lesion[15,16].

However, there is one group of glial tumours which differs from the rest. These are the juvenile pilocytic astrocytomas arising around the third ventricle. These tumours are well defined, and would seem to extend hardly at all beyond their macroscopic limits. On the other hand, most of them are inaccessible for radical resection, because of their location.

The purpose of the current study was to examine the proposition that pilocytic astrocytomas are suitable targets for Gamma Knife treatment. In addition, some attempt has been made to define suitable treatment parameters for this group of tumours.

Material and Methods

8 tumours were treated in 7 patients. The patients were referred with clinical records together with either CT and/or MRI pictures. They were accepted on the basis of these pictures. Histological evidence of the diagnosis was highly desirable. However, if the tumour were demonstrated to be very slow-growing and in a situation where biopsy was considered unacceptably risky, because of small tumour volume and critical location, it was accepted without histology. The patients were all treated with the Gamma Knife, using CT for target localisation and the KULA system (Elekta Instrument AB, Stockholm) for dose planning. Where necessary, general anaesthesia was used for the duration of the treatment; because of the young age of some of the patients. Follow-up was

assessed on the basis of clinical reports from the referring physician, together with post-operative CT or MRI taken at 6 monthly intervals.

Results

There were 7 patients, 4 males and 3 females. The age range was 7.5 to 33 years with a mean of 18 years. Mean follow-up was 21 ± 12 months. 4 tumours had been reduced in volume by an open internal decompression procedure (Fig. 1a–c). It should be explained that there were two tumours in one little boy, because after the decompression there were isolated remains of tumour related to the third and fourth ventricles respectively. In a 5th patient a stereotactic biopsy had been taken. In all patients where it was available, the histology was reported to be consistent with the diagnosis of juvenile type pilocytic astrocytoma. In 2 patients there was no biopsy. In one of these there was a significant increase in tumour volume, when the pre-treatment CT images were compared with the treatment images. The time between these two examinations was about 3 months. Thus, this tumour was

assumed to be more aggressive than is usual for juvenile type astrocytomas. This resulted in this patient receiving a higher radiation dose.

3 of the tumours were located in the pineal region, 2 were in the hypothalamus just behind the optic chiasm. 2 extended laterally from the posterior third ventricle wall into the thalamus and one was in the wall of the fourth ventricle.

7 of the 8 tumours were treated with 12 Gy to the tumour edge and 40 Gy to the tumour centre. All the tumours were well localised radiologically. The 8th tumour received a dose of 20 Gy to the edge and 66.7 Gy to the centre. This higher dose was a consequence of the demonstrated tumour growth between CT examinations during 3 months, as mentioned above.

In 3 tumours there was no change in volume. In 4 there was a reduction in tumour volume and in 1 the tumour disappeared (Fig. 1b–e and Fig. 2a and b). One of the tumours which reduced in volume was the one which showed active growth prior to treatment and which received a higher dose. In no case has any increase in tumour volume occurred so far.

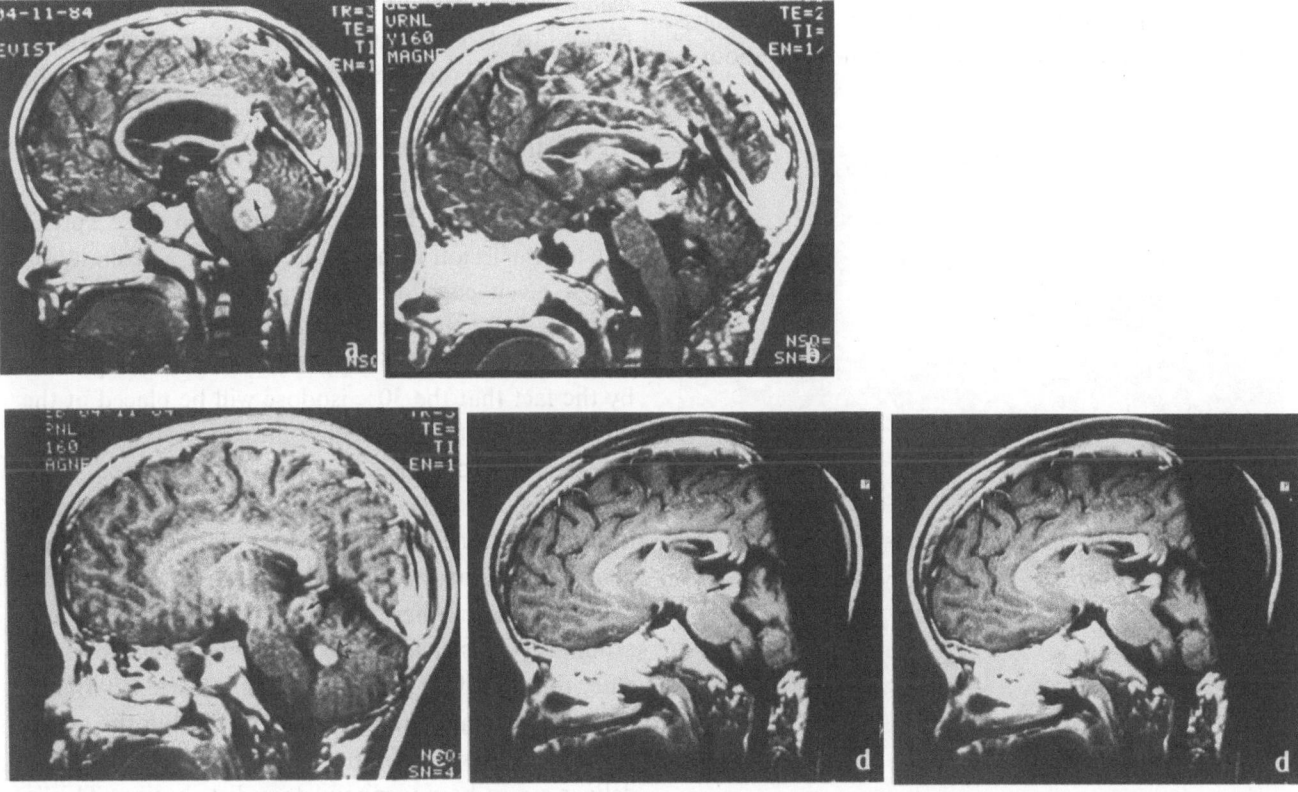

Fig. 1. (a) Pineal region glioma with caudal extension to the 4th ventricle (arrow). Pre-surgery mid-sagittal MRI. (b) Post-surgery mid sagittal MRI–same patient. Tumour volume is reduced but there is still much remaining in the pineal region (arrow). (c) Post-surgery right parasagittal MRI at the level of the lateral recess of the 4th ventricle (arrowhead) as well as in the pineal region (arrow). (d) Post-Gamma Knife treatment MRI equivalent to (b). Note the reduction in tumour volume (arrow). (e) Post-Gamma Knife treatment MRI equivalent to (c). Note reduction in volume of the pineal region tumour component and the absence of the 4th ventricle component

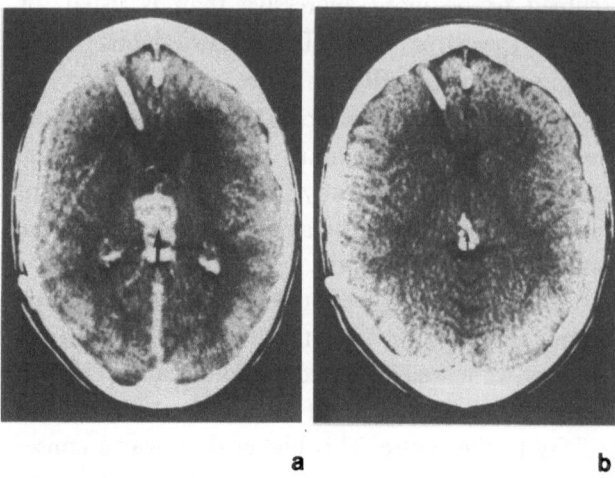

Fig. 2. (a) Pineal region glioma (arrow) before Gamma Knife treatment. (b) Same tumour 6 months after treatment. Note the marked reduction in volume

The dose plans were designed to ensure that the optic chiasm and tracts received no more than a maximum of 10 Gy. No case of visual deterioration has been observed to date. With the pineal region tumours, it was possible to design the dose so that it followed the contour of the tumour, sparing where possible the quadrigeminal plate; as shown in Fig. 3. However, 2 patients with pineal region tumours have suffered diplopia, which lasted in both cases about 6

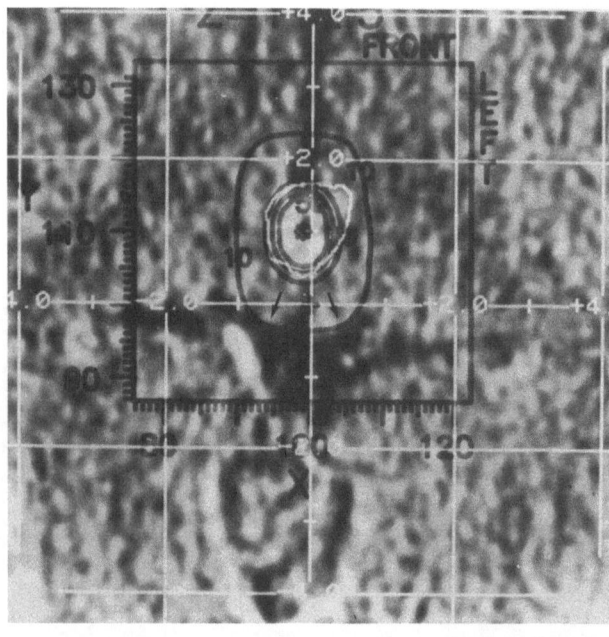

Fig. 3. One CT slice from a dose plan for a pineal region tumour. An extension of the tumour is shown into the peri-aqueductal grey matter (white contour). Note how the dose conforms to the tumour with relative sparing of the tectal plate and the remaining mesencephalon

months. In one the latency from treatment to diplopia was 6 months. In the other it was 3 months, and this was the tumour which had received the higher dose. At the time of writing there is no case in whom diplopia has not resolved.

Discussion

The study design is retrospective with some weaknesses for that reason. The greatest of these is the lack of biopsy in 2 cases. This seems an unavoidable problem, since important ethical matters relating to the risk of biopsy are involved and the tumour would have been treated irrespective of the result of the biopsy, because its location made any other surgical approach inappropriate. The non-biopsied tumours all occurred in children and were radiologically characteristic for the diagnosis, as far as that is possible to determine. The follow-up is short, particularly for interpreting the significance of tumours which have not changed in size, when it is remembered that these tumours are very slow growing.

The radiosurgical technique in this study is somewhat unconventional. In Gamma Knife surgery it is usual to place the 50% isodose or higher at the edge of the target. This results in the sharpest fall in dose and dose-rate outside the lesion, as a result of the construction of the unit[20]. In this study it has been argued that if the edge dose is low enough, then the gradient of the dose fall outside is less crucial. Moreover, it can be shown that the difference in dose spread outside the lesion is much the same for a given lesion and a given edge dose, irrespective of whether the 30% or 50% isodose is used (Thorsen and Ganz unpublished data). This apparent paradox is explained by the fact that the 30% isodose will be placed at the target edge using a smaller collimator size than if the 50% were used. Since the dose fall is sharper with smaller collimators, the dose spread around the target, is much the same for the two dose-planning strategies, provided the same edge dose is used. On the basis of experience with other tumour categories, an edge dose around 12 Gy is preferred for essentially benign lesions[5]. After the edge dose is determined it has seemed logical to deposit as much radiation energy within the target volume as possible. Gamma Knife dose plans always deliver a non-homogeneous dose distribution. This is inherent to the technique. While theoretically undesirable, the practical success of the method justifies its use[5]. There is no useful information concerning the significance of dose homogeneity in single dose radiosurgery. However, our group has been able to demonstrate useful results with the sort of dose strategy outlined above, for skull base lesions such as acoustic neurinomas and meningiomas[4,5]. This type of dose-planning has been considered inappropriate for malignant tumours and arteriovenous malformations, because of the higher edge dose required and because of the short-term risks associated with these lesion categories.

The role of radiosurgery for malignant gliomas, both with the LINAC and the Gamma Knife, has now been reviewed a number of times[1-3,19]. There seems to be a broad agreement that the role is that of a booster, rather than of a definitive treatment. The current results may indicate that the Gamma Knife may have a more significant role for the pilocytic astrocytomas. Even so, as reported here, surgical debulking may be required in many cases, if the problems related to the radiosurgical treatment of larger lesions are to be avoided. The appropriateness of radiosurgery for pilocytic astrocytomas as opposed to other gliomas is related to differences in the biology of these tumours. The size, malignancy and inadequate radiological definition of glioblastomas and malignant astrocytomas make these essentially very difficult radiosurgical targets. The doses that could reasonably be expected to give an adequate therapeutic result, would be associated with a high rate of complications. On the other hand with pilocytic astrocytomas, whatever lesion is demonstrated on the images is far closer to the true extent of the tumour. It is the location of these tumours which defeats the surgeon and it is this which also makes them such attractive radiosurgical targets. They can of course be treated by conventional radiotherapy. However, the risks of radiation to larger volumes of developing brain is of course to be avoided[6,7]. Nonetheless, the experience of the Gamma Knife in the treatment of Cushing's Disease in a paediatric age group makes it most likely that hypothalamic disorders of growth failure and disturbances of sexual development may well follow the use of radiosurgery aimed at lesions in the anterior part of the diencephalon. It is too early to report on this in the current series.

Conclusions

1. Gamma Knife radiosurgery may represent a most useful new therapeutic modality for juvenile astrocytomas of the diencephalon.
2. An inhomogeous dose with 12 Gy to the tumour edge and 40 Gy to the centre appears to provide a useful therapeutic effect with a very low rate of complications.
3. There is a risk of temporary diplopia for astrocytomas close to the pineal gland.
4. Pre-radiosurgery tumour debulking is desirable to maximise the advantages of radiosurgical technique.

References

1. Alexander E, Coffey RJ, Loeffler JS (1993) Radiosurgery of gliomas. In: Alexander E, Loeffler JS, Lunsford LD (eds) Stereotactic radiosurgery. McGraw Hill, New York, pp 207–219
2. Coffey RJ, Lunsford LD, Flickinger JC (1992) The role of radiosurgery in the treatment of malignant brain tumours. Neurosurg Clin N Am 3: 231–244
3. Dempsey PK, Kondziolka D, Lunsford LD, Coffey RJ, Flickinger JC (1992) The role of stereotactic radiosurgery in the treatment of glial tumours. In: Lunsford LD (ed) Stereotactic radiosurgery update Elsevier, New York, pp 407–410
4. Ganz JC, Myrseth E, Thorsen F, Backlund E-O (1992) Acoustic schwannoma: early results of radiosurgical treatment. In: Tos M, Thomsen (eds) Acoustic neuroma. Kugler, Amsterdam, pp 301–304
5. Ganz JC, Backlund E-O, Thorsen FA (1993) The results of gamma knife surgery for meningiomas, related to size of tumour and dose. Stereotact Funct Neurosurg 61: 23–25
6. Inoue HK, Nakamura M, Ono N, Kohga H, Kakegawa T (1993) Long-term follow-up study of conventional irradiation for brain tumours in children: role of radiosurgery. Acta Neurochir (Wien) 122: 163
7. Inoue HK, Nakamura M, Ono N, Kawashima Y, Hirato M, Ohye C (1993) The long-term clinical effects of radiation therapy for primitive gliomas and medulloblastomas: a role for radiosurgery. Stereotact Funct Neurosurg 61: 51–58
8. Kilhström L, Karlsson B, Lindquist C (1992) Gamma knife surgery in brain metastases. In: Lunsford LD (ed) Stereotactic radiosurgery update. Elsevier, New York, pp 4429–434
9. Kilhström L, Karlsson B, Lindquist C (1993) Gamma knife surgery for cerebral metastases. Implications for survival based on 16 years experience. Stereotact Funct Neurosurg 61: 65–90
10. Kondziolka D, Lunsford LD (1992) Radiosurgery of meningiomas. Neurosurg Clin N Am 3: 219–230
11. Linskey ME, Lunsford LD, Flickinger JC, Kondziolka D (1992) Stereotactic radiosurgery for acoustic tumours. Neurosurg Clin N Am 3: 191–205
12. Lunsford LD, Kondziolka D, Bissonette DJ, Maitz AH, Flickinger JC (1992) Stereotactic radiosurgery of brain vascular malformations. Neurosurg Clin N Am 3: 79–98
13. Norén G, Arndt J, Hindmarsh T (1988) Stereotactic radiosurgical treatment of acoustic neurinomas. In: Lunsford LD (ed) Modern stereotactic neurosurgery. Martinus Nijhoff, Boston, pp 481–489
14. Norén G, Arndt J, Hindmarsh T (1983) Stereotactic radiosurgery in cases of acoustic neurinoma: further experiences. Neurosurgery 13: 12–22
15. Rubinstein L (1979) Tumours of the central nervous system. In: Firminger HI (ed) Atlas of tumour pathology. Second series, Fascicle 6. Castle House, Tunbridge Wells, pp 1–50
16. Scherer HJ (1938) Structural development in gliomas. Am J Cancer 34: 333–351
17. Steiner L, Lindquist C (1987) Radiosurgery in cerebral arteriovenous malformations. In: Tasker RR (ed) Neurosurgery: state of the art reviews. Stereotactic surgery. Hanley and Belfus, Philadelphia, pp 329–336

18. Steiner L, Lindquist C, Steiner M (1991) Meningiomas and gamma knife radiosurgery. In: Al-Mefty O (ed) Meningiomas. Raven, New York, pp 263–272

19. Sturm V, Kimmig B, Wowra B, Voges J, Schabbert S, Schlegel W, Pastyr O, Treuer H, Lorenz WJ (1992) Radiosurgery in malignant intracranial tumours. In: Steiner L, Lindquist C, Forster D, Backlund E-O (eds) Radiosurgery: baseline and trends. Raven, New York pp 155–160

20. Thorsen FA, Ganz JC (1993) Dose planning with the Leksell gamma knife: the effect on dose volume of more than one shot at the same target point. Stereotact Funct Neurosurg 61: 151–163

Correspondence: J. Ganz, M.A., Ph.D., FRCS, Department of Neurosurgery, Haukeland Hospital, University of Bergen, N-5027 Bergen, Norway.

Acta Neurochir (1994) [Suppl] 62: 67–71
© Springer-Verlag 1994

Long-Term Follow-up of Gliomas Treated with Fractionated Stereotactic Irradiation

H. J. Landy, J. G. Schwade, P. V. Houdek, A. M. Markoe, and **L. Feun**

Departments of Neurological Surgery, Radiation Oncology, and Medicine, Sylvester Comprehensive Cancer Center, University of Miami School of Medicine, Miami, FL, U.S.A.

Summary

Eighteen patients have been treated for gliomas with fractionated stereotactic linear accelerator (LINAC) irradiation. A plastic halo ring secured with skull pins allows daily attachment of the patient to the stereotactic frame mounted on the linear accelerator. The patients received 9–31 fractions of 1.8–3 Gy/fraction over periods of 20–49 days. Total doses delivered stereotactically where 16–60 Gy (90% isodose) delivered to 3–7 cm diameter tumors. The six patients with glioblastoma had a median survival of 16 months (range 7–60 months). The two patients with anaplastic astrocytoma survived 7 and 78 months. Most of the patients with high grade tumors also received other adjuant treatments. Of the ten patients with low grade gliomas, one expired 66 months after treatment, and the remainder are alive 22–82 months after treatment. One pediatric patient displayed evidence of focal radiation injury with visual loss. No patient developed initial recurrence of tumor outside the focally irradiated field. Stereotactic localization of irradiation protects surrounding brain tissue; fractionation improves the therapeutic ratio.

These extended follow-up data indicate that stereotactic restriction of radiation fields in treatment of gliomas does not result in deterioration of survival results. Further investigation is warranted into the use of higher focal fractionated radiation doses to attempt to improve local control and survival.

Keywords: Brain tumor; glioma; radiosurgery; radiotherapy.

Introduction

Ionizing radiation is the most important adjuvant treatment for intracranial neoplasms that cannot be cured surgically. While radiation can kill tumor cells or arrest their growth, it may also injure surrounding normal tissue. In the nervous system, death of normal tissue is not followed by effective regeneration, and the sequelae may be devastating.

In order to deliver radiation to the brain with relative safety, two principles should be considered. The first principle is localization of the radiation. Gliomas are usually relatively localized tumors with recurrence generally noted within 2 cm of the original lesion; multifocality is observed in only 5–6% of patients[9]. In current practice, radiotherapy for gliomas is generally restricted to the region of radiographically involved brain, and whole-brain radiation is avoided[9,17]. Modern neuroimaging techniques, primarily computerized tomography (CT) and magnetic resonance imaging (MRI), allow visualization of the extent of such tumors, and image guided stereotactic techniques allow direction of radiation beams at these visualized targets.

This stereotactic administration of radiation has been termed radiosurgery and has been performed with particle beams, multisource cobalt devices (gamma knife), and linear accelerators (LINAC)[3,5,7,8,12,14–16,18,20–22,24,27,29,30,32,33,35]. These devices produce focal radiation fields with steep dose gradients that minimize radiation exposure of critical neural structures adjacent to the irradiated lesions.

The second principle to be considered in discussing efficacy and safety of tumor irradiation is fractionation of the radiation dose. The therapeutic ratio of a given dose of radiation is improved by dividing the dose into smaller fractions that are administered at intervals. Such fractionation improves tumor cell killing while decreasing normal tissue damage. Particular stages of the cell cycle (G2 and M) are more sensitive to radiation damage than others; if radiation is given at different times, more cells may be injured at radiosensitive phases than if a single dose is administered. Tumor cells that are hypoxic are less sensitive to radiation; death of some tumor cells during a course of fractionated treatment may allow other marginally oxygenated cells to become better oxygenated and more radiosensitive.

Fractionation of the radiation dose allows normal tissue to repair sublethal damage between doses; tumor cells have less capacity to repair sublethal damage[6].

The size of a lesion that may be treated with a single dose is limited. The larger the volume irradiated, the higher the risk of a given single dose of radiation[26]. Fractionation allows larger targets to be treated with higher doses.

Most stereotactic radiosurgery, whether by particle beam, gamma unit, or LINAC, has been administered as single-dose treatment that has been directed at vascular malformations, acoustic neuromas, pituitary adenomas, and a variety of other tumors. In the treatment of neoplasms, accepted radiobiological principles, as discussed above, suggest that fractionated radiation delivery may be safer and more effective.

In this center, development of radiosurgery has concentrated on techniques for delivering fractionated radiation in a stereotactic fashion[10–12,18,19,30,34,35]. The current system employs a halo ring that the patient wears throughout the course of treatment; the ring attaches to a stereotactic frame for each daily fraction.

This report discusses the long-term results of stereotactic fractionated irradiation of gliomas.

Materials and Methods

Stereotactic Equipment and Technique

The fundamental requirement for delivery of stereotactic radiation in a fractionated manner is ability to accurately reproduce head positioning. As in most stereotactic procedures, fixation to the skull provides the most secure maintenance of position. The device must allow replacing the head in the stereotactic frame as many times as desired. The system employs a halo ring which secures to the skull and then mates to the stereotactic frame. Three or four standard skull pins are used; pin locations are chosen to avoid prior craniotomy wounds. The halo is applied using local anesthesia and remains in place on the patient's head throughout the course of treatment. The halo is attached to the stereotactic frame for each dose or radiation.

The halo is fabricated of radiolucent Delrin plastic (Commercial Plastic & Supply Corp., Cornwells Heights, PA, USA) with threaded metal inserts to carry the skull pins. The current version of the ring has three holes into which adapter posts insert for interface with the frame. The posts project from a horseshoeshaped bracket which attaches to the base of the frame.

The first version of the stereotactic frame carried a quadrilateral plastic grid that produced reference markings on the CT slices; these markings were used to derive target coordinates directly from the films[34]. These coordinates were then set on a phantom target mounted on a frame attached to the linear accelerator couch. The couch and frame were then adjusted to place the target at the isocenter of rotation of the linear accelerator. The phantom was then replaced by the patient with the halo attached to the frame on the LINAC couch. The first system allowed treatment with rotation of the beam in a single plane; the newer system allows more flexibility in treatment planning.

The current frame is based on the use of a dedicated CT simulator (CT-SIM/0600, Medical High Technology International, Inc., Clearwater, FL, USA) that is directly interfaced to the radiation planning computer (Theraplan L, Theratronix, Kanata, Ontario, Canada). A magnetic field positioning system is employed to facilitate daily patient positioning[12]. The halo is attached to the stereotactic frame on the CT table, and the frame is adjusted to allow comfortable positioning of the head. CT scanning is performed, and target coordinates are derived from the CT computer. Reference marks are placed on the halo using the laser positioning system of the scanner.

The CT slices appear on the radiation planning computer monitor. Dose planning is performed with simulation of rotation of the LINAC beam on the monitor. Treatment may be designed with single rotational arcs, multiple convergent arcs, fixed ports, wedged fields, or combinations of these techniques to produce the best coverage of the lesion while providing maximal possible radioprotection of the brain.

The magnetic field positioning system (Polhemus Inc., Colchester, VT) is used to facilitate daily setup for treatment and to monitor consistency of head position; this system has previously been described in detail[12] and will be summarized here. A low frequency magnetic field source is mounted on the LINAC; the magnetic field detector is mounted on the halo and interfaced to a personal computer. The detector digitizes coordinates of its position in the magnetic field yielding six coordinates: three cartesian coordinates (x, y, and z) and three Euler angles (azimuth, elevation, and roll). This system provides verification of consistency of head position during treatment.

The patient's halo is attached to the frame on the LINAC couch with the target at the isocenter; the laser of the LINAC is used in positioning. The magnetc field detector is attached to the halo and connected to its computer. Port films are also periodically used to check positioning. The positioning and treatment procedure is repeated on a daily basis. The LINAC currently in use with the system is the Varian Clinac 2500C (Varian Associates, Inc., Palo Alto, CA) which provides both 6MV and 24MV beam capability. The overall precision of the system has been measured with phantom targets to be 1.5 mm maximum difference between target and dose distribution centers[12].

Patients

The 18 patients were aged 8–63 years; 11 patients were male, and 7 were female. Gliomas treated included low grade hemispheral astrocytomas, hypothalamic gliomas, oligodendragliomas, anaplastic astrocytomas, and glioblastomas (Table 1).

All patients received fractionated treatement. The ranges of the dosimetric parameters are listed in Table 2. The target sizes listed refer to the tumor diameters. Treatment included appropriate margins beyond image identifiable tumor with larger fields used at the beginning of treatment and decreased field sizes later in treatment. In general, initial fields extended approximately 2 cm outside the

Table 1. *Gliomas Treated with Stereotactic Fractionated Irradiation*

Tumor	n
Hypothalamic glioma	3
Astrocytoma	5
Anaplastic astrocytoma	2
Glioblastoma	6
Oligodendroglioma	2
Total	18

Table 2. *Radiation Dose Planning Ranges of Parameters in 18 Patients*

Tumor diameter	3–7 cm
Total dose	1600–6000 cGy
Fraction dose	180–300 cGy
Number of fractions	9–31
Duration of treatment	20–49 days

Doses are specified at the 90% isodose line.

limit of CT or MRI visualized peritumoral edema with boost fields decreased to the size of the tumor. Doses listed in Table 2 refer to doses delivered with the stereotactic system. Two of the patients received only the small field boost portion of their treatment using the stereotactic system in order to boost the total dose of the enhancing tumor margin to 7900 cGy. One patient received stereotactic treatment for a recurrent tumor previously irradiated conventionally. Another patient received two courses of stereotactic treatment, 5.5 years aparts; the second course was for recurrence of anaplastic asytrocytoma.

Results

Placement of the halo and the mechanics of daily treatment were generally tolerated well. The elasticity of the Delrin maintains stable pin pressure, and periodic tightening of pins was only occasionally necessary. One patient insisted on removal of the halo due to psychological stress after less than one third of the planned treatment for a small low grade astocytoma. Only one halo has become dislodged during treatment. This occurred in the case of a hemiparetic patient with a small anaplastic astrocytoma. The patient was not ambulatory and was inadvertently dropped by transport personnel directly on the halo resulting in dislodgment of the halo.

One patient suffered apparent radiation injury. The patient was 9 years old and was treated for a hypothalamic glioma. Six months after treatment, stepwise visual loss occurred. MRI showed increased signal consistent with edema in the optic chiasm and tracts without evidence of tumor progression. The patient received a hypofractionated course of treatment with 18 fraction of 300 cGy over 29 days. No visual recovery occurred; treatment with anticoagulation and hyperbaric oxygen was not beneficial.

The five patients with hemispheral low-grade astrocytomas are alive with mean follow-up of 53 months (range 21–82 months). Four of those patients have had clinically and radiographically stable disease; one patient had recurrence of tumor and has been retreated with surgery and chemotherapy. The two patients with oligodendroglioma have stable disease with follow-up periods of 65 and 68 months. One patient with hypothalamic glioma expired 66 months after treatment;

the other two are alive with follow-up of 22 and 70 months.

The patients with high-grade gliomas have had multimodality treatment including chemotherapy regimens; therefore, survival results are affected by many factors. Of the two patients with anaplastic astrocytoma, one survived 78 months with treatment that included two courses of stereotactic radiation. The other patient expired of systemic medical problems 7 months after treatment. Median survival of the glioblastoma patients was 16 months (range 7–60 months, one patient remaining alive at 13 months).

None of the patients with tumor recurrence developed initial recurrence outside the irradiated fields, although, with further progression, tumor later extended outside initially treated fields.

Discussion

The prognoses for most patients with intracranial gliomas remain poor. In a recent large survey, five year survival rates were reported to be 5.5% for glioblastoma, 18.2% for anaplastic astrocytoma, and 32.5% for astrocytoma[25]. The survival data in this study suggest that stereotactic restriction of radiation fields in treatment of gliomas does not result in deterioration of survival results. Fractionated stereotactic irradiation is a modality that has theoretical advantages. Further investigation of this type of treatment with delivery of higher boost doses to restricted fields is warranted.

The addition of a stereotactic frame to technology widely available in major medical centers allows precision focal irradiation while maintaining the capability of delivering fractionated treatment. The use of bony fixation to the skull offers greater accuracy and reliability than conventional radiotherapy head holders employing ear bars, nose bridges, and bite blocks. As compared to conventional fractionated radiotherapy, the stereotactic technique allows use of radiation fields more closely conforming to the size and shape of the target.

Single-dose radiosurgery systems provide focal delivery of radiation with steep dose gradients near the margins; however, neural structures included within the treatment fields or immediately adjacent to treatment margins still receive significant radiation doses. Although stereotactic systems produce tight control of radiation delivery, the dose to adjacent structures through which the beams must pass is not reduced to zero. A measure of protection of these structures is afforded by fractionation of the radiation dose.

The advantage of radiation dose fractionation in protection of normal tissue was first demonstrated in experiments designed to sterilize animals by testicular irradiation[6]. Fractionation of a given dose of radiation reduces its biological effect both for normal tissue and neoplastic tissue; however, normal tissue has a greater ability to repair sublethal damage than tumor tissue. Tumor tissue that is reproducing faster will traverse radiosensitive phases of the cell cycle more than slowly cycling normal tissue. Loss of radiation injured tumor cells will allow marginally oxygenated tumor cells to become better oxygenated and more radiosensitive. These factors combine to produce preferential injury of tumor cells as compared to normal tissue; that is, the therapeutic ratio of a given dose of radiation is improved by dividing the dose into fractions[6]. This effect of fractionation is the reason that most radiotherapy of neoplastic disease in human medicine is delivered in a fractionated fashion.

Data reported after treatment of acoustic neuromas with the gamma knife illustrate the risk of single dose irradiation of neural structures[22]. Delayed onset of facial nerve deficits occurred in 34% of patients, and trigeminal nerve deficits were observed in 32% of patients. Useful hearing preservation was reported in 38% one year after treatment. These results were found to be similar to a matched group of patients treated surgically[4].

With a single dose of radiation, the size of the lesion that may be safely irradiated with a given dose is limited[26]. With single dose radiosurgery, the targets are generally limited to approximately 2.5–3.5 cm diameter. As target diameter increases, the dose delivered is reduced. With fractionated treatment, larger targets may be taken to higher doses. With larger targets, use of stereotactic techniques may reach a point of diminishing returns; however, a 5 cm diameter spherical target represents only approximately 5% of the brain volume. Even with such a relatively larger target, stereotactic delivery of radiation may be advantageous in protecting the rest of the brain.

One patient in this series had apparent radiation injury of optic pathways included in the radiation field for treatment of a hypothalamic glioma. This patient received a hypofractionated dose regimen, and the patient was 9 years old. Pediatric patients are more sensitive to radiation than adults; although, by age 9, the differences in normal tissue sensitivity from the adult may be small. This patient illustrates the risks involved in straying from conventional generally safe dose regimens. Both fraction size and total dose seem to be important factors affecting risk of radiation injury of nervous tissue[1].

Increasing doses of radiation produce improvement in survival of patients with malignant gliomas[28,36]; however, the dose that may be delivered is limited by the risk of radiation injury[31]. In the treatment of primary brain tumors, limitation of the size of the radiation fields may avoid significant adverse effects on brain tissue that is not affected by tumor. Avoidance of iatrogenic brain injury imposed by radiation may allow improved quality of life, and perhaps the patient might better tolerate further treatment at the time of tumor recurrence. Serial treatment with repeat tumor resection, focal reirradiation, and chemotherapy may be better tolerated if uninvolved brain tissue has been spared excessive radiation exposure.

Studies correlating radiographic findings with biopsy and autopsy data have shown that high grade gliomas are relatively localized neoplasms[9,13]. Recurrence is usually located in the original tumor bed or within a short distance of the original lesion[9]. Because of the relatively localized nature of the disease, aggressive local therapy is appropriate. However, biopsy data indicate that tumor cells may be found infiltrating beyond the margin of obvious tumor[13], therefore treatment must also be directed at peripheral areas. Use of the stereotactic teletherapy system allows customized radiation fields to be designed to cover these areas. During the course of the fractionated treatment, radiation fields may be varied to deliver different total doses to the macroscopic tumor and the area of possible microscopic invasion.

Radiosurgical techniques may produce focal irradiation with fields similar to interstitial sources without the requirement for implantation of sources. Thus, the risks of intracranial hemorrhage and infection related to implantation are eliminated. However, the radiobiological differences between brachytherapy and radiosurgery may be significant. Brachytherapy delivers low dose rate continuous radiation over a period of time[2]. This is more likely to be advantageous in tumor treatment than single dose radiosurgery techniques because of the exploitation of the radiobiological principles underlying dose fractionation. Continuous radiation over a prolonged period of time is, in essence, extreme fractionation. Both brachytherapy and fractionated radiosurgery techniques theoretically may be more efficacious in tumor control than single dose radiosurgery. One report of recurrence after brachytherapy suggests that with higher local radiation dose delivery, local recurrence is replaced by recurrence farther removed from the original lesion[23]. Radiobiological differences between the low dose rate continuous radiation of brachytherapy and the fractionated high dose rate radiation of fractionated radiosurgery may be of significance and require further investigation.

References

1. Aristizabal S, Caldwell WL, Avila J (1977) The relationship of time-dose fractionation factors to complications in the treatment of pituitary tumors by irradiation. Int J Radiat Oncol Biol Phys 2: 667–673

2. Bernstein M, Gutin PH (1981) Interstitial irradiation of brain tumors: a review. Neurosurgery 9: 741–750

3. Betti OO, Derechinsky VE (1984) Hyperselective encephalic irradiation with linear accelerator. Acta Neurochir (Wien) [Suppl] 33: 385–390

4. Camarata PJ, Haines SJ, Lunsford LD, Levine SC, Erickson DL (1991) Cranial nerve preservation after treatment of acoustic neurilemmomas: a comparison of microsurgical excision and radiosurgery. Presented at the 59th Annual Meeting of the American Association of Neurological Surgeons

5. Colombo F, Benedetti A, Pozza F, Avanzo RC, Marchetti C, Chierego G, Zanardo A (1985) External stereotactic irradiation by linear accelerator. Neurosurgery 16: 154–160

6. Hall EJ, Cox JD (1989) Physical and biologic basis of radiation therapy. In: Moss WT, Cox JD (eds) Radiation oncology. Mosby, St Louis, pp 1–57

7. Hartmann GH, Schlegel W, Sturm V, Kober B, Pastyr O, Lorenz WJ (1985) cerebral radiation surgery using moving field irradiation at a linear acceleration facility. Int J Radiat Oncol Biol Phys 11: 1185–1192

8. Heifetz MD, Wexler M, Thompson R (1984) Single-beam radiotherapy knife. A practical theoretical model. J Neurosurg 60: 814–818

9. Hochberg FH, Pruitt A (1980) Assumptions in the radiotherapy of glioblastoma. Neurology 30: 907–911

10. Houdek PV, Van Buren JM, Fayos JV (1983) Dosimetry of small radiation fields for 10 MV x-ray. Med Phys 10: 333–336

11. Houdek PV, Fayos JV, Van Buren JM, Ginsberg MS (1985) Stereotaxic radiotherapy technique for small intracranial lesions. Med Phys 12: 469–472

12. Houdek PV, Schwade JG, Serago CF, Landy HJ, Pisciotta V, Wu X, Markoe AM, Lewin AA, Abitbol AA, Bujnoski JL, Marienberg ES, Fiedler JA, Ginsberg MS (1991) Computer controlled stereotaxic radiotherapy system. Int J Rad Onc Biol Phys 22: 175–180

13. Kelly PJ, Daumas-Duport C, Kispert DB, Kall BA, Scheithauer BW, Illig JJ (1987) Imaging-based stereotaxic serial biopsies in untreated intracranial glial neoplasms. J Neurosurg 66: 865–874

14. Kjellberg RN, Shintani A, Frantz AG, Kliman B (1968) Proton-beam therapy in acromegaly. N Engl J Med 278: 689–695

15. Kjellberg RN, Hanamura T, Davis KR, Lyons SL, Adams RD (1983) Bragg-peak proton-beam therapy for arteriovenous malformations of the brain. N Engl J Med 309: 269–274

16. Kondziolka D, Lunsford LD, Coffey RJ, Flickinger JC (1991) Stereotactic radiosurgery of meningiomas. J Neurosurg 74: 552–559

17. Kun LE (1989) The brain and spinal cord. In: Moss WT, Cox JD (eds) Radiation oncology. Mosby, St Louis, pp 597–639

18. Landy HJ, Houdek PV, Schwade JG, Egnor M (1991) Fractionated stereotactic radiation for skull base tumors. Abstract. Skull Base Surg [Suppl] 11

19. Landy HJ, Schwade JG, Houdek PV, Feun L, Rodriguez M (1992) Fractionated stereotactic radiation for glioma. In: Lunsford LD (ed) Stereotactic radiosurgery update. Elsevier, New York, pp 421–424

20. Leksell L (1951) The stereotaxic method and radiosurgery of the brain. Acta Chir Scand 102: 316–319

21. Leksell L (1983) Stereotactic radiosurgery. J Neurol Neurosurg Psychiatry 46: 797–803

22. Linskey M, Lunsford LD, Flickinger JC (1991) Stereotactic radiosurgery for acoustic tumors: three year experience. Presented at the International Stereotactic Radiosurgery Symposium, Pittsburgh, PA, June 19–21

23. Loeffler JS, Alexander E, Hochberg FH, Wen PY, Morris JH, Schoene WC, Siddon RL, Morse RH, Black PM (1990) Clinical patterns of failure following stereotactic interstitial irradiation for malignant gliomas. Int J Radiat Oncol Biol Phys 19: 1455–1462

24. Lunsford LD, Kondziolka D, Flickinger JC, Bissonette DJ, Jungreis CA, Maitz AH, Horton JA, Coffey RJ (1991) Stereotactic radiosurgery for arteriovenous malformations of the brain. J Neurosurg 75: 512–524

25. Mahaley MS, Mettlin C, Natarajan N, Laws ER, Peace BB (1989) National survey of patterns of care for brain-tumor patients. J Neurosurg 71: 826–836

26. Marks LB, Spencer DP (1991) The influence of volume on the tolerance of the brain to radiosurgery. J Neurosurg 75: 177–180

27. Podgorsak EB, Olivier A, Pla M, Lefebvre PY, Hazel J (1988) Dynamic stereotactic radiosurgery. Int J Radiat Oncol Biol Phys 14: 115–126

28. Salazar OM, Rubin P, Feldstein ML, Pizzutiello R (1979) High dose radiation therapy in the treatment of malignant gliomas: final report. Int J Radiat Oncol Biol Phys 5: 1733–1740

29. Saunders WM, Chen GTY, Austin-Seymour M, Castro JR, Collier JM, Gauger G, Gutin P, Phillips TL, Pitluck S, Walton, RE, Zink SR (1985) Precision high dose radiotherapy. II. Helium ion treatment of tumors adjacent to critical central nervous system structures. Int J Radiat Onclo Biol Phys 11: 1339–1347

30. Schwade JG, Houdek PV, Landy HJ, Bujnoski JL, Lewin AA, Abitbol AA, Serago CF, Pisciotta VJ (1990) Small-field stereotactic external-beam radiation therapy of intracranial lesions: fractionated treatment with a fixed-halo immobilization device. Radiology 176: 563–565

31. Sheline GE, Wara WM, Smith V (1980) Therapeutic irradiation and brain injury. Int J Radiat Oncol Biol Phys 6: 1215–1228

32. Sturm V, Kober B, Hover KH, Schlegel W, Boesecke R, Pastyr O, Hartmann GH, Schabbert S, Winkel KZ, Kunze S, Lorenz WJ (1987) Stereotactic percutaneous single dose irradiation of brain metastases with a linear acceleration. Int J Radiat Oncol Biol Phys 13: 279–282

33. Thoren M, Rahn T, Guo W, Werner S (1991) Stereotactic radiosurgery with the Cobalt-60 gamma unit in the treatment of growth hormone-producing pituitary tumors. Neurosurgery 29: 663–668

34. Van Buren JM, Houdek P, Ginsberg M (1983) A multipurpose CT-guided stereotactic instrument of simple design. Appl Neurophysiol 46: 211–216

35. Van Buren JM, Landy HJ, Houdek PV, Ginsberg MS (1986) CT directed stereotactic fractionated rotational radiotherapy by linear accelerator. Abstract. Neurosurgery 19: 149

36. Walker MD, Strike TA, Sheline GE (1979) An analysis of dose-effect relationship in the radiotherapy of malignant gliomas. Int J Radiat Oncol Biol Phys 5: 1725–1731

Correspondence: Howard J. Landy, M.D., Department of Neurological Surgery, University of Miami, 1501 NW 9 Avenue, Miami, Florida 33136, U.S.A.

Acta Neurochir (1994) [Suppl] 62: 72–76
© Springer-Verlag 1994

Linac Radiosurgery in Brain Metastases

J. Voges[1], H. Treuer[1], J. Erdmann[1], W. Schlegel[2], O. Pastyr[2], R. P. Müller[3], and V. Sturm[1]

[1] Department of Stereotactic and Functional Neurosurgery, University of Cologne, [2] Department of Radiotherapy, German Cancer Research Center, Heidelberg, and [3] Department of Radiotherapy, University of Cologne, Cologne, Federal Republic of Germany

Summary

Brain metastases are usually well-circumscribed and more or less spherical lesions. These conditions meet the criteria for radiosurgery (RS). A pilot study initiated by our group in 1983, demonstrated the effectiveness of Linac-RS in the treatment of solitary brain metastases with low radiosensitivity.

A second trial including patients with 1–3 metastases started in 1990. By April 1993, 46 patients had been treated in this series. The radiation doses delivered to the tumour margin ranged from 10 to 25 Gy, and were chosen with respect to size, number and location of the tumours or previous whole brain radiotherapy (WBRT), decreasing mainly with increasing tumour volumes. 34/46 patients had a follow-up of more than 12 weeks. In 7/46 patients the disease progressed rapidly during the first weeks after RS and follow-up examinations were not performed. 5/46 patients had a follow-up of less than 6 weeks and follow-up CT/MR-examinations were not available. 14/46 patients received WBRT before RS. The regularly performed follow-up examinations (clinical status, CT-/MR-examinations in 6 or 12 weekly intervals) revealed tumour progression in 5/34 patients. Permanent cessation of the growth (11/34), tumour shrinkage (18/34) and decrease of surrounding oedema together with clinical amelioration have been observed a few weeks after radiosurgery. The median follow-up was 50 weeks. 14/46 patients died due to generalized progression of their disease. In 4 other patients death was most probably caused by raised intracranial pressure due to local tumour recurrence (2 patients) or the occurrence of new cerebral metastases (2 pat.). There was no treatment related mortality. In 2 patients worsening of their neurological condition was due to the treatment.

Keywords: Cerebral metastases; multiple metastases; radiosurgery; Linac radiosurgery; results.

Introduction

In about 50% of cancer patients, brain metastases are found at autopsy[14]. With a rate of 43% of all intracranial tumours, they constitute a major neurosurgical problem[9]. The incidence of intracranial metastatic lesions has been estimated to be 8.5 per 100,000[21]. Zülch stated, that the average frequency of brain metastases varies widely (range: 3.2%–37%) depending on the different populations of clinical patients evaluated[23]. The increasing incidence of some of the primaries (e.g. lung cancer) is likely to increase the significance of this problem. As expected, reviews of epidemiological, clinical and autopsy studies, revealed, that the number of metastatic brain tumours is increasing[5,15].

Solitary, surgically accessible lesions can be extirpated with microsurgical techniques. The combination with external fractionated irradiation can prolong the survival of these patients significantly[20]. Radioresistant metastases localized in functionally important areas of the brain or multiple tumours are hardly treatable by conventional methods.

Different from primary malignant brain tumours, metastases are usually more or less spherical, well circumscribed and relatively small. They thus are potentially treatable with radiosurgery, i.e. stereotactically guided percutaneous single dose irradiation. High accuracy and steep dose gradients enable the application of highly focussed single radiation-doses to the target volumes and to optimally spare surrounding healthy tissue.

In 1983 we inaugurated the use of radiosurgery for the treatment of solitary inoperable brain metastases with low radiosensitivity[19]. Although this treatment schedule has meanwhile been adopted by most radiosurgery groups, there is still uncertainty regarding its combination with conventional treatment schedules, the influence of treatment volume and/or histological diagnosis on the response to RS as well as radiobiological effects of high single doses to tumour and healthy tissue.

Methods and Materials

Stereotactic Irradiation

The patient's head was fixed in a modified, CT-compatible Riechert-Mundinger stereotactic frame[18] under general or local anaesthesia. After administration of contrast medium (Solutrast 300[R]) a CT-examination with a stereotactic localiser was performed[18]. CT-data were stored on a magnetic tape and transferred to a computer (VAX station VS 3500, Digital Equip, Corp., USA) The tumour borders were outlined manually on the computer screen in every horizontal CT-slice[16].

By use of special computer programmes, target point, width of the collimator and depth dose distribution were calculated. The treatment plan was controlled by the displaying of any interesting isodose line to the stereotactic CT-images[17] (2- and 3-dimensionally). In our system[6,12] beam-convergence is achieved by use of 10 arcs of Linac-table rotation in steps of 18° and rotation of the gantry from 20°–160°. With a set of easily changeable tungsten collimators, spherical fields from 5–54 mm in diameter can be irradiated with dose gradients from 10% (large fields) to 20% (small fields) per mm distance from the tumour surface.

The treatment parameters of the evaluated patients are listed in Table 1. In most patients the therapeutic dose (isodose-surface covering the treatment volume) was 70% or 80% of the dose, given to the target point (41/46 pat.). In 1/46 we chose the 75% and in 2/46 the 40% or 50% isodose level respectively. In 4/14 patients with more than one lesion the treatment was performed in two sessions with intervals of some days. The dose given to each metastasis was reduced in patients with tumour volumes exceeding 10 ml with multiple lesions of larger volumes and/or if WBRT had been applied in the first place. In tumours located in the cerebellum or brain stem the doses were reduced as well.

Additional Treatment and Follow-up

Immediately before and during the first hours after radiosurgery dexamethasone was administered (dose: 0.4–0.5 mg/kg/24 hours). After discharge from the hospital (1 day after treatment), the dexamethasone dosage was reduced stepwise commensurate with the neurological condition and/or the result of CT/MR-examinations.

6, 12, 18 weeks postoperatively and later on at 12-weekly intervals CT and MR-investigations (without and with contrast-medium) as well as neurological examinations were carried out.

Survival was defined as the time interval between treatment and the end of retrospective analysis (April 1993) or the patient's death.

Patients

46 consecutive patients treated with radiosurgery from July 90 to April 93 for single or multiple (total number treated: 66 lesions) cerebral metastases have been analysed retrospectively. The median age of these patients was 56 years (range: 22–75 years), the female/male ratio 18/28. The Karnofsky performance status [8] evaluated before radiosurgery ranged from 50% to 100% (median: 90%).

28 patients with known primary cancer presented with a characteristic clinical course as well as typical CT- and MR-images. In these cases the risk of a biopsy was assumed to be higher than the risk of a radiosurgical treatment based on clinical and imaging findings. These patients were treated without histological verification of the intracerebral tumour. In the other patients the histological diagnosis was confirmed before radiosurgery by microsurgical tumour extirpation (17 pat.) or stereotactic biopsy (1 pat.).

The histological diagnoses were as follows: adenocarcinoma of the lung (9 pat.) or intestine (1 pat.), melanoma (8 pat.), squamous cell cancer of the lung (7 pat.), renal cell carcinoma (7 pat.), breast cancer (7 pat.), ovarian cancer (1 pat.), urethral carcinoma (1 pat.) and squamous cell cancer of the base of the tongue (1 pat.). In another 4 patients the histological diagnosis "metastasis of unknown origin" was yielded by microsurgical extirpation or stereotactic biopsy.

49/66 metastases were located in the cerebral hemispheres (14 of this group in critical cortical areas and 5 close to the midline). 5 tumours were located in the basal ganglia-diencephalon region, 5 in the brainstem and 6 metastases in the cerebellum. In one patient a small skull metastasis was treated together with two intracerebral tumours.

In 32/46 patients cerebral metastases were treated before Linac-radiosurgery either by microsurgical tumour extirpation (18 patients) or conventional fractionated radiotherapy (14 patients). The treatment parameters of the radiotherapy-group are listed in Table 2.

Results

46 patients with single or multiple cerebral metastases, treated from 1990 to April 1993 with Linac-radiosurgery have been analysed retrospectively. 34/46 patients had follow-up times of 12 weeks and more, 12/46 patients a follow-up of less than 12 weeks. In 7 of these 12 patients, who died during the first 6 weeks after radiosurgery, no imaging studies could be performed. The other 5 patients were alive at the end of the retrospective analysis, but due to short follow-up times no imaging data were available.

In patients with a follow-up of at least 12 weeks the tumour volume, re-assessed on follow-up CT- or MR-

Table. 1. *Treatment Parameters of 46 Patients, Treated with Linac-Radiosurgery*

Tumour volume (no. lesions)	
0–10 ml	43
10.1–20 ml	14
20.1–30 ml	4
>30 ml	5
median	4.8
range	0.5–69
Dose (Gy)	
median	20
range	10–25
Field diameter (mm)	
median	23.1
range	7.8–46.3
Targets (no.)	80

Table 2. *Treatment of Cerebral Metastases prior to Linac-Radiosurgery*

Extirpation (no. pat.)	17
WBRT (no. pat.)	15
dose to whole brain (Gy):	
median	38
range	10–57
time interval from WBRT to RS (wks.)	
median	16
range	1–113

images, was compared with the intra-operatively calculated tumour volumes. 3–6 months after radiosurgery the tumour volume decreased in 18/34 patients, was stable in 11 patients and increased in 5 cases. This is an initial tumour control rate of 85%.

In order to assess the impact of histology on the initial tumour response, the pre-operative tumour volumes were set as 100% and compared with the mean value of the reassessed tumour volume. The mean relative volume reduction was 23% in melanoma patients, 27% in renal cell cancers, 53% in breast cancers, 60% in adenocarcinomas and 77% in patients with squamous cell cancer of the lung (Fig. 1).

In 24/34 patients the pre-operative images documented space occupying peritumoural oedema. After radiosurgery the area of oedema decreased in 12/24 (50%), remained stable in 9/24 (37.5%) and increased in 3/24 (12.5%) patients.

3 months after radiosurgery the neurological status had improved in 10/34 patients, had been unchanged in 18/34 patients (including 14 patients, which had been free of symptoms at the date of radiosurgery) and worsened in 6 patients.

Figure 2 is a graph of survival data estimated with the Kaplan-Meier method[7] for all evaluated patients. With a mean follow up time of 50 ± 35 weeks (range: 1–146 weeks) the mean estimated survival probability is 60 weeks. 28/46 patients were alive at the end of retrospective analysis. The actuarial median survival is 24 weeks.

7/18 patients died during the first 3 months after radiosurgery. The death of these patients was caused by rapid progress of their systemic disease. Clinical data and autopsy reports of 11/18 patients with a follow-up exceeding 12 weeks revealed, that in 7 cases the death was most probably caused by generalized

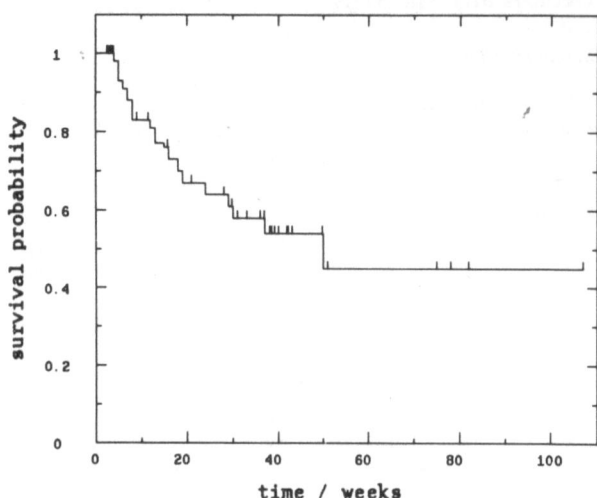

Fig. 2. Kaplan-Meier representation of the probability of survival after Linac-RS of cerebral metastases. Ticks: represent censored patients

progression of the disease. Only 4/18 patients died due to raised intracranial pressure from local tumour recurrence (2 pat.) or the occurrence of new cerebral metastases (2 pat.).

Radiosurgery caused no mortality and with two exceptions no worsening of the neurological status. In one patient with a metastasis of renal cell cancer (vol: 7.6 ml) the tumour responded initially very well to the treatment (22 Gy, normalized to the 75% isodose). 10 months after radiosurgery the patient was referred to our department with more marked hemiparesis. The MR-examination revealed an increasing ringshaped contrast enhancement with newly developed peritumoural oedema. A PET-examination (^{18}FDG-PET) confirmed the diagnosis of radiation induced necrosis. In another patient with metastasis (renal cancer) located in the brain stem (pons), no tumour was visible 3 months after RS, but a dose of 22 Gy applied to the tumour surface (volume: 1.2 ml) caused some tissue damage and consequent worsening of a pre-existing hemiparesis.

Discussion

In this series of 46 retrospectively analysed patients, an initial response to radiosurgery (tumour shrinkage or growth control) has been achieved in 29 patients with a follow-up of at least 12 weeks or more. Thus the primary objective of RS for cerebral metastases, i.e. local control of the disease, has been achieved in 85% of the cases. This value is comparable to response rates reported in the literature (range: 71%–100%,

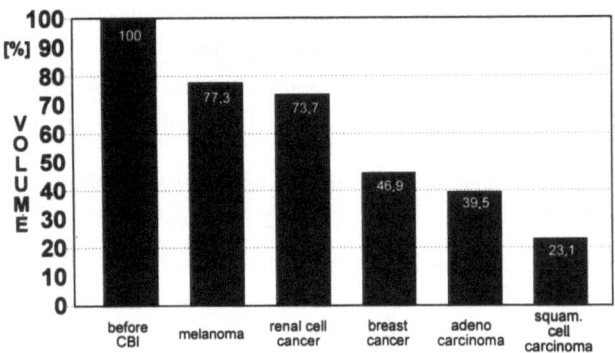

Fig. 1. Relative volume reduction: the tumour volumes were reassessed on follow-up CT- and MR-images 3–6 months after Linac-RS and compared with the treated volume

technique used: Gamma-Knife RS or LINAC-RS) for single[3,10] or multiple[1,4,11] lesions.

WBRT performed before RS does not seem to influence the initial tumour response rate significantly. Coffey *et al.* treated 24 patients with small solitary metastases (range of tumour volume: 0.3–10 ml), where Gamma-Knife RS was applied as a boost immediately after WBRT. For 17/18 evaluated patients tumour growth control was reported[3]. Loeffler *et al.* evaluated 18 patients with a total of 21 recurrent metastases. Their patients underwent WBRT (30–49 Gy) 1–146 months (median: 10 months) before RS. With a median follow up of 9 months, all tumours have been controlled locally[10]. These results are comparable to our experience with our first series, in which solitary brain metastases were treated exclusively with radiosurgery (tumour control rate: 100%)[21] and to the data of our second series (tumour control rate: 85%), including 15 patients, who were treated with WBRT prior to RS.

The median actuarial survival of our patients (24 weeks) is in the same range as the data reported in the literature. With 28/46 patients still under observation the mean survival probability of 60 weeks indicates, that with ongoing follow-up time the median survival value will increase. Mehta *et al.* found a median survival of 22 weeks in 40 patients (total number of treated metastases: 58). The mean follow-up was 6.5 months and 8/40 patients were alive at the end of the analysis[11]. In the series of Fuller *et al.* 47 tumours were treated in 27 patients. The median actuarial survival was 33 weeks and 9/27 patients were still under observation[4].

In our series, 14/18 patients died of progressive systemic cancer and only 4/18 as a consequence of intracranial spread of the disease. In the series of Fuller *et al.* the ratio of "systemic generalization" versus "intracerebral generalization" was 15:3 patients[4]. The percentage of patients, who died from progression of their brain tumours after WBRT is about 50%[1,22]. Compared to this series, in which RS was used as an up-front treatment this value is relatively high.

In our series 14/46 patients had more than one cerebral metastasis, in 25/46 patients the tumour volume exceeded 10 ml and in 15/46 WBRT had already been performed before RS. Despite dose reduction in patients, who had large tumour volumes, multiple lesions and/or who had previously undergone WBRT, a higher incidence of persisting or increasing oedema has been found in follow-up CT- and/or MR-examinations.

Dose reduction cannot conclusively explain the failures of treatment in our series, as only 3/5 nonresponders belong to this group. Also the histological diagnosis of the primary seems to influence the tumour response. Mainly patients with malignant melanoma had a less pronounced tumour volume reduction.

Radiosurgery caused no mortality and in only two of our patients deterioration of the neurological condition. The short hospitalisation time (2 days) and the benignity of the described procedure are of special importance for patients with brain metastases and a short life expectancy. Therefore RS is an attractive modality for palliative treatment of brain metastases. Compared with fractionated radiotherapy and/or surgery it has clear advantages: As shown by our own results and the experiences of others[3,4,10,11,19], stereotactically guided, highly focussed irradiation of single or multiple metastases with doses between 10 and 25 Gy is well tolerated and accompanied by an extremely low rate of side effects. Arrest of growth or shirnkage of the tumour is achieved in 85%–100% of the cases, even in multiple lesions or metastases, previously considered "radioresistant".

Besides the histological diagnosis the most important prognostic factors are size, shape and number of the tumours. Small single metastases of spherical shape are optimally amenable to radiosurgery.

It is clear, that micrometastases, undetectable by modern imaging methods, would be missed, if WBRT is eschewed. On the other hand, in our series most patients died from systemic disease and not from newly occurring brain metastases. Regarding the limited possibilities to increase survival by all available means, optimal palliation, i.e. survival under the best possible conditions, must be a major aim of treatment. We think radiosurgery to be an excellent tool to achieve this aim and use it as primary treatment for brain metastases with low radiosensitivity for up to 3 lesions. If new metastases occur during follow-up, radiosurgery, which requires minimal hospitalisation time, could be repeated or followed by WBRT.

References

1. Adler JR, Cox RS, Kaplan I, Martin DP (1992) Stereotactic radiosurgical treatment of brain metastases. J Neurosurg 76: 444–449
2. Cairncross JC, Kim JH, Posner JB (1980) Radiation therapy for brain metastases. Ann Neurol 7: 529–541
3. Coffey RJ, Flickinger JC, Bissonette DJ, Lunsford LD (1991) Radiosurgery for solitary brain metastases using the Cobalt-60 gamma unit: methods and results in 24 patients. Int J Rad Oncol Biol Phys 20: 1287–1295

4. Fuller BG, Kaplan ID, Adler J, Cox RS, Bagshaw MA (1992) Stereotaxic radiosurgery for brain metastases: the importance of adjuvant whole brain irradiation. Int J Rad Oncol Biol Phys 23: 413–418

5. Gercovich R, Luna M, Gottlieb J (1975) Increased incidence of cerebral metastasis in sarcoma patients with prolonged survival from chemotherapy. Report of cases of leimyosarcoma and chondrosarcoma. Cancer 36: 1843–1851

6. Hartmann GH, Schlegel W, Sturm V, Bernd K, Pastyr O, Lorenz WJ (1985) Cerebral radiation surgery using moving field irradiation at a linear accelerator facility. Int J Rad Oncol Biol Phys 11: 1185–1192

7. Kaplan EL, Meier P (1958) Nonparametric estimation from incomplete observations. J Am Statist Assoc 53: 457–481

8. Karnofsky DA, Abelmann WH, Carver LF, Burchenal JH (1948) The use of nitrogen mustards in the palliative treatment of carcinoma with particular reference to bronchogenic carcinoma. Cancer: 634–656

9. Karrer K, Fleischmann E, Hochpöchler F (1984) Site of primary intracranial metastases. Adv Neurosurg 12: 10–14

10. Loeffler JS, Kooy HM, Wen PY, Fine HA, Cheng CH-W, Mannarino EG, Tsai JS, Alexander III E (1990) The treatment of recurrent brain metastases with stereotactic radiosurgery. J Clin Oncol 8: 576–582

11. Mehta MP, Rozental JM, Levin AB, Mackie TR, Kubsad SS, Gehring MA, Kinsella TJ (1992) Defining the role of radiosurgery in the management of brain metastases. Int J Rad Oncol Biol Phys 24: 619–625

12. Pastyr O, Hartmann GH, Schlegel W, Schabbert S, Treuer H, Lorenz WJ, Sturm V (1989) Stereotactically guided convergent beam irradiation with a linear accelerator: localization-technique. Acta Neurochir (Wien) 99: 61–64

13. Patchell RA (1991) Brain metastases. Neurol Clin 9: 817–824

14. Pickren JW, Lopez G, Tzukada Y (1983) Brain metastases. An autopsy study. Cancer Treat Symp 2: 295–313

15. Posner J (1980) Brain metastasis: a clinician's view. In: Weiss L, Gilbert H, Posner J (eds) Brain metastasis. Martinus Nijhoff, The Hague

16. Schlegel WJ, Scharfenberg H, Sturm V, Penzholz H, Lorenz WJ (1981) Direct visualization of intracranial tumours in stereo-tactic and angiogrpahic films by computer calculation of longi-tudinal CT-sections: a new method for stereotactic localization of tumour outlines. Acta Neurochir (Wien) 58: 27–35

17. Schlegel W, Scharfenberg H, Doll J, Hartmann G, Sturm V, Lorenz WJ (1984) Three dimensional dose planning using tomographic data. In: IEEE Comp. Society (eds) Proc of the Eighth International Conference on the Use of Computers in Radiation Therapy. Silver Spring, IEEE Comp Soc Press, pp 191–196

18. Sturm V, Pastyr O, Schlegel W, Scharfenberg H, Zable HJ, Netzeband G, Schabbert S, Berberich W (1983) Stereotactic computer tomography with a modified Riechert-Mundinger device as the basis for integrated neuroradiological investi-gations. Acta Neurochir (Wien) 68: 11–17

19. Sturm V, Kober B, Höver KH, Schlegel W, Boesecke R, Pastyr O, Hartmann G, Schabbert S, Zum Winkel K, Kunze S, Lorenz WJ (1987) Stereotactic percutaneous single dose irradiation of brain metastases with a linear accelerator. Int J Rad Oncol Biol Phys 13: 279–281

20. Sundaresan N, Galicich JH (1985) Surgical treatment of brain metastases. Clinical and computerized tomography evaluation of the results of treatment. Cancer 55: 1382–1388

21. Survey of intracranial neoplasms (1977) Office of Biometry and Epidemiology, National Institute of Neurological and Communicative Disorders and Stroke, NIH, Bethesda, MD USA

22. Zimm S, Wampler GL, Stablein D, Hazra T, Young HF (1981) Intracranial metastases in solid tumour patients: natural his-tories and results and treatment. Cancer 48: 384–394

23. Zülch KJ (1979) Histological typing of tumours of the central nervous system. WHO, Geneva

Correspondence: J. Voges, M.D., Neurochirurgische Universitäts-klinik, Abteilung für Stereotaxie und funktionelle Neurochirugie, Josef-Stelzmann-Strasse 9, D-50931 Köln, Federal Republic of Germany.

Acta Neurochir (1994) [Suppl] 62: 77–82
© Springer-Verlag 1994

Gamma Knife Radiosurgery of a Series of Only Minimally Selected Metastatic Brain Tumours

H. Jokura[1,2], **K. Takahashi**[1,2], **T. Kayama**[2], and **T. Yoshimoto**[2]

[1] Jiro Suzuki Memorial Clinic, Gamma House, Furukawa, and [2] Division of Neurosurgery, Institute of Brain Diseases, Tohoku University, Sendai, Japan

Summary

From December 1991 to October 1992, 77 lesions in 25 consecutive patients were treated with Gamma Knife radiosurgery. Thirteen patients (52%) had multiple metastases up to sixteen lesions and twelve patients had a single metastasis. The volume of the largest tumour treated was 12.5 cm³. Karnofsky performance status (KPS) of the patients was 20–90% (mean 70). Marginal tumour dose given was 18 to 35 Gy (mean 26.1 Gy) in 30 to 90% isodose line according to the tumour volume and site.

All but two patients were followed by MRI or CT scan repeatedly for a minimum of 6 month or to death. All but one of the tumours were locally controlled. Seventeen patients died during follow up and in four death was due to remote CNS metastases. The median survival for this minimally selected group of patients was 8.5 months, and the median survival for the patients with a single metastasis was 10.5 months. In patients with multiple metastases the median survival reached only 2.5 months but in 11 patients out of 13 patients neurological symptoms and signs improved or stabilized shortly after radiosurgery.

Keywords: Brain metastasis; Gamma Knife; radiosurgery.

Introduction

The short treatment time required and minimal invasiveness are the advantages of radiosurgery. These characteristics of this treatment modality will be of great benefit to patients with metastatic brain tumours whose life expectancy is limited and who often are in bad physical condition. Radiosurgery has been used mainly for single metastasis for several years with[1,2,5,7] or without [3,4,10] whole brain radiation therapy (WBRT). It is reported from several institutes that the local control rate is as high as 80–100%[1,2,5,7,10]. Therefore radiosurgery is now gaining a steady following in the treatment of metastatic brain tumours.

In this study, we explore the value of radiosurgery for a series of patients with only minimally selected metastatic brain tumours including multiple lesions with low quality of life (QOL).

Methods and Materials

25 consecutive patients with 77 lesions were treated from December 1991 to October 1992. To be eligible, the largest tumour in a patient had to be less than 3 cm in mean diameter, surgical removal of tumour with acceptable morbidity had to be impossible or the patient refused open surgical removal, and neurological symptoms and signs from brain metastases had to be the dominant factor of a deteriorating QOL.

Nineteen patients were male and six were female. The age ranged from 24 to 76 and the mean was 63 years. Fifteen patients achieved a Karnofsky performance status (KPS) of more than 70, but ten patients had a performance scale of less than 60 due to their neurological condition (Mean 70). Thirteen patients (52%) had multiple metastases, up to sixteen lesions, and twelve patients had a single metastasis (Fig. 1).

The volume of the largest tumour in a patient ranged from 0.6 cm³ to 12.5 cm³ and the mean was 6.5 cm³. Most of the following tumours in patients with multiple lesions were less than 4 cm³ and many were less than 1 cm³ (Fig. 2). Primary sites are shown in Fig. 3.

Prior to radiosurgery two patients were treated by surgical removal alone. In one case a new single lesion appeared and in the other, tumour recurred locally with seven new lesions four months later. Only in the latter, gave we a planned combination of 40 Gy WBRT after gamma knife surgery, because we doubted that CSF dissemination occurred during surgical removal.

One patient received surgical removal followed by WBRT of 50 Gy and the tumour locally recurred six month later.

In 22 cases, 88% of this series, Gamma Knife radiosurgery was the sole treatment for brain metastases. In four patients, repeated gamma knife surgery was performed for new lesions appeared during the follow-up. In one case referring doctor gave 50 Gy WBRT for new lesions three months after radiosurgery.

Image acquisition for dose planning was done exclusively by super conductive magnet MRI (MRVectra, Yokogawa Medical Systems, Tokyo, Japan). Gadolinium-enhanced 4 mm axial and coronal short TR images with an intersection gap of 1 mm throughout the brain were used. Using the Leksell Gamma Knife type B (Elekta Instrument AB, Stockholm, Sweden), we gave 18 to 35 Gy (mean 26.5) to the margin of the tumour. Our standard dose to the periphery

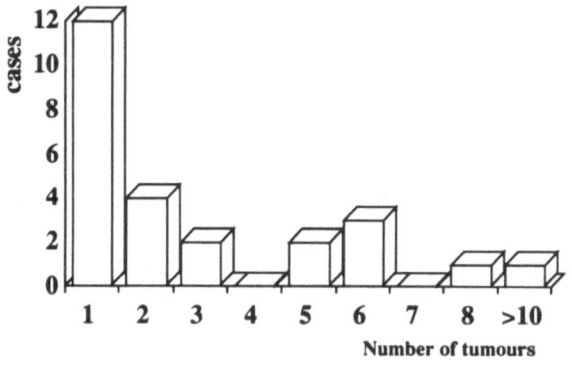

Fig. 1. Patient distribution according to number of tumours

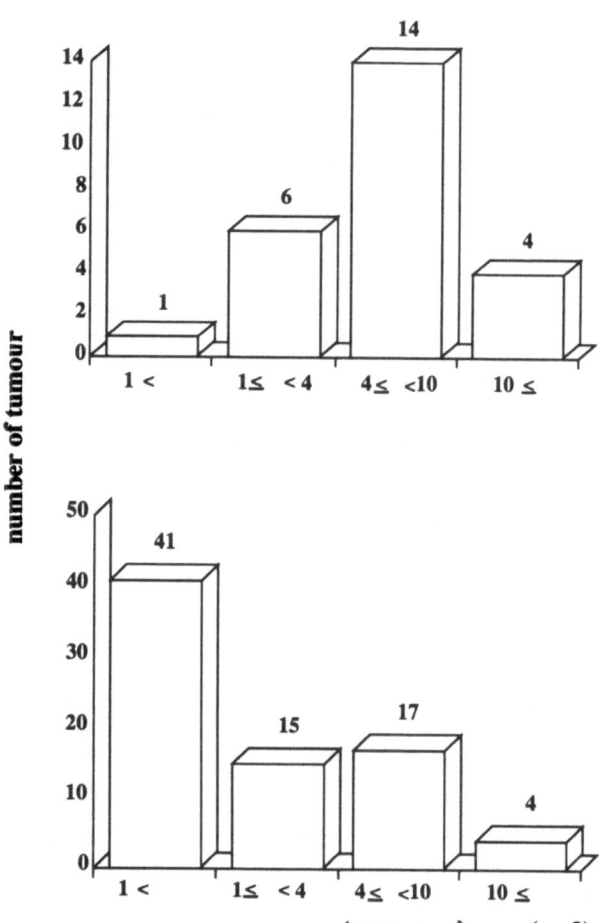

Fig. 2. Volume distribution of tumours. Upper: volume of largest tumour in a patient. Lower: whole tumours treated by radiosurgery

was 25 Gy, but according to the tumour volume and site, we decreased or increased doses. Covering isodose used, ranged from 30–90% (mean 51.2%). Number of shots required for the largest tumour in a patient ranged from 1 to 10 (mean 3.7).

All the patients were followed for a minimum of 6 months or to death and QOL was assessed in terms of KPS. Follow up scans for evaluating lesions were available in 23 cases and repeated except in two cases who died 0.5 month and one month after radiosurgery.

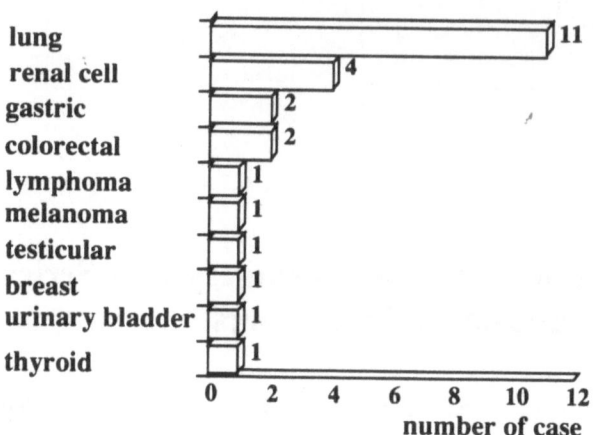

Fig. 3. Primary site of tumours

Results

There was no treatment related mortality or acute morbidity. Figure 4 shows the course of the largest tumours in a patient after gamma knife surgery. All but one tumour regressed considerably and in many cases regression of tumours was detected as early as two weeks after radiosurgery (Fig. 5). When prior imaging study suitable for volume measurement was available we plotted its value. Growing of the tumours was very rapid in many cases and indicated the importance of earliest possible treatment. In this volume analysis we excluded second and third largest and follow the tumours next in size in a patients with multiple metastases, because many of them had volumes less than 1 cm^3 and furthermore CT or MRI available from referring doctors were not appropriate for evaluating the volume of all these small tumours. Only one adenocarcinoma from the lung of 7.8 cm^3 close to the motor cortex treated with 20 Gy to the periphery enlarged continuously after treatment with some loss of enhancement in the center. Dramatic improvement of perifocal oedema was observed with the regression

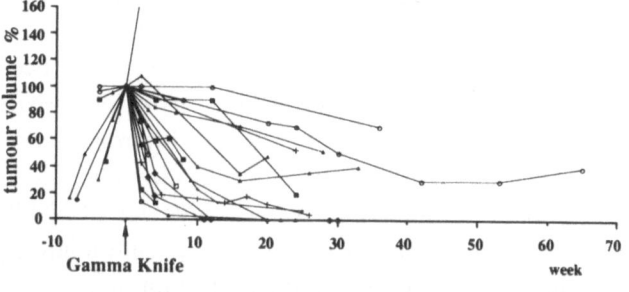

Fig. 4. Response of tumour volume to radiosurgery. The volume at the time of radiosurgery is plotted as 100%

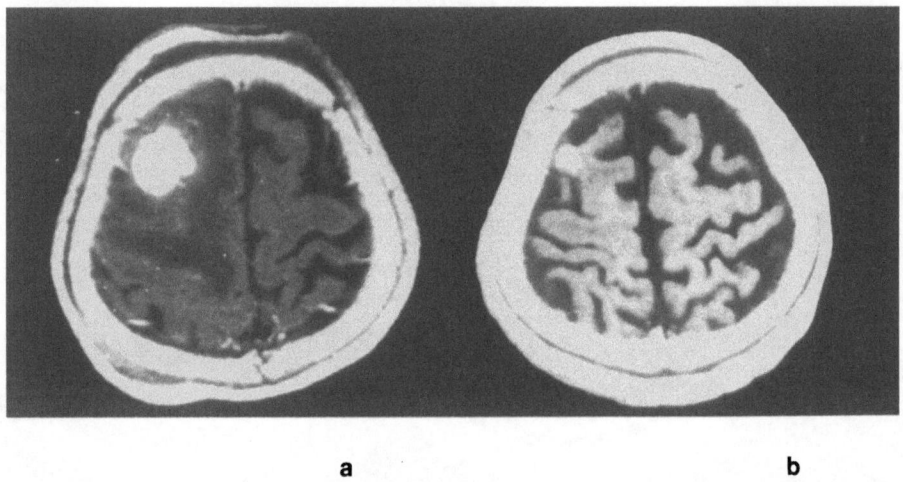

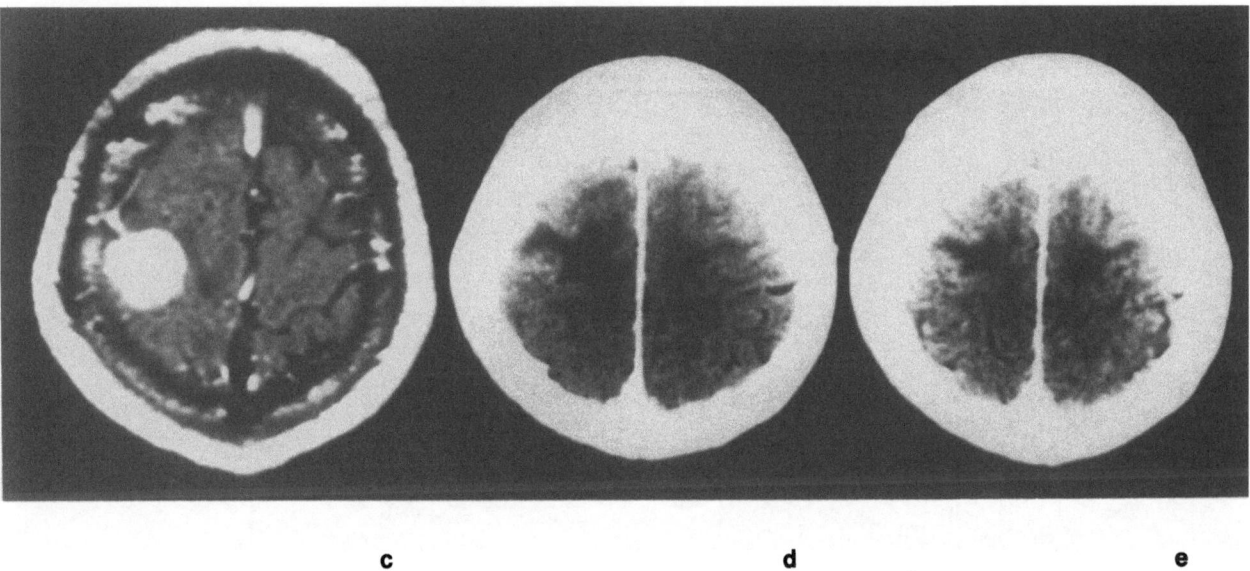

Fig. 5. (a) Gadolinium-enhanced T1 weighted image during radiosurgery showing metastatic transitional cell carcinoma in the right frontal lobe in a 65-year-old man. Tumour was treated with 21 Gy to the periphery. (b) MRI performed one month later showed dramatic regression of tumour. (c) Gadolinium-enhanced MRI of metastatic adenocarcinoma in a 46-year-old man at radiosurgery (25 Gy to the periphery). Contrast-enhanced CT scan at four weeks (d) and ten weeks (e) after radiosurgery

of tumours and this was associated with improvement of the neurological condition (Figs. 6 and 7). KPS was stabilized in 12/25, or improved in 11/25 for some period during follow up and in two deteriorated continuously after radiosurgery.

We cannot find any difference in response to radiosurgery on the basis of the histology of the tumour.

Seventeen patients died during follow up. In four (24%) death was due to CNS lesions. Two were from tumour dissemination into CSF space, one from multiple spinal metastases and one due growth of an untreated tumour. During the follow-up, new CNS lesions appeared in 8 cases (32%). Table 1 shows the details of these cases. There were two with single and

six with multiple metastases at the time of initial radiosurgery. Four patients had repeated radiosurgery for new lesions and two patients had WBRT (one planned). No patient died of brain lesions who had secondary radiosurgery. In two patients who were alive at the last follow up after second radiosurgery, systemic disease had progressed considerably and it seemed that brain disease would not be a limiting factor of QOL and survival.

Median survival of whole series, in which more than half the patients (52%) had multiple metastases, was 8.5 months. Median survival was 10.5 months in cases with single metastases and 2.5 months in cases with multiple metastases (Fig. 8). The median survival of

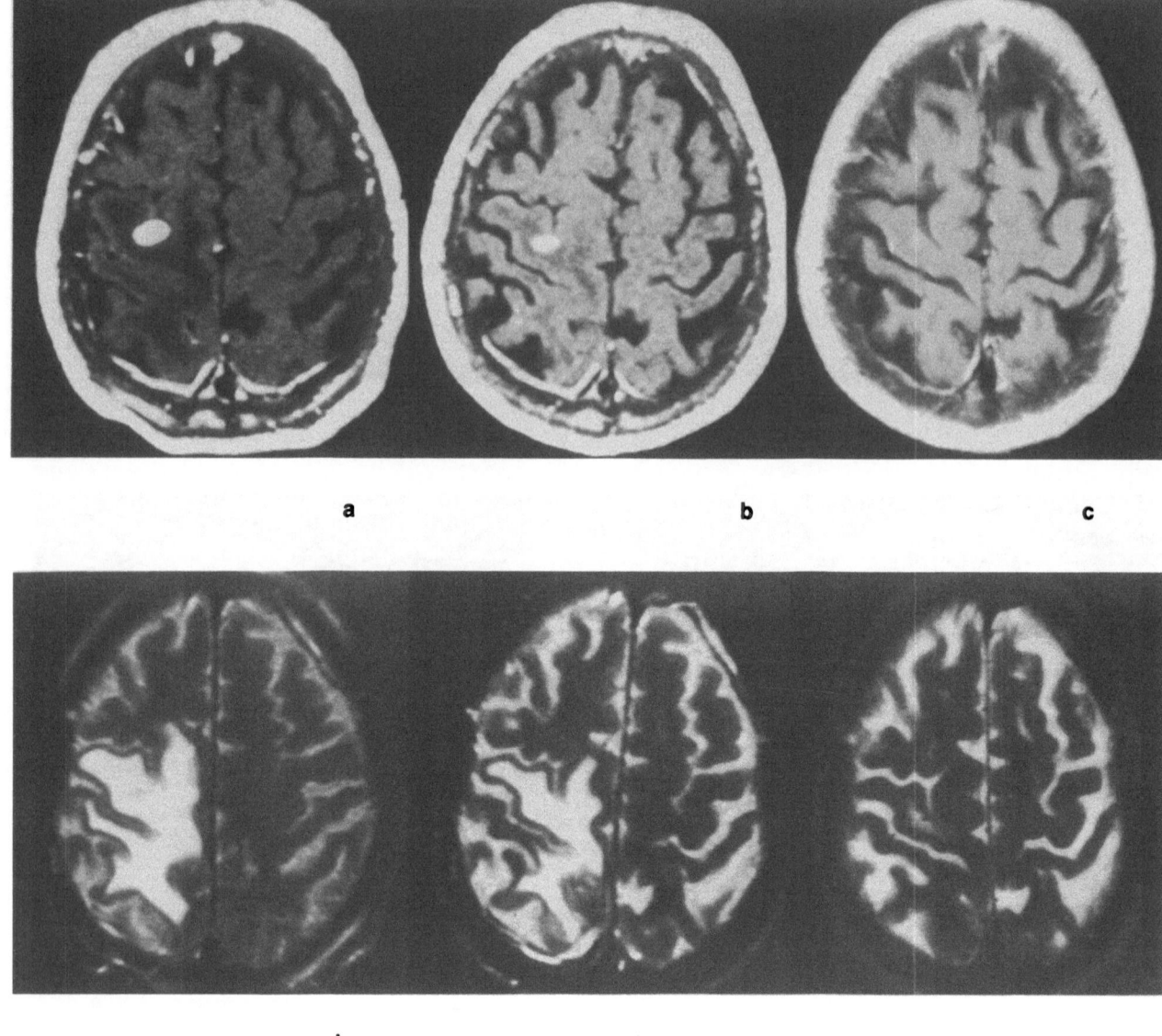

Fig. 6. Gadolinium-enhanced T1 images and T2 images of metastatic renal cell carcinoma in a 74-year-old man at radiosurgery (a, d), one month (b, e), and three month after (c, f) radiosurgery. Tumour was treated with 33.3 Gy to the periphery. Improvement of perifocal oedema was associated with regression of tumour and the patient's hemiparesis had completely relieved

Table 1. *Patients with New Lesions During Follow-up*

Case	Primary	Single or multiple	2nd treatment	Survival (month)	Dead or alive	Cause of death
1	lung	s	WBRT	6	d	primary + visceral meta.
2	lung	s	—	10.5	d	CSF dissemination
3	melanoma	m	gamma	8.5	d	pirmary + visceral meta.
4	lung	m	—	10	d	primary + visceral meta.
5	lung	m	WBRT	5	d	spinal meta.
6	renal cell	m	gamma	8	a	—
7	renal cell	m	gamma	2	d	pneumonia
8	rectal	m	gamma	6	a	—

s single metastasis at initial radiosurgery, *m* multiple metastasis at initial radiosurgery, *d* dead, *a* alive at last follow up.

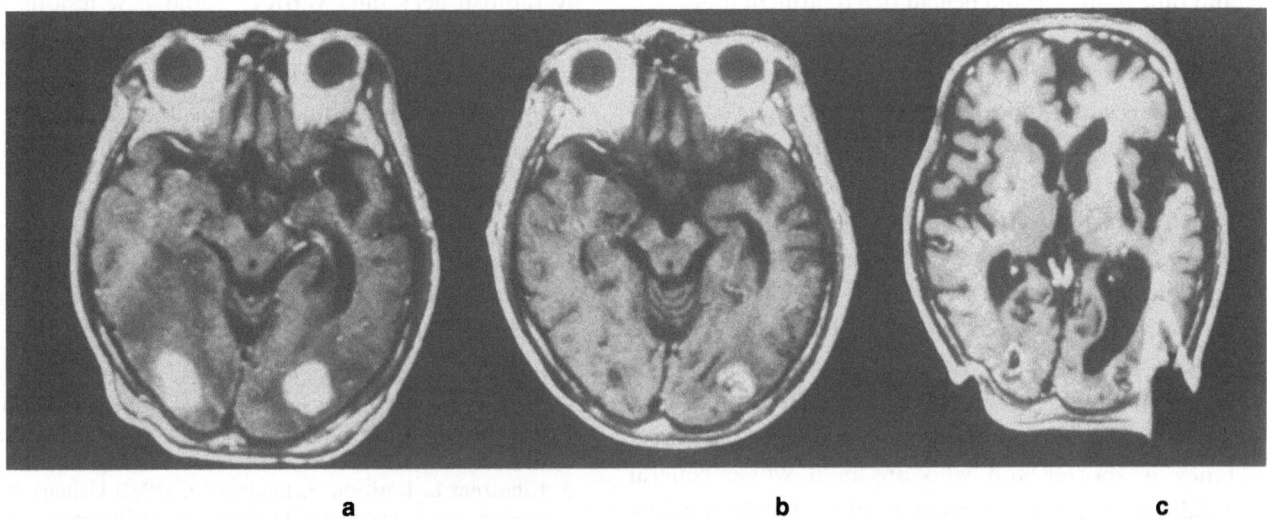

a   b   c

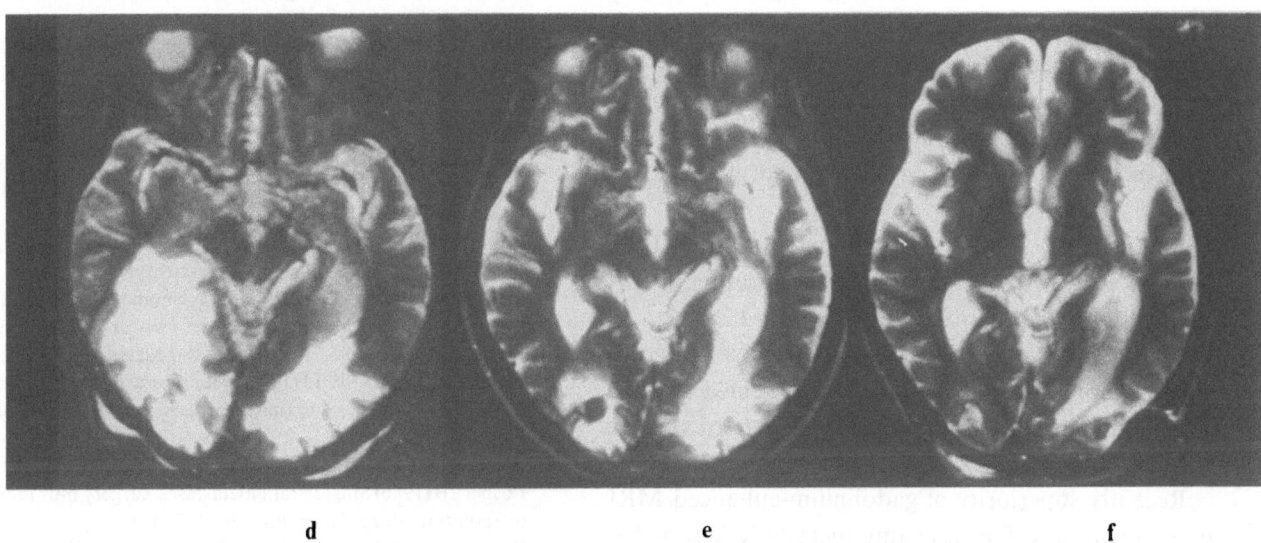

d   e   f

Fig. 7. 66-year-old patient with uncontrolled renal cell carcinoma and multiple visceral metastases. Gadolinium-enhanced MRI at radiosurgery (a) shows tumours in both occipital lobes. T2 image (d) shows diffuse perifocal oedema and by which he was deprived of his vision. We gave 25 Gy to the periphery of these tumours respectively and treated three other small tumours simultaneously. One month later he recovered his vision almost completely. Images three months after radiosurgery (b, e) and at second radiosurgery for new lesions six month after the initial radiosurgery (c, f)

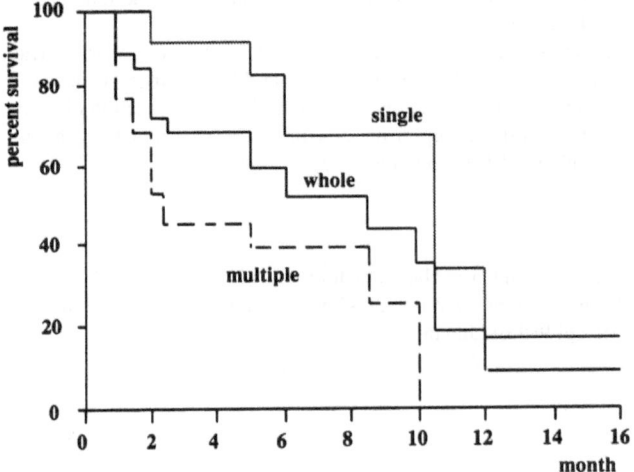

Fig. 8. Actual survival (Kaplan-Meier) of all patients, patients with single metastases, and with multiple metastases

the patients with multiple metastases was not satisfactory, but eleven patients out of thirteen experienced improvement or stabilization of the neurological condition resulting from very rapid regression of tumour and perifocal oedema.

Discussion

Cerebral metastases are not an independent disease but a manifestation of disseminated systemic malignant disease which is very difficult to cure and in many cases life is limited. Any treatment for brain metastases is principally palliative and the aim of a treatment is to improve or maintain QOL and to avoid death caused by metastatic brain tumours. We should be very careful about the balance of cost, i.e. invasion and time required, and benefit of a treatment modality. Surgical removal followed by WBRT gives the best result but it is indicated in only a very limited number of patients with surgically accessible and well controlled primary disease[6,8,9,11]. There is some benefit from WBRT, but to attain median survival of 3–6 months[6,8] patients have to stay in hospital for a few weeks. Radiosurgical treatment of metastases has great advantages in this respect. The treatment finishes within several hours with very little impact on the general condition of patients. We think the advantage of this treatment modality should be more appreciated by the patients with multiple metastases whose life expectancy is shorter and who are in a worse general condition. In our series, median survival of the patients with multiple metastases was not satisfactory mainly due to death from systemic disease, within 2 month after radiosurgery. It shows the difficulties in estimating of progression of the systemic disease. Nevertheless, in most cases QOL was stabilized or improved shortly after treatment and the aim of treatment was accomplished.

Radiosurgery is used in combination with WBRT in many institutes with the hope of eradicating microscopic tumour not visible on imaging studies[1,2,5,7]. In this series patients were principally treated by radiosurgery alone and new lesions which seemed to have some influence on QOL and survival were treated by repeated radiosurgery.

Recently superiority of gadolinium-enhanced MRI over enhanced CT in detecting metastatic lesions became apparent[12]. In our series, in order to decrease "new lesions" during follow-up, we made great efforts, not to miss minute tumours using thin sliced enhanced MRI throughout the brain in all cases at the time of dose planning. We believe tumours of a few mm in diameter would never missed by our scan protocol. If there should be some tumours less than that it would take at least a few months before they became symptomatic and could be treated by repeated radiosurgery which takes only a few hours. In four cases, for whom we repeated radiosurgery, no one died of new metastatic brain lesions and the impact of new lesions on the QOL and survival was very small. In our series median survival of patients with single metastases was 10.5 months which is comparable with that of cases treated

by radiosurgery plus WBRT[2,7] and new lesions appeared only in 2/12. We feel that only a very limited number of patients receive benefit from the combination with WBRT if image acquisition at the time of radiosurgery was done by enhanced thin-sliced MRI.

References

1. Adler JR, Cox RS, Kaplan I, Martin DP (1992) Stereotactic radiosurgical treatment of brain metastases. J Neurosurg 76: 444–449
2. Coffey RJ, Flickinger JC, Bissonette DJ, Lunsford LD (1991) Radiosurgery for solitary brain metastases using the cobalt-60 gamma unit: methods and results in 24 patients. Int J Rad Oncol Biol Phys 20: 1287–1295
3. Kihlström L, Karlsson B, Lindquist C (1992) Gamma Knife surgery in brain metastases. In: Proceedings of the International Symposium on Radiosurgery, Pittsburgh. Elsevier, New York, pp 429–434
4. Lindquist C (1989) Gamma knife surgery for recurrent solitary metastasis of a cerebral hypernephroma: case report. Neurosurgery 25: 802–804
5. Loeffler JS, Kooy AM, Wen PY, Fine HA, Cheng C-W, Mannarino EG, Tsai JS, Alexander E III (1990) The treatment of recurrent brain metastases with stereotactic radiosurgery. J Clin Oncol 8: 576–582
6. Mandell L, Hilaris B, Sullivan M, Sundresan N, Nori D, Kim H, Martini N, Fuks Z (1986) The treatment of single brain metastasis from non-oat cell lung carcinoma. Surgery and radiation versus radiation therapy alone. Cancer 58: 641–649
7. Mehta MP, Rozental JM, Levin AB, Mackie TR, Kubsad SS, Gehring MA, Kinsella TJ (1992) Defining the role of radiosurgery in the management of brain metastases. Int J Rad Oncol Biol Phys 24: 619–625
8. Patchell RA, Cirrincione C, Thaler HT, Galicich JH, Kim JH, Posner JB (1986) Single brain metastases: surgery plus radiation or radiation alone. Neurology 36: 447–453
9. Patchell RA, Tibbs PA, Walsh JW, Dempsey RJ, Maruyama Y, Kryscio RJ, Markesbery WR, Macdonald JS, Young B (1990) A radomized trial of surgery in the treatment of single metastases to the brain. N Engl J Med 322: 494–500
10. Strum V, Kober B, Häver KH, Schlegel W, Boesecke R, Pastyr O, Hartmann GH, Schabbert S, Winkel K, Kunze S, Lorenz WJ (1987) Stereotactic percutaneous single dose irradiation of brain metastases with linear accelerator. Int J Radiat Oncol Biol Phys 13: 279–282
11. Sundaresan N, Galicich JH, Beattie EJ (1983) Surgical treatment of brain metastases from lung cancer. J Neurosurg 58: 666–671
12. Sze G, Milano E, Johnson C, Heier L (1990) Detection of brain metastasis: Comparison of contrast-enhanced MR with unenhanced MR and enhanced CT. AJNR 11: 785–791

Correspondence: Hidefumi Jokura, M.D., Jiro Suzuki Memorial Clinic, Gamma House, 3-1-3-5, Minamimachi; Furukawa-City, Miyagi 989-61, Japan.

Acta Neurochir (1994) [Suppl] 62: 83–87

Long-Term Follow-up Study of Conventional Irradiation for Brain Tumours in Children: A Role for Radiosurgery

H. K. Inoue[1], **H. Kohga**[1], **M. Nakamura**[1], **N. Ono**[1], **T. Kakegawa**[1], **M. Hirato**[1], **C. Ohye**[1], **T. Shibazaki**[2], and **Y. Andou**[2]

[1] Department of Neurosurgery, Gunma University School of Medicine, Maebashi, and [2] Gamma Unit Center, Hidaka Hospital, Takasaki, Japan

Summary

21 younger patients (less than 10 years of age) with brain tumours, treated by conventional irradiation, were followed 5 to 20 years (mean 12), using CT scan and/or MR imaging, in order to evaluate adverse effects on the developing brain.

Pathological changes such as brain atrophy, lesions in the white matter, calcifications in the brain, and angiopathy were observed in 13 (62%) out of 21 cases. The incidence of abnormalities was related to the age at treatment and the follow-up period. All six cases treated at or under 5 years old and followed more than 10 years showed pathological changes in the brain.

In order to minimize the radiation damage, 5 patients with brain tumours less than 5 years old were treated by gamma knife surgery. The early results encourage further trials. Radiosurgery may play a role as an alternative treatment or as a component of future multidisciplinary treatment for brain tumours is children.

Keywords: Brain tumour; radiation; long-term side effects; children; radiosurgery.

Introduction

Conventional fractionated radiation therapy is effective treatment and commonly used in children for brain tumours such as gliomas, medulloblastomas, germinomas, and craniopharyngiomas. The efficacy of this treatment is demonstrated by the disappearance of tumours (medulloblastoma and germinoma) and by the control rate of recurrence (glioma and craniopharyngioma). However, radiation therapy may bring about long-term side effects with regard to brain function even in adults[1,6,16].

In children, short stature, poor school performance, pituitary dysfunction and cranial nerve disturbances have been reported as long-term side effects of irradiation[4,5,7,13,15]. They have been most obvious in cases with whole brain irradiation, especially in younger children under 5 years of age. In a study of long-term survivors with medulloblastomas and primitive gliomas, we found several pathological changes in the brain on CT scan and/or MR imaging[10]. The adverse effects of radiation therapy were observed not only in respect of cerebral function but also in relation to the morphology of the developing brain. A multidisciplinary treatment should be considered for these tumours.

The development of radiosurgery has increased the therapeutic options for brain tumours. It may also play an important role in the multidisciplinary treatment of brain tumours in children. This study discusses the long-term effects of conventional radiation therapy on the developing brain and suggests a role for radiosurgery based on the early results of Gamma Knife surgery.

Patients and Methods

Children under 10 years of age with brain tumours, who received conventional fractionated radiation therapy were studied by CT scan and/or MR imaging at 5 to 20 years after treatment. The types of brain tumour were germ-cell tumours, astrocytomas, craniopharyngiomas, medulloblastomas, and primitive gliomas. Germ-cell tumours followed for more than 5 years were all germinomas. The site of the tumours were pineal, suprasellar, and in the basal ganglia. Most cases had whole brain irradiation. The astrocytomas were in the optic pathways, the 3rd ventricle, and the cerebellum. All patients received local irradiation. Craniopharyngiomas were all cystic and were resected partially or subtotally before local irradiation. Patients with medulloblastomas or primitive gliomas were treated by whole brain and spinal irradiation. CT scan and/or MR imaging were compared before and after radiation therapy from sequential studies of the each case.

Recently 5 children under 5 years of age were treated by radiosurgery using a Gamma Unit. These cases were patients with recurrent tumours after conventional irradiation and patients whose parents refused open surgery or were eager for minimum invasive treatment.

Results

Long-Term Effects of Conventional Irradiation

There were 21 cases, 13 males and 8 females, from 1 to 10 years of age (mean 5.8). These tumours were 6 germinomas, 5 astrocytomas, 4 craniopharyngiomas, 4 medulloblastomas, and 2 primitive gliomas. The radiation dose was 30 Gy to 60 Gy (mean 47.9) except is one patient who received a second course of radiation therapy because of recurrence. The mean follow-up period was 12 years.

Twelve patients received whole brain irradiation. They are listed in Table 1. Six patients with germinomas (case 1 to 6) were 8 to 10 years old (mean 9) and received 40 Gy to 60 Gy (mean 52.3). Pathological changes appeared in three cases 5 to 7 years after treatment. These were focal brain atrophy and lesions in the white matter (Fig. 1). Six cases with embryonal tumours (case 7 to 12), 4 medulloblastomas and 2 primitive gliomas, were 1 to 8 years old (mean 3) and received 43 Gy to 99 Gy (mean 57.7). Five of them were followed more than 10 years and all had abnormalities in the brain. These were spotty calcifications, massive calcifications (Fig. 2), atrophy of the brain, and intracerebral haemorrhage due to angiopathy (Fig. 3).

Nine patients received local irradiation. They are listed in Table 2. Four cases with craniopharyngiomas (case 1 to 4) were 5 to 9 years old (mean 6.5) and received 50 Gy to 60 Gy (mean 55). Two cases showed abnormalities (brain atrophy and calcification) from 2 to 7 years after radiation therapy (Figs. 4 and 5). Five patients with astrocytomas (case 5 to 9) were 2 years to 6 years of age (mean 4.2) and received 30 Gy to 55 Gy (mean 35). Three of them showed lesions in the

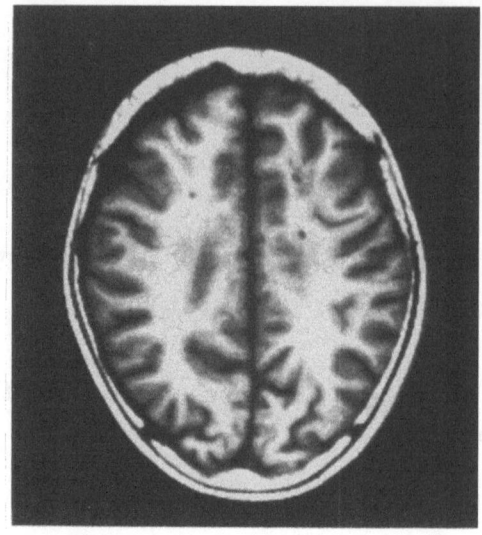

Fig. 1. MR imaging of an 18-year-old male who received whole brain irradiation at 8 years of age. Multiple low intensity lesions reocgnized in the white matter by T1-weighted imaging

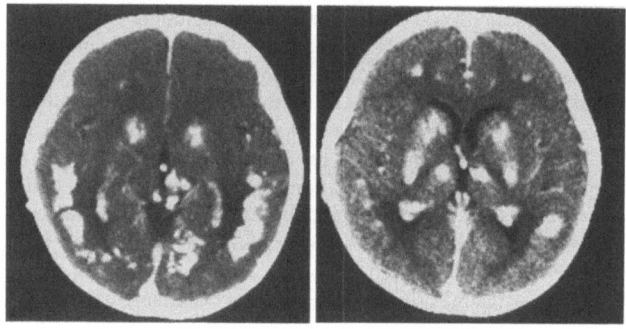

Fig. 2. CT scans of a 12-year-old male showing massive calcifications in the brain. He received whole brain irradiation twice at the time of 1 and 2 years of age

Case	Age	Sex	Radiation (Gy)	follow-up (ys)	Changes
1	10	M	40	17	focal atrophy
2	10	M	60	13	
3	8	M	60	12	low intensity
4	9	M	50	9	
5	10	M	60	8	
6	8	F	44	7	focal atrophy
7	2	F	43	19	calcification, atrophy
8	8	M	52	18	spotty calcification
9	5	F	51	17	spotty calcification
10	1	M	48, 51	14	massive calcification
11	1	F	51	10	angiopathy
12	3	M	50	7	

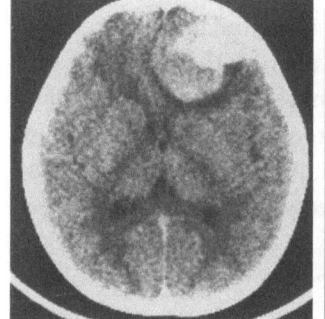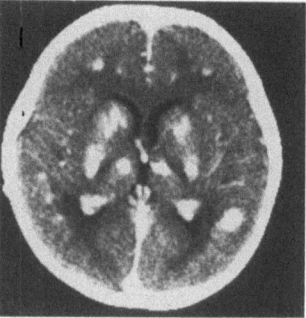

Fig. 3. A CT scan of 6-year-old female showing a large high density lesion in the left frontal lobe (left). A CT scan of the same patient at the age of 10 shows a high density lesion in the left temporal lobe (right). She had whole brain irradiation at the age of one

Table 2. *Long-Term Follow-up of 9 Patients Treated by Local Irradiation*

Case	Age	Sex	Radiation (Gy)	follow-up (ys)	Changes
1	6	F	52	17	atrophy
2	5	F	58	16	calcification
3	5	M	60	8	
4	9	M	50	5	
5	5	M	55	20	spotty calcification
6	6	F	30	9	
7	2	F	30	9	
8	5	F	30	5	low intensity
9	3	M	30	5	focal atrophy

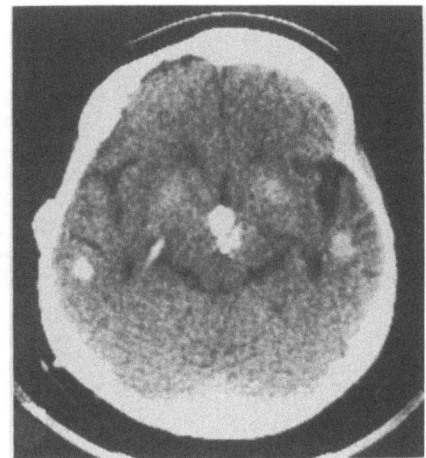

Fig. 5. A CT scan of a 19-year-old female who received local irradiation at 5 years old. A calcified tumour in the 3rd ventricle and high density lesions in both basal ganglia and both temporal lobes may be seen

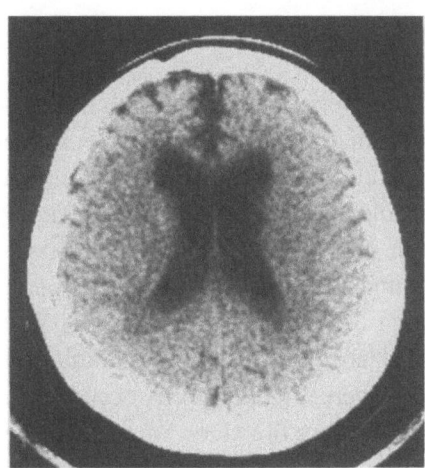

Fig. 4. A CT scan of a 17-year-old female showing brain atrophy. She had radiation therapy at the age of 6

white matter, focal brain atrophy, and spotty calcification, respectively 4 to 19 years after treatment.

Abnormal changes in the brain were found in 13 (62%) of 21 cases. Correlation between the type of change, the period after treatment, and the radiation dose was not obvious. However, the incidence of abnormality was related to the age at treatment and the follow-up period. In younger patients, under 5 years of age, 73% (8 out of 11) showed abnormalities. 10 of 11 cases (91%) followed more than 10 years had changes and all six cases (100%) treated at under 5 years old and followed for longer than 10 years showed abnormalities in the brain.

Early Results of Radiosurgery

There were five patients, 3 males and 2 females, from 3 to 4 years of age (Table 3). Three patients had recurrent tumours 1 to 2 years after resection and conventional irradiation. The other 2 cases were treated by radiosurgery following resection in one case and as the sole treatment in the other. Maximum doses were 30 Gy to 42 Gy and marginal doses were 6.6 Gy to 20 Gy depending on the tumour size and the surrounding structures. Two of the recurrent cases developed tumour dissemination in spite of the local control achieved by radiosurgery. One patient with a cerebral astrocytoma showed large cysts and required open surgery 9 months after radiosurgery. One patient with a tumour arising from the floor of the 4th ventricle

Table 3. *Summary of 5 Patients Treated with Radiosurgery*

Case	Age	Sex	Histology	Radiosurgery (Gy) max/marginal	Early results
1	4	F	unknown	40/20	good response
2	3	M	embryonal	42/21	(dissemination)
3	3	M	ependymoma	33/7	(short term follow-up)
4	3	M	ependymoma	34/10	(dissemination)
5	3	F	astrocytoma	30/9	cyst formation

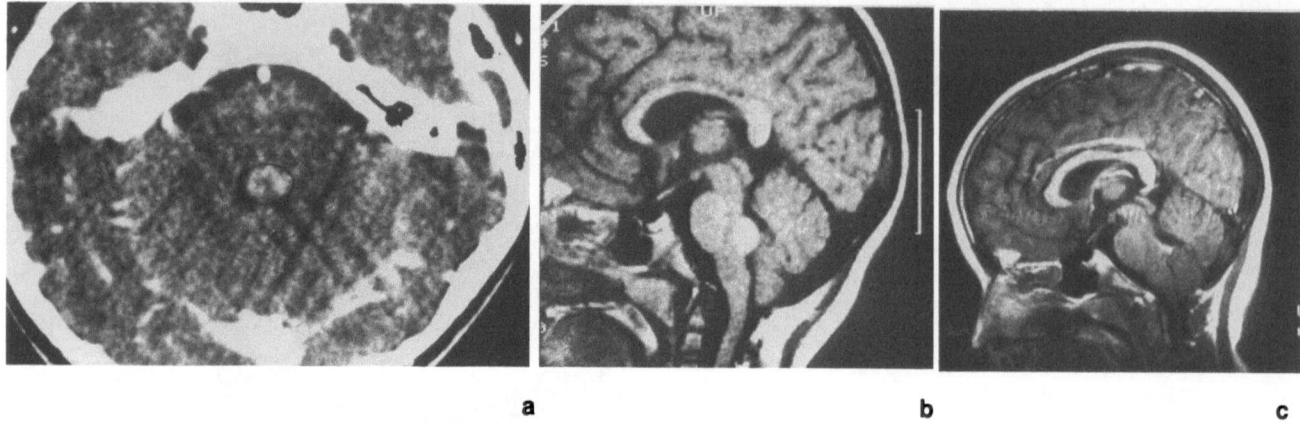

Fig. 6. (a) Contrast enhanced CT scan of a 4-year-old female during gamma knife surgery. The tumour was treated to the 50% isodose, with 20 Gy as the marginal dose. (b, c): Pre- (b) and post-treatment (c) MR imaging. The tumour volume decreased markedly 14 months after radiosurgery

was treated only by radiosurgery (Fig. 6a, b). The tumour decreased gradually and no regrowth has been observed 14 months after treatment (Fig. 6c).

Discussion

In a previous report, we have described the long-term clinical effects of conventional irradiation for embryonal tumours. We recorded that pathological changes in the brain appeared after the passage of many years in addition to the clinically adverse effects, such as physical, intellectual, and endocrine disturbances[10]. Though conventional irradiation is effective for brain tumours in children, an exact evaluation of the adverse effects is essential.

In this study, we could not find any correlations between the type of change, the period after treatment, the type of radiation field, and the radiation dose. However, we found pathological changes in 62% of patients who had received radiation therapy under the age of 10 and followed for more than 5 years and in 91% of patients followed for more than 10 years. Furthermore, all patients under 5 years old at the time of radiation and followed for more than 10 years had abnormalities in the brain. The results indicate that it is important to consider protecting the normal brain from therapeutic irradiation in children, especially those under 5 years of age. Radical resection followed by low-dose neuroaxis radiation therapy has been reported recently, with a view to reducing radiation toxicity[9]. However, a long-term follow-up is required even in cases treated with low-dose irradiation.

An understanding of the mechanism of radiation-induced brain damage is important for the protection

of normal brain. Many reports have shown that radio-necrosis is caused by small vessel occlusion[3,8,12]. Large vessel occlusion has also been described after cranial irradiation and histological studies have shown endo-thelial proliferation, fibrous thickening and hyalini-zation of the subintima, with thickening and disruption of the elasticic lamina[2]. Mineralizing micro-angiopathy is found in childhood leukemia after cranial irradiation and it has been reported that all lesions occurred in children who were 10 years of age or younger at the time of irradiation. Moreover, the prevalence of lesions among patients who were less than 5 years old was highly significant[14]. Though the patients were treated with a combination of chemotherapy, the results were quite similar to our experience. It is suggested that vessels in the developing brain are more sensitive than those in the adult brain. Brain atrophy and lesions in the white matter described here may also be caused by angiopathy though other damage such as neuronal degeneration and demyelination may exist. Longer survival of brain tumour patients and the increasing use of MR imaging in the follow-up study will probably increase the recognition of pathological changes secon-dary to cranial irradiation. With increasing data a better understanding of the mechanism of brain damage is to be expected.

We started radiosurgery using a Gamma Unit to minimize the radiation damage to the developing brain in patients with recurrent tumours following conven-tional irradiation and patients with minor symptoms. The early results are encouraging enough to suggest the need for further trials. Radiosurgery may play a role as one modality in multidisciplinary treatment for recurrent tumours and as an alternative treatment for primary tumours with minor symptoms. However, a long-term follow-up is required for the evaluation of the long-term effects and of the adverse effects to the developing brain. Experimental sudies using an animal model are also important for understanding the mechanism of radiation effects and for protecting the normal brain[11].

Acknowledgement

We thank Dr. Jeremy C. Ganz for reviewing the manuscript and checking the English.

References

1. Al-Mefty O, Kersh JE, Routh A, *et al* (1990) The long-term side effects of radiation therapy for benign brain tumours in adults. J Neurosurg 73: 502–512

2. Brant-Zawadzki M, Anderson M, DeArmond SJ, *et al* (1980) Radiation-induced large intracranial vessel occlusive vasculopathy. AJR 134: 51–55

3. Brismar J, Roberson GH, Davis KR (1976) Radiation necrosis of the brain. Neuroradiological considerations with computed tomography. Neuroradiology 12: 109–113

4. Cohen ME, Duffner PK (1984) Brain tumours in children. Principles of diagnosis and treatment. Raven, New York, pp 308–327

5. Darendeliler F, Livesey EA, Hindmarsh PC, *et al* (1990) Growth and growth hormone secretion in children following treatment of brain tumours with radiotherapy. Acta Paediatr Scand 79: 950–956

6. DeAngelis LM, Delattre J-Y, Posner JB (1989) Radiation-induced dementia in patients cured of brain metastases. Neurology 39: 789–796

7. Diffner PK, Cohen ME, Thomas PRM, *et al* (1985) The long-term effects of cranial irradiation on the central nervous system. Gancer 56: 1841–1846

8. Eyster EF, Nielsen SL, Sheline GE, *et al* (1974) Cerebral radiation necrosis simulating a brain tumour. J Neurosurg 39: 267–271

9. Halberg FE, Wara WM, Fippin LF, *et al* (1991) Low-dose cranial radiation therapy for medulloblastoma. Int J Radiat Oncol Biol Phys 20: 651–654

10. Inoue HK, Nakamura M, Ono N, *et al* (1993) Long-term clinical effects of radiation therapy for primitive gliomas and medulloblastomas: a role for radiosurgery. Stereotact Funct Neurosurg 61: 51–58

11. Inoue HK, Kohga H, Hirato M, *et al* (1994) Neurobiological effects of radiosurgery: immunohistochemical and electron microscopic studies of a rat model. Stereotact Funct Neurosurg 62/63: in press

12. Mikhael MA (1978) Radiation necrosis of the brain. Correlation between computed tomography, pathology and dose distribution. J Comput Assist Tomogr 2: 71–80

13. Oberfield SE, Allen JC, Pollack J, *et al* (1986) Long-term endocrine sequelae after treatment of medulloblastoma: prospective study of growth and thyroid function. J Pediatr 108: 219–223

14. Price RA, Birdwell DA (1978) The central nervous system in childhood leukemia. III. Mineralizing microangiopathy and dystrophic calcification. Cancer 42: 717–728

15. Riva D, Milani N, Pantaleoni C, *et al* (1991) Combined treatment modality for medulloblastoma in childhood: effects on neuropsychological functioning. Neuropediatrics 22: 36–42

16. Taphoorn MJB, Heimans JJ, Snoek FJ, *et al* (1992) Assessment of quality of life in patients treated for low-grade glioma: a preliminary report. J Neurol Neurosurg Psychiatry 55: 372–376

Correspondence: Hiroshi K. Inoue, M.D., Ph.D., Department of Neurosurgery, Gunma University School of Medicine, Showamachi 3-39-22, Maebashi 371, Japan.

Acta Neurochir (1994) [Suppl] 62: 88–92

Stereotactic Radiosurgery of Vestibular Schwannomas with a Linear Accelerator

F. Martens[1], **L. Verbeke**[2,3], **M. Piessens**[2], and **M. Van Vyve**[1]

Departments of [1]Neurosurgery and [2]Radiotherapy, OLV Ziekenhuis, Aalst and [3]Department of Radiotherapy University Hospital Ghent, Ghent, Belgium

Summary

The authors describe their initial experience with stereotactic radiosurgery of 22 cases with vestibular schwannomas using a linear accelerator. 14 of them with a follow-up of at least one year were studied. 6–9 months after treatment 86% had central tumour necrosis, 71% tumour shrinkage and none of them evidence of tumour growth 3 patients developed reversible facial nerve impairment, 2 had permanent facial numbness. Hearing diminished in one case out of three with normal hearing and in two out of three with already diminished hearing.

Although there is a general consensus[11] that microsurgery is the treatment of choice for these benign tumours, stereotactic radiosurgery challenges this opinion. Stereotactic radiosurgery not only proves to be a valuable alternative for selected cases not suitable for microsurgery, but it is conceivable that it will become the treatment of choice for small vestibular tumours. Tumour control can be obtained in the majority of treated patients with fewer complications and with a higher rate of cranial nerve sparing.

This series indicates that linear accelerators can achieve results similar to the Gamma Unit in the treatment of vestibular schwannomas.

Keywords: Acoustic neurinoma; vestibular schwannoma; stereotactic radiosurgery; stereotactic technique.

Introduction

Stereotactic radiosurgery has gained considerable attention from neurosurgeons and radiation oncologists during the last decade. Many clinical studies have confirmed the efficiency of gamma units and linear accelerators in the treatment of small intracranial lesions, particularly inoperable cerebral arteriovenous malformations and solitary brain metastases. The discussion concerning the superiority of the gamma unit versus linear accelerators has abated and an increasing number of groups is working with one or the other device[22].

The use of stereotactic radiosurgery for treatment of vestibular schwannomas meets much scepticism from the microneurosurgical experts. Nevertheless the clinical results obtained with the gamma knife confirm the validity of this application and offer new therapeutical possibilities to patients. At this moment the number of vestibular schwannomas treated with linear accelerators is limited and there are no large series of patients available. We present our initial experience in the treatment of vestibular schwannomas with a linear accelerator.

Methods and Material

Twenty-two patients were treated with stereotactic radiosurgery for vestibular schwannomas. The treatment procedure was as follows. In the first 14 patients detailed below, the stereotactic frame (Fischer, Germany) was attached to the skull after mild sedation (diazepam 10 mg IM) and local anaesthesia (lidocaine 2%) were administered. With the appropriate CT localisers, multiple CT images needed for tumor visualisation and treatment planning were obtained. Target coordinates calculation and isodose calculation were then performed using software developed locally. The isocentre of the linear accelerator (Philips SL) and the target(s) were aligned and stereotactic radiosurgery was performed using 5 or 7 converging arcs of 160° in 5 or 7 different table rotations. More recently patients are treated with a Leksell G frame, specific localisers and a Siemens Mevatron (KD) linear accelerator adapted with a floor-stand (3D-Line, Italy). Dedicated three-dimensional software running on a graphic workstation (Silicon Graphics) is used for planning and isodose calculation.

The prescribed dose to the 70% isodose contour was 20 Gy in the first 12 patients, the dose was lowered to 16 Gy later on, following the experience of other radio-surgical centres.

Fourteen patients (8 male, 6 female) with a follow-up of at least one year were studied. The mean follow up was 19 months (12–24 months) and the mean age was 51 years (range 24–79 years). The indications were as follows. Four patients were in poor medical condition and the surgical risk was considered unacceptable. One patient with neurfibromatosis 2 was operated earlier for bilateral neurinomas and was irradiated for a recurrence on the side with facial preservation. The other patients preferred stereotactic radiosurgery as an alternative to surgery for personal reasons. The mean lesion size was 15.3 mm (range 7–30 mm), excluding one large lesion (50 mm) that was treated in an 79-year old women.

The patients were discharged the day after the treatment and could eventually go back to work in a few days. Follow-up CT scans and/or MRI and audiometry were obtained every three months in feasible.

Results

Radiological changes were observed on CT scan and MRI (Figs. 1 and 2). Evidence of central necrosis could be established 6 to 9 months after stereotactic radiosurgery in all but two patients. Until now shrinkage of the tumour occurred in four patients with a follow up of more than fourteen months. No patient had evidence of tumour growth until now.

Two patients developed a facial paresis 6 months and one patient had a paralysis 8 months after irradiation. The complete paralysis recovered partially 15 months later to a House Grade II, patients with a partial paralysis recovered completely.

Two patients had facial numbness that persisted until now but this was not considered troublesome.

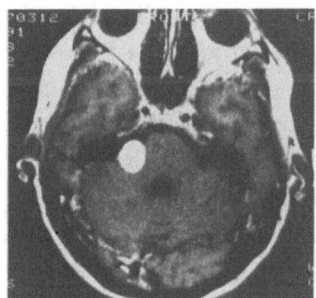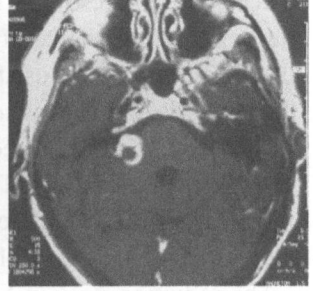

Fig. 1. 65 y old female. Transversal MRI before (left), and 11 months later showing a central necrosis (right)

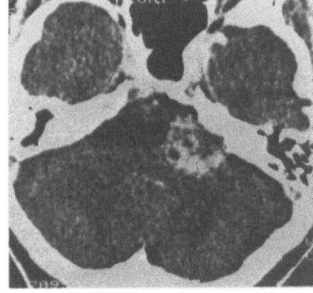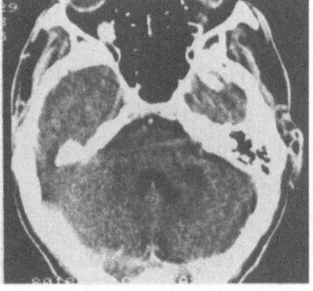

Fig. 2. 55 y old male. CT scan before (left) and 14 months (right) after radiosurgery (20 Gy on the 70% isodose) with central necrosis and diminished volume

Most of the patients (8/14) were deaf at the time of the diagnosis. Three patients had normal hearing of which one had a diminishing of 10 dB six months after irradiation, the two others had unchanged audition 14 and 18 months later. Three patients had diminished hearing not considered serviceable. Two of them had further hearing loss on audiometry.

There was no mortality.

Discussion

The approved management of vestibular schwannoma is either conservative or surgical[11]. The conservative attitude is based on the knowledge that vestibular schwannomas usually grow slowly and that at least a fraction does not increase at all. In a series of 70 untreated neurinomas, Bederson et al.[5] reported an average increment of 2 mm per year, but 40% of the tumours had no detectable growth. Rapid growth or clinical deterioration required surgery in 13%. Also evident spontaneous regression occurred in 6% of the studied tumours. Other authors observed growth in approximately 90% of untreated tumours[6]. A few exceptionally fast growing neurinomas are known with enlargement of the diameter from 2 to 3 cm in 3 month's time[17]. These cases justify frequent CT or MRI controls during the first year if a conservative treatment is considered. The habitually slow tumoral growth incited to treat a number of patients, with advanced age or poor medical condition, 'conservatively'[2,8]. However this attitude is debatable as the tumour growth is variable and at least proportion of elderly patients will experience serious symptoms in their remainder life[25]. Poor surgical morbidity and mortality rates at that moment can be expected.

The microsurgical removal of vestibular schwannoma focused its efforts at first on preservation of facial nerve function, but with increasing expertise the saving of the cochlear nerve became the prime target in patients with serviceable hearing[10,12,24,28]. Samii reported sparing of the facial nerve in almost all patients and preservation of 'serviceable hearing' in 57% in cases of very small intracanalicular tumours[28]. Despite these astounding results due to the refinement of microsurgical techniques and use of sophisticated electrophysiological monitoring[14] there still is a relatively high complication rate reported in the literature. This is principally related to the size of the tumour[6]: when tumours larger than 2 cm are operated with the suboccipital route there is a mortality of 1.5–2.8% and a morbidity of 4–28.5%[10,12]. There is some discussion about the best operative approach but on the whole in patients with medium to large tumours, if hearing preservation is not an issue, the results obtained by either the translabyrinthine, middle fossa or suboccipital ways are virtually identical: the operative mortality is approximately 2%, total tumour excision is achieved in 95% of the patients and the facial nerve is anatomically preserved in 74% of the cases[23]. If sparing of hearing is attempted the suboccipital approach is mandatory as the translabyrinthine approach invariably destroys hearing. To evaluate if patients can benefit from the attempt to preserve hearing, it is fundamental to establish the degree of preoperative auditory impairment on the tumour side as well as on the contralateral ear.

It is worthwhile to remember the study of the 'Acoustic Neuroma Society'[30] in 1989 that reports the results of vestibular schwannoma surgery from the patient's point of view. Although probably biased toward patients who have poor outcomes and significant problems the data cannot be ignored. The following postoperative complications in a series of 541 patients were recorded: meningitis in 6%, cerebrospinal fluid fistula in 7% and a high percentage of cranial nerve lesions. Total hearing loss was present in 94%, partially in 4%. Only 1% of the patients had normal postoperative hearing. Eightly per cent had a temporary or permanent facial paralysis and 19% had a normal facial nerve function.

Stereotactic radiosurgery for vestibular schwannomas was introduced in 1969 by Leksell[18]. The knowledge that heavy focal radiation doses could create tissue changes in inoperable arteriovenous malformations[29] incited to treat benign tumours. This histological changes in neurinomas after irradiation were studied in organ cultures by Anniko *et al.*[3,4]. Both the Schwann cells and the intercellular substance revealed time- and dose-dependent degenerative changes. There was a limited number of surviving cells in specimens treated with as much as 150 Gy, indicating a wide range of radiosensitivity among individual tumour cells, which in part may be related to different phases of the cell cycle at the time of irradiation. The greater majority of the cells reacted rather uniformly to the ionising irradiation with progressive signs of degeneration and ultimate cell death. These findings agree with those observed in a tumour excised 10 months after stereotactic radiosurgery for persisting growth. The central part contained a few cells only, mainly fibroblasts, in contrast to the periphery that was exposed to a lower dose and showed considerably more normal Schwann

cells. These surviving cells had either been exposed to a sublethal dose or had been able to repair the damage. Another important point is the role of primary damage to the vascular supply of the tumour tissue. Experimental studies in brain tissue show that the vascular and brain tissue damage is parallel phenomena, temporally inseparable from each other. In the cases of delayed radiation necrosis, it is believed that the brain damage is preceded by blood vessel abnormalities. Recently radiobiological models were developed[20] using xenografts in the subrenal capsule of athymic mice. These will give better understanding of the histological outcome of these tumours, but longer periods of observation are needed for definite conclusions.

The largest groups of patients have been treated with the gamma units of the Stockholm Karolinska Hospital[26] and the Pittsburgh Medical Centre[19]. Their results can be summarised as follows.

The Stockholm group performed 336 radiosurgical procedures for vestibular schwannomas in 325 patients until December 1990. The authors have detailed the results of 227 procedures with a follow up of at least 12 months.

Hundred-and-one patients have been treated with the Pittsburgh Gamma Unit. The size of the tumours treated by both groups is limited to 30 mm diameter.

Whereas in Stockholm stereotactic radiosurgery is the treatment of choice of neurinomas, the following selection criteria were used in Pittsburgh: a tumour of 30 mm diameter or less and a patient with (1) 75 years of age or more and/or a medical history with unacceptable operative risk, (2) Tumour localisation in the only hearing ear, (3) bilateral tumours, (4) recurrence after surgery, (5) refusal of microsurgical excision.

The radiation dose in Stockholm was initially 25–35 Gy at the periphery of the tumour but it could gradually be decreased to 10–15 Gy, with the lowest dose delivery on the largest tumours. The same experience was reported in Pittsburg where the dose was lowered from 18–20 Gy to 15–16 Gy.

The effect of stereotactic radiosurgery was best observed on CT and MRI. In Stockholm in 70% of the cases there is a diminished contrast enhancement or signal intensity after 6 to 12 months. Shrinkage occurred in 31% during the first 24 months, but this increases to 58% later on. Growth was observed on consecutive CT scans in 79 neurinomas before treatment. Of these enlarging tumours, 53% decreased in size, 28% had growth arrest after stereotactic radiosurgery. In Pittsburgh 55% decreased in size after one year, 42% remained unchanged, one patient had tumour growth, central necrosis was present in 62%. In both centers tumour control could be obtained in 80–90% of the cases and this high success rate was confirmed by long term follow-up[27].

Complications of radiosurgery are damage to the fifth, seventh and eight cranial nerve, hydrocephalus and treatment failure.

In Stockholm the incidence of facial weakness after treatment was 16%, with a latency period of 6–8 months. The paresis was temporary in all patients, even when a complete paralysis occurred (4%). Recovery was completed in 6–12 months. Synkinesis was sometimes seen after reinnervation. Slight facial numbness occurring after 6–8 months was seen in 12% and usually recovered.

The incidence of trigeminal or facial neuropathy in Pittsburgh was respectively 37% and 33%. The recovery of normal facial function required 1 to 9 months. No patient regained normal facial function if the grade at onset was worse than House grade III. The trigeminal neuropathy recuperates even more slowly. This group found more trigeminal and facial lesions than previously described. As mentioned before this led to decreasing of the radiation dose at the periphery of the tumour to 15–16 Gy.

Twenty-four percent of the patients in Stockholm had conserved no changes (22%) or improvement (2%) hearing, 53% experienced slight impairement and 23% had serve impairment or complete hearing loss. After 5 years the percentage of patients with unchanged hearing is about the same indicating that hearing is well preserved over the years after gamma knife stereotactic radiosurgery. In Pittsburgh preoperative useful hearing was present in 22%, 46% of these patients conserve their hearing after one and two years. Improvement occurred in 2 patients.

Hydrocephalus could be observed in 8% of the patients in Stockholm and required a shunt operation. This disturbance in CSF circulation is attributed to an increased protein concentration.

Treatment failure occurred in seven patients in Stockholm of which four were operated and three others were irradiated again, resulting in tumours control in two and persisting growth in one, which was removed surgically.

There was no mortality in both series.

These results suggest that stereotactic radiosurgery is a good alternative to surgical removal of vestibular schwannomas sized up to 30 mm. In selected cases (e.g. in bilateral tumours in neurofibromatosis type II or patients with interfering medical illness) it is the treat-

ment of choice. If the tumour presents persisting growth, stereotactic radiosurgery can be repeated and in the occurrence of fast growth surgical excision is still quite possible. If consecutive imaging cannot prove growth after stereotactic radiosurgery, one must be cautious to interpret this as a favourable response to stereotactic radiosurgery because some series do not observe growth in 40% of untreated tumours[5].

Conversely to the treatment of arteriovenous malformations and cerebral metastases[7,9,15,16], the actual experience of stereotactic radiosurgery of vestibular schwannomas with linear accelerators is limited. The preliminary reports of this and other small series[1,13] do not permit statistical analysis and comparison with the results of the gamma unit. However the observed radiological changes on CT scan and MRI and complication rates of facial and trigeminal dysfunction are comparable. In the present study 28% of the vestibular schwannomas with a follow up of 14 to 20 months have a decrease in volume, while 77% present characteristic radiological changes. There were slightly more facial nerve complications (30%), related to the relative high dose delivery (20 Gy) but all recovered. It is obvious that larger groups of patients and more uniformity in dose prescription on linear accelerators are needed to confirm this first clinical impression.

Conclusion

The advantages of stereotactic radiosurgery are well-known: the technique is minimally invasive, shortens hospitalisation time and inability to work to a minimum, spares cranial nerves more consistently and has fewer complications than open surgery. Large series indicate that the rate of tumour arrest obtained by microneurosurgery can be equalled or surpassed by stereotactic radiosurgery. It must also be stressed that if stereotactic radiosurgery does not obtain growth arrest, microsurgery can still be applied without increased technical difficulties.

It will take longer follow up to establish definitively if stereotactic radiosurgery is the treatment of choice of vestibular schwannomas with limited volume for all patients. At the present time it certainly offers a therapeutic window for patients unsuitable for microsurgery. Therefore 'watchful waiting' is no longer indicated as it is not justified not to mention stereotactic radiosurgery as a treatment possibility to patients with vestibular schwannomas of limited size. These preliminary results indicate that results obtained in the treatment of vestibular schwannomas with linear accelerators will probably be similar to those of the Gamma Unit.

References

1. Alexander III E, Loeffler JS (1992) Radiosurgery using a modified linear accelerator. Neurosurgery Clin North Am 3: 167–191
2. Anand VT, Kerr AG, Byrnes DP, Smyth GD (1992) Non-surgical management of acoustic neuromas. Clin Otolaryngol 17: 406–410
3. Anniko M, Aendt J, Noren G (1981) The human acoustic neurinoma in organ culture II. Tissue changes after gamma irradiation. Acta Otolaryngol (Stockh) 91: 223–235
4. Anniko M, Noren G (1981) The human acoustic neurinoma in organ culture I. Methodological aspects. Acta Otolaryngol (Stockh) 91: 47
5. Bederson JB, von Ammon K, Wichmann WW, Yasargil MG (1991) Conservative treatment of patients with acoustic tumors. Neurosurgery 28: 646–651
6. Bentivoglio P, Cheeseman AD, Symon L (1988) Surgical management of acoustic neurinomas during the las five years. Part I. Surg Neurol 29: 197–204
7. Betti O, Derechinsky V (1986) Hyperselective encephalic irradiation with linear accelerator. Acta Neurochir (Wien) [Suppl] 33: 385–390
8. Clark WC, Moretz WH, Acker JD, Gardner LG, Eggers F, Robertson (1985) Nonsurgical management of small and intracanalicular acoustic tumours. Neurosurgery 16: 801–803
9. Colombo F, Benedetti A, Pozza F, Avanzo RC, Marchetti C, Chierego G, Zanardo A (1985) External stereotactic irradiation by linear accelerator. Neurosurgery 16: 154–60
10. Ebersold MJ, Harner SG, Beatty CW, Harper CM, Quast LM (1992) Current results of the retrosigmoid approach to acoustic neurinoma. J Neurosurg 76: 901–909
11. Eldridge R, Parry D (1992) Summary: vestibular schwannoma (acoustic neuroma) consensus development conference. Neurosurgery 30: 962–964
12. Fisher G, Fisher C, Rémond J (1992) Hearing preservation in acoustic neurinoma surgery. J Neurosurg 76: 910–917
13. Friedman WA, Bova FJ, Spiegelmann R (1992) Linear accelerator radiosurgery at the University of Florida. Neurosurgery Clin North Am 3: 141–166
14. Harper CM, Harner SG, Slavit DH, Litchy WJ, Daube JR, Beatty CW, Ebersold MJ (1992) Effect of BAEP monitoring on hearing preservation during acoustic neuroma resection. Neurology 42: 1551–1553
15. Hartmann GH, Schlegel W, sturm V, Kober B, Pastyr O, Lorenz W (1985) Cerebral radiation surgery using moving field irradia-
tion at a linear accelerator facility. Int J Radiat Oncol Biol Phys 11: 1185–1192
16. Hitchcock E, Kitchen G, Dalton E, Pope B (1989) Stereotactic LINAC radiosurgery. Br J Neurosurg 3: 305–312
17. Laasonen EM, Troupp H (1986) Volume growth of acoustic neurinomas. Neuroradiology, 28: 203–207
18. Leksell LA (1971) Note on the treatment of acoustic tumours. Acta Chir Scand 137: 763–765
19. Linskey ME, Lunsford DL, Flickinger JC, Kondziolka (1992) Stereotactic radiosurgery for acoustic tumors. Neurosurg Clin North Am 3: 191–206
20. Linskey ME, Martinez AJ, Kondziolka D, Flickinger JC, Maitz AH, Whieside T, Lunsford LD (1993) The radiobiology of human acoustic schwannoma xenografts after stereotactic radiosurgery evaluated in the subrenal capsule of athymic mice. J Neurosurg 78: 645–653
21. Loeffler JS, Siddon RL, Wen PY, Nedzi LA, Alexander E III (1990) Stereotactic radiosurgery of the brain using a standard linear accelerator: a study of early and late effects. Radiother Oncol 17: 311–321
22. Lundford LD (1993) Stereotactic radiosurgery: at the threshold or at the crossroad? Neurosurgery 32: 799–804
23. Moskowltz N, Long DM (1991) Acoustic neurinomas. Historical review of a century of operative series. Neurosurgery Quarterly 1: 2–18
24. Nadol JB Jr, Chiong CM, Ojemann RG, McKenna MJ, Martuza RL, Montgomery WW, Levine RA, Ronner SF, Glynn RJ (1992) Preservation of hearing and facial nerve function in resection of acoustic neuroma. Laryngoscope 102: 1153–1158
25. Nedzelski JM, Canter RJ, Kassel EE, Rowed DW, Tator CH (1986) Is no treatment good treatment in the management of acoustic neuromas in the elderly? Laryngoscope 96: 825–829
26. Norén G, Greitz D, Hirsch A, Lax I (1992) Gamma knife radiosurgery in acoustic neurinoma. In: Steiner L (ed) Radiosurgery baseline and trends. Raven, New York pp 141–148
27. Norèn G, Hirsch A, Mosskin M (1993) Long-term efficacy of gamma-knife radiosurgery in vestibular schwannoma. Acta Neurochir (Wien) 122: 135–184
28. Samii M, Matthies C, Tatagiba M (1991) Intracanalicular acoustic neurinomas. Neurosurgery 28: 189–199
29. Steiner L, Leksell L, Forster DMC, Greitz P, Backlund EO (1974) Stereotactic radiosurgery in intracranial arteriovenous malformations. Acta Neurochir (Wien) 21: 195–209
30. Wiegand DA, Fickel V (1989) Acoustic neuroma – the patient's perspective subjective assessment of symptoms, diagnosis, therapy and outcome in 541 patients. Laryngoscope 99: 179–187

Correspondence: Martens F., M.D., Department of Neurosurgery, OLV Ziekenhuis Aalst, Moorselbaan 164, B-9300 Aalst, Belgium.

Acta Neurochir (1994) [Suppl] 62: 93–97

The Early Effects of Gamma Knife on 40 Cases of Acoustic Neurinoma

T. Kobayashi, T. Tanaka, and **Y. Kida**

Department of Neurosurgery, Gamma Knife Center, Komaki City Hospital, Jobushi, Komaki City, Japan

Summary

Early results of gamma radiosurgery on 44 cases of acoustic neurinoma were studied by follow-up MRIs and changes of neurological signs every 3 months. Mean follow-up period was 12 (3 to 20) months. Enhanced MRI revealed that the central low intensity signal area (LISA) appeared at 3 to 6 months after the treatment, which was re-enhanced at 6 to 9 months, then the tumours begun to decrease in size at 9 to 12 months, which observation was noted in 11 out of 44 cases (25%). The other tumours were unchanged in size. Regarding the side effects, facial palsy appeared in 7 cases (16%) after the treatment, of whom 3 cases have improved. Trigeminal nerve palsy was found in 3 cases (7%). Deterioration of hearing was found in 11 out of 21 cases (52%) who had hearing disturbances before treatment.

The pathological study of a treated tumour at 11 months revealed that central LISA was found as complete necrosis and degeneration of tumour cells and vessels with thickening walls found at the margin of the tumour. MRI is not only useful for the dose planning of radiosurgery but valuable for the follow-up study of treated tumours.

Keywords: Gamma Knife; gamma radiosurgery; acoustic neurinoma; von Recklinghausen disease; MRI.

Introduction

Since the first treatment of acoustic neurinoma using the Gamma Knife by Lars Leksell in 1969[4], several series with good results have been published in the literature[1,3,5-7]. However only a few reports have mentioned details of the early changes of treated tumours.

The early effects of the use of the Gamma Knife in 44 out of 66 cases of acoustic neurinomas which were followed-up for more than 3 months were evaluated in minute detail by repeated MRIs and neurological studies.

Materials and Methods

386 cases of intracranial lesions have been treated by Leksell Gamma Unit at Komaki City Hospital since May 1991 through December 1992. There were 207 cases of brain tumours (53%); of these 66 (32%) were intracranial neurinomas. 44 out of 66 cases were acoustic neurinomas and were followed up for more than 3 months after the treatment. Mean age of the patients was 53 years. Male to female ratio was 16:28. Four bilateral tumours (von Recklinghausen disease) were included. Prior Surgical treatment had been performed in 10 cases (23%). Gamma knife was the initial treatment in 34 cases (77%).

Different grades of hearing disturbance were found in 21 cases (48%) and deafness in 23 cases (52%).

Dose planning was made by 3 mm sllices of T1 weighted enhanced images of axial and coronal planes using Micro Vax computer system. Multi-isocenters were used to cover the whole tumour using mostly 50% isodose line. The mean diameter of the tumour was 21.0 mm and the volume 6.2 cu cm. The tumours were treated by the Leksell Gamma Unit with a mean maximum dose of 29.9 Gy and a marginal dose of 14.8 Gy using mean numbers of isocenter of 4.9 (Table 1). The early effects of gamma radiosurgery were evaluated in great detail by the changes in repeated MRIs and neurological examinations every 3 months. The volume measurement of treated tumour and central low intensity signal area (LISA) was made on MRI by computer analysis.

Results

Repeated MRIs revealed that the characteristic changes were found in the tumours with mean follow-up periods of 12 (3 to 20) months. Diffusely enhanced tumour on T1 weighted images before treatment became central LISA at 3 to 6 months, which was re-enhanced at 6 to 9 months. Then the tumour began to decrease its size 9 to 12 months after the treatment. These characteristic changes were found in 11 cases (25%). Most of the other tumours showed central LISA without decrease in size in 29 cases (66%), in whom re-enhancement of the tumour was found in 8 cases (18%). The other 4 cases were unchanged (Table 2). The volume of the tumours had a tendency to increase slightly up to 6 months, then decreased to its previous size by 12 months which was not statistically significant but the volume of LISA significantly increased by 6

Table 1. *Characteristics of Acoustic Neurinomas*

Cases (n = 44)		Dosimetry		
Age:	52.5	mean diameter:	21.0	mm
Sex M:F = 16:	28	mean volume:	6.2	cm^3
NF-2	4	< 1 cm^3	5	
Prior Surgery	10	1 ~ 4	13	
Initial Treat.	34	4 ~ 10	17	
Hearing disturb.	21	> 10 cm^3	9	
Deafness	23			
		max. dose:	29.9	Gy
		marginal. d:	14.8	Gy
		% isodose	54.8	%

Table 3. *Changes in Neurological Signs of Acoustic Neurinoma*

changes in Neurological signs: (44 cases)

Hearing disturb:21	{ unchanged	9
	improved	1
	deteriorated	11
Facial palsy:8	{ improved	1
	deteriorated	7
	(later improvement/4)	
Trigeminal palsy:4	{ improved	1
	deteriorated	3

Table 2. *MRI Changes of Acoustic Neurinomas*

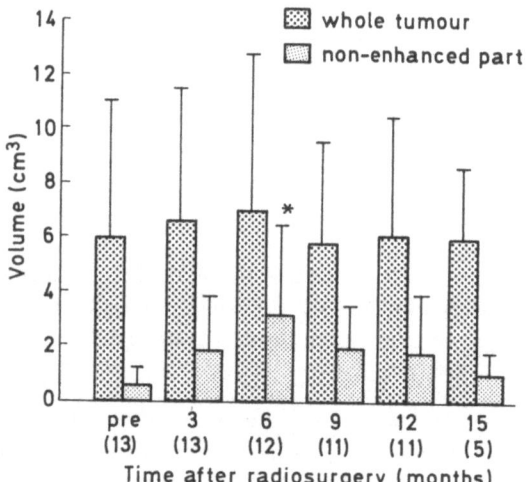

MRI. changes:44 cases

Perifocal oedema: symptomatic 2
Hydrocephalus: symptomatic 2

Fig. 1. Computer analysis of changes of tumour volume and volume of non-enhanced part

found in two cases and a ventriculo-peritoneal shunt was necessary.

The changes in neurological signs were as follows: Hearing of treated ear showed further deterioration in 11 out of 21 cases (52%). Hearing improved in one and remained unchanged in 9 cases. Facial palsy was found in 7 cases (16%) of whom four were freshly sustained and three showed progression of the palsy at 6 to 9 months after treatment. Four cases improved within two months with the use of steroids and glycerol. Facial numbness was found in three patients which also was temporary (Table 3).

Case Presentation

Case 1. 42 year-old male, Right acoustic neurinoma. This patient began to notice hearing disturbance in his right ear two years ago, which progressed to deafness. Facial numbness on the same side appeared in April 1991, then loss of taste was found in May. He was found to have a cerebello-pontine angle tumour on CT scan in July and was referred to Komaki City Hospital for gamma knife treatment. The mean diameter of his tumour was 33.5 mm; the tumour was treated by Gamma Knife with a maximum dose of 28 Gy and a marginal dose of 14 Gy using 10 isocenters on August 8 (PRE). The tumour showed central LISA on MRI at 6 months (6 M), and re-enhancement at 11 months (11 M), and finally decreased in size at 16 months (16 M) (Fig. 2). His loss of taste and facial numbness improved within the 12 months.

Case 2. 61 year-old female, von Recklinghausen disease. This patient had a history of craniotomy for a parasagittal meningioma in July 1984, which was followed by posterior fossa craniectomy for the total removal of her left acoustic neurinoma in February 1985. Patient also had had a laminectomy for spinal cord glioma at the level of C3 to C4. Left facial and trigeminal palsy were found and hearing loss of below 70 dB was found postoperatively. Because of the deterioration of hearing and increasing size, her right C-P angle tumour was treated by gamma knife on May 29, 1991. The mean diameter of the tumour was 23 mm and the tumour was irradiated with a maximal dose of 30 Gy and a marginal dose of 15 Gy using 6 isocenters. The tumour showed central LISA at 6 and 9 months (Fig. 3, 6 M–9 M), which was followed by re-enhancement and decrease in size at 13 months (13 M). Her hearing on the right side gradually deteriorated at 6 and 9 months after the treatment (Fig. 3).

Case 3. 51 year-old female, Right acoustic neurinoma. This patient complained of facial numbness and hearing loss on the right side

months and then decreased gradually (Fig. 1). The other finding on MRIs was perifocaledema found on T2 weighted image in 20% of cases but only two cases became symptomatic, who were controlled by the use of steroids. Finally communicating hydrocephalus was

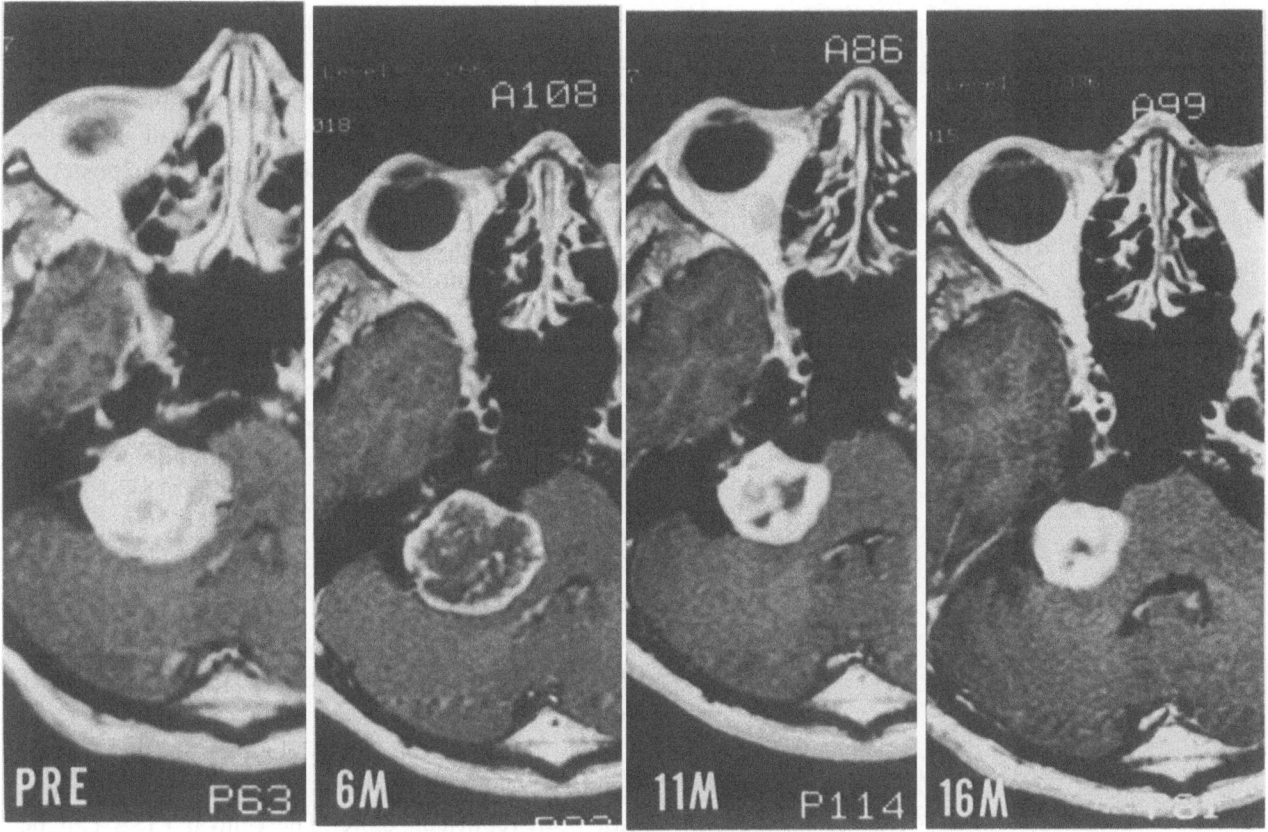

Fig. 2. Characteristic changes of acoustic neurinoma on repeated MRI (case 1)

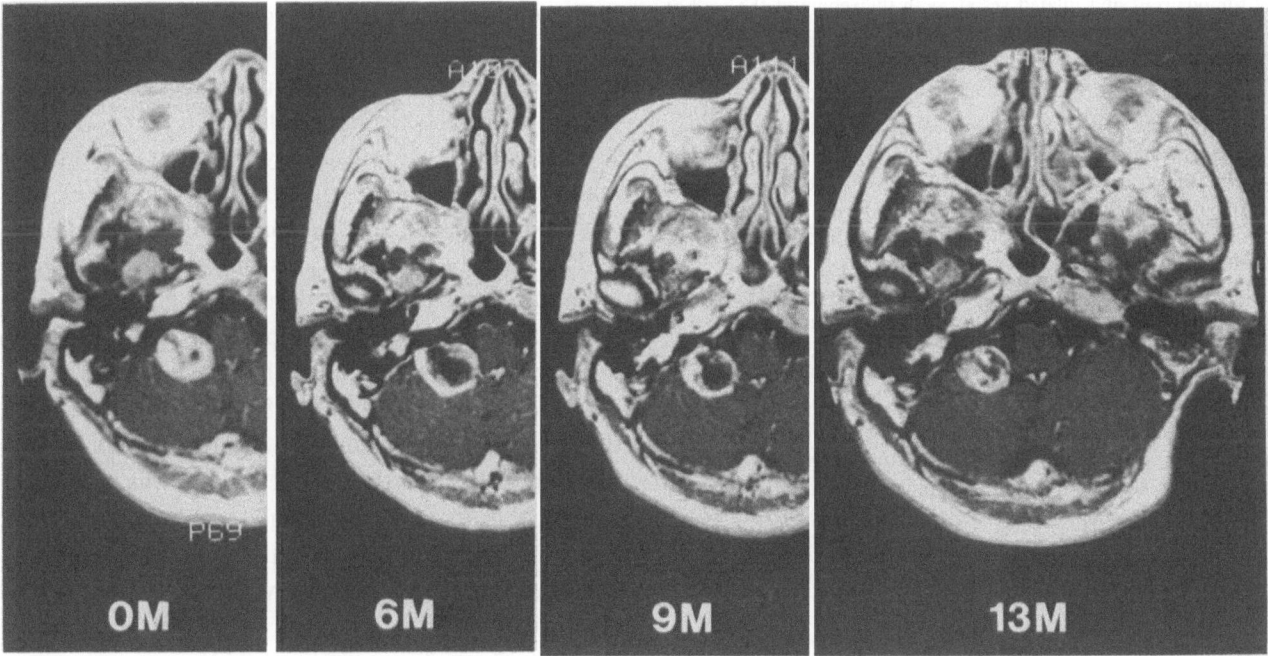

Fig. 3. MRI changes of tumours of von Recklinghausen's disease (case 2)

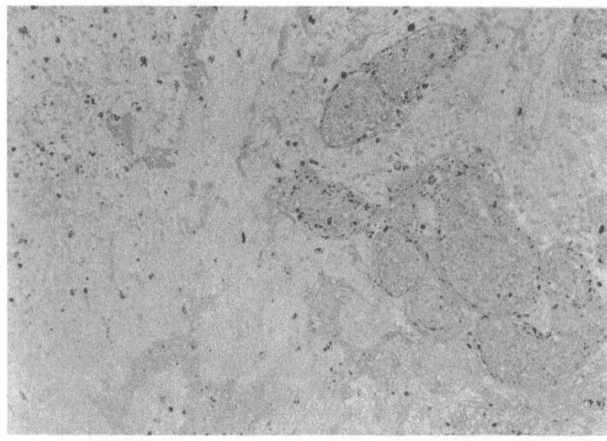

a

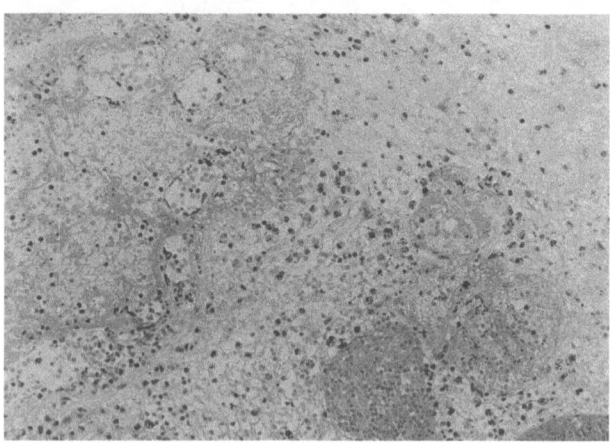

b

Fig. 4. The pathological findings of treated tumour: complete necrosis of tumour tissue at the center of the tumour (a) and degeneration of tumour cells and dilated vessels with thickening of the wall at the periphery of the tumour (b) were found

for two months. CT revealed enhanced mass in her right C-P angle. Because of her refusal of operation, the tumour was treated by gamma knife on January 14, 1992. The mean size of the tumour was 33 mm in diameter and volume of 18.8 cu cm. The maximum dose was 27 Gy and the tumour margin was covered by 45% isodose line (12.15 Gy) using 12 isocenters.

She was noticed to have communicating hydrocephalus at 5 months after the treatment and a ventriculo-peritoneal shunt was inserted.

At 11 months, she was operated on her irradiated mass because of its increasing size and the onset of an abducens palsy in spite of showing central LISA. The pathological study of this tumour revealed complete necrosis of tumour tissue at the center of the tumour (Fig. 4a), degeneration of tumour cells and dilated vessels with thickening of the wall at the periphery of the tumour (Fig. 4b).

Discussion

It has been reported that 1475 cases of acoustic neurinoma (13%) out of 11300 cases of all intracranial

lesions have been treated using the gamma knife in the world during 1968 to 1992[2]. In Japan, 268 cases of acoustic neurinoma (16%) out of 1722 cases of intra cranial lesions were treated during the last 27 months.

We always use MRI for dose planning and follow-up study of acoustic neurinoma, because of its higher resolution compared to CT scan especially in posterior fossa tumours.

Regarding the effects of gamma radiosurgery on acoustic neurinoma, Noren[6] reported that tumour shrinkage was obtained in 114 (50%); volume remained unchanged in 79 (35%) and enlarged in 34 (15%) out of 227 cases treated, and the tumour control rate was 85% with a mean follow-up period of 54 months. From an analysis of unilateral tumour and bilateral tumour (NF 2) groups, the control rate of unilateral group was significantly higher than that of bilateral tumours. Flickinger *et al.*[1] also reported that their tumour control rate was 92% from the series of 40 cases with follow-up of more than one year. Our control rate was 96% which is comparable with both papers, but further follow-up study is necessary.

The characteristic, early changes in the treated tumours which were found on repeated MRI, have not been reported before. The central LISA can be understood as radiation necrosis of tumour tissue as shown by the pathological findings in case 3. It is also interesting that the volume of LISA became maximal at 6 months after the treatment and decreased thereafter in good correlation with the tumour volume. However the meaning of re-enhancement which occurred at 6 to 9 months is not well understood. It may be assumed that the revascularization of necrotic tissue. fibrous tissue replacment or vascular changes induced by radiation are playing some role.

As side effects of radiosurgery, facial nerve and trigeminal nerve palsy are frequently found. Dan Leksell[3] reported that facial and trigeminal palsies were found in 15% and 17% of the cases but all of them were temporary and improved. Flickinger *et al.*[1] also reported that they found facial palsy in 31% and trigeminal palsy in 29%. Our results showed facial palsy in 16% and trigeminal palsy in 8% which is better than those reports. Regarding the hearing preservation, Flickinger reported that useful hearing was preserved in 46% of cases and surprisingly no hearing loss was found in small tumours less than 1 cm in diameter. Our results were comparable with Flickinger's series in that hearing was preserved in 10 out of 21 cases (48%) at 12 months.

References

1. Flickinger JC, Lunsford LD, Coffey RJ, Linsky ME, Bissonette DJ, Maitz AH, Konziolka D (1991) Radiosurgery of acoustic neurinoma. Cancer 67: 345–353
2. Gamma Knife Users Meeting (1992) Annual report
3. In: Leksell DG (1987) Stereotactic radiosurgery. Neurol Res 9: 60–68
4. Leksell L (1971) Stereotaxis and radiosurgery: an operative system. Thomas, Springfield
5. Linsky ME, Lunsfoed LD, Flickinger JC, Kondziolka D (1992) Stereotactic radiosurgery for acoustic tumours. Stereotactic Radiosurgery 3: 191–205
6. Noren G, Greitz D, Hirch A, Lax I (1992) Gamma knife radiosurgery in acoustic neurinoma. In: Steiner L (ed) Radiosurgery. Raven, New York, pp 141–148
7. Steiner L, Lindquist C, Steiner M (1992) Radiosurgery. In: Symon L (ed) Advances and technical standards in neurosurgery, Vol 19. Springer, Wien New York. pp 73–75

Correspondence: T. Kobayashi, M.D., Department of Neurosurgery, Gamma Knife Center, Komaki City Hospital, 1-20 Jobushi, Komaki City, Aichi Pref. 485, Japan.

Acta Neurochir (1994) [Suppl] 62: 98–100

Quality Assurance Programme on Stereotactic Radiosurgery

G. H. Hartmann

German Cancer Research Center, Department of Radiological Diagnostics and Therapy, Heidelberg, Federal Republic of Germany

Summary

In order to achieve a high level of quality in radiosurgical procedures, a quality assurance programme (QAP) has to be worked out. An informal "Quality Assurance Task Group" is currently preparing a QAP for that purpose. The concepts that have been worked out and critically discussed by the members of the task group are presented. The final version of the QAP is expected to be completed at the end of 1993.

Keywords: Stereotactic radiosurgery; quality assurance.

Introduction

Stereotactic radiosurgery is (mostly single and focal) irradiation of an incranial target localized by an imaging compatible device. It is a multidisciplinary treatment modality containing elements from neurosurgery, radiation therapy, neuroradiology and other disciplines. Therefore, in addition to reports dealing with quality assurance in one of these disciplines such as conventional radiotherapy[1,2,4], there is a need to specifically address the problems involved in quality assurance for stereotactic radiosurgery.

One of the main concerns is that normal tissue, and especially normal brain tissue, is more sensitive to a high irradiation dose when applied in one or a few fractions compared to conventional fractionation, since there are ample possibilities and, accordingly, a certain risk of missing a small cranial target by a single focused irradiation. Inaccurate radiosurgical irradiation however means that either the target can be severely understood or the normal tissue can receive an extremely large dose compared to the tissue tolerance dose. It follows that the question of the spatial accuracy of dose delivery and the methods for providing and guaranteeing maximum accuracy have to be one of the main topics in a QAP as far as the technical and physical aspects are considered.

The ultimate aim of a QAP in radiosurgery should be that patients will profit from this treatment modality. Since stereotactic radiosurgery is still not a universally established procedure, its efficacy has still to be explored. Therefore, it is of the utmost importance that clinical studies will be performed within the framework of protocols, the results of which will be compared among different institutions, and will be based on a common high and standardized level of quality, including clear instructions and standardized parameters for the main procedures in stereotactic radiosurgery.

In recent times, several documents on quality assurance (QA) in Radiosurgery have appeared or will appear[3,7,8]. This paper describes the state of QAP in stereotactic radiosurgery which is currently worked out by a "Quality Assurance Task Group". The informal group was established at the end of an international workshop on proton and narrow beam therapy in Oulu, Finland, June 1989. Members are: Jürgen N. Arndt, Stockholm, Sweden; Bernhard Bauer-Kirpes, Veenendaal, The Netherlands; Robert, Boesecke, Freiburg, Germany; Giorgio Chierego, Vicenza, Italy; Igor Ermakov, St. Petersburg, Russia; Günther H. Hartmann (Chairman), Heidelberg, Germany; Wendell Lutz, Tucson, AR, USA; Christina Marchetti, Venezia-Mestre, Italy; Mark H. Phillips, Seattle, WA, USA; Ervin B. Podgorsak, Montreal, Canada; Christopher F. Serago, Boston, MASS, USA; Lothar Schad, Heidelberg, Germany; Harald Treuer, Köln, Germany; Stanislav M. Vatnitsky, Loma Linda, CA, USA. So far, two full meetings have taken place in Heidelberg, one in October 1991 and the second in May this year in order to outline and prepare the document. The principal objective of this quality assurance programme on stereotactic radiosurgery is to give recommendations based on the view of experienced experts in radiosurgery. The recommendations apply to physical and technical aspects of the radiosurgery facility itself, as well as to all procedures and additional equipment involved. The document, however, is not intended to cover any matters of clinical judgement in the management of patients.

The Quality Assurance Programme

In the document an attempt is made to adopt a synoptic view of the three main radiosurgical methods currently in use, the Gamma Knife, the linac-based methods and the use of changed particles. The document will be limited to the technical and physical aspects of stereotactic radiosurgery, not addressing problems like patient records and forms, treatment policies and medical treatment planning, or review and audit programmes.

Due to the still uncompleted status of the document, details cannot be given. The main structure of the report, however, may be seen from Table 1. In order to meet the requirement of a clear conceptual approach and, at the same time, of being practical, the document is structured into two parts: into a conceptual part to be found in the introductory chapter which is dealing with definitions and requirements in Stereotactic Radio-

Table 1. *Structure of QAP Quality Assurance Programme for Stereotactic Radiosurgery*

Contents

1. Introduction
    1.1 Objective of the quality assurance programme
    1.2 Definitions
    1.3 Requirements and limitations
    1.4 Main subjects and key parameters in stereotactic radiosurgery
    1.5 Tolerance of key parameters

2. General Quality Assurance Programme
    2.1 Stereotactic components and procedures
    2.2 Dose delivery
    2.3 Dosimetry and Treatment planning
    2.4 Complete system integration

3. Quality assurance programme for each treatment (execution)
    3.1 Preparation of collimator and machine compounds
    3.2 Verification of treatment set-up
    3.3 Safety checks
    3.4 Use of a check list

4. Additional Practical Considerations and Methods

5. Appendix
    Glossary of terms

surgery, and into a part of practical tests. These tests are also split into two groups: The first series refer to the general QAP which are necessary before one can start with this treatment modality at a specific facility, whereas the second series refer to the tests which are necessary prior to each patient treatment. Each test is follows a common guide line of issues: the problem which is addressed, the aim of the test, the method used, the expected results and the frequency of application.

Within the conceptual part, in the section of definitions, an attempt is made to give a precise description of the terms which are frequently used in stereotactic radiosurgery. Examples are such apparently obvious terms like target point and isocenter. According to the recent ICRU Report 50[5], a distinction is made between the clinical target volume, the planning target volume, and the treated volume. The concept which is behind the use of terms of accuracy and precision is also addressed.

The final version of the QAP is expected to be completed at the end of this year and to be published as a booklet by Springer-Verlag.

Concept of Spatial Accuracy and Precision

Figure 1 is intended to examplify the concept of spatial accuracy and precision in radiosurgery in the QAP. For simplification, a two-dimensional scale is used. The position of the target point is given in the figure as a black dot. Now the irradiation procedure is repeated several times. The actual position of each center of the administered radiation may then be distributed in different patterns around the target point as shown in the two cases on the left and on

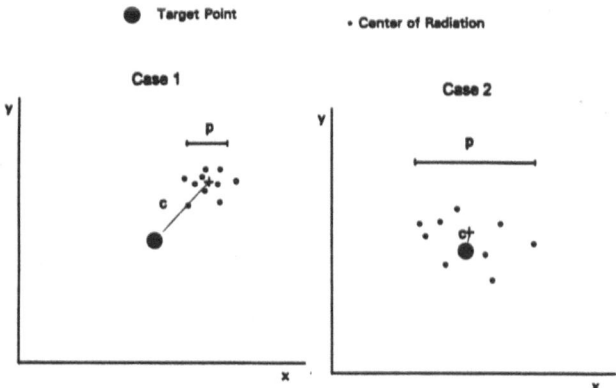

Fig. 1. Different patterns of accuracy and precision when a focal irradiation is given to a target point several times. The mean position of the center of irradiation is represented by a cross

the right side of the figure represented by small dots. The obvious difference can be quantitatively described[6] by the definition of the two following terms and the parameters c and p:

Accuracy of the mean = the closeness, c, of agreement between the target point and the mean position of the centers of irradiation which would be obtained by applying the irradiation procedure a large number of times. c is expressed by the spatial deviation between the mean position and the target point.

Precision = the closeness, p, of agreement between the positions of the center of radiation obtained by applying the irradiation procedure several times under prescribed conditions. p is expressed by the standard deviation of all single deviations.

Probability, that the "Treated Volume" does not deviate from the "Planning Target Volume" by more than:		
1 mm	1.5 mm	2.0 mm
c = 0.5 nm p = 0.25 mm		
94.9%	99.98%	99.99%
c = 0.5 mm p = 0.5 mm		
59.5%	92.7%	99.4%
c = 0.5 mm p = 1.0 mm		
18.5%	44.3%	70.2%

Fig. 2. Risk of inaccurate irradiation when the accuracy and precision parameter c and p are known

Once the parameters c and p have been quantitatively assessed, they can serve to estimate the risk of possible deviations between the planning target volume and the actual treated volume at a specific patient treatment. Examples of such estimates are shown in Fig. 2.

References

1. AAPM Report No 13 (1984) Physical aspects of quality assurance in radiation therapy, AAPM Task Group 24, American Institute of Physics, NY
2. Brahme A (ed) (1988) Accuracy requirements and quality assurance of external beam therapy with photons and electrons. Acta Oncol [Suppl] 1
3. Drzymala RE (1991) Quality assurance for linac-based stereotactic radiosurgery. In: Starkschall G, Horton J (eds) Proceedings of an American College of Medical Physics Symposium, pp 121–129
4. ICRU Report 24 (1976) Determination of absorbed dose in a patient irradiated by beams of x or gamma rays in radiotherapy procedures. International Commission on Radiation Units and Measurements, Washington
5. ICRU Report 50 (1993) Prescribing, recording, and reporting photon beam therapy. International Commission on Radiation Units and Measurements, Washington
6. International Standard Organisation (ISO) (1977) Statistics. Vocabulary and symbols. International Standard ISO 3534-1977, Geneva
7. Larson DA, Bora F, Eisert D, Kline R, Loeffler J, Lutz W, Mehta M, Palta J, Schewe K, Schultz C, Shaw E, Wilson F, Lunsford LD, Alexander E, Chapman P, Coffey R, Friedman W, Harsh G, Macinnas R, Olivier A, Steinberg G, Walsh J (1994) Consensus statement on stereotactic radiosurgery quality improvement. Int J Radiation Oncology Biol Phys 28: 527–530
8. Tsai JS, Buck BA, Goran RT, Svensson K, Alexander III E, Cheng C-W, Mannarino EG, Loeffler JS (1991) Quality assurance in stereotactic radiosurgery using a standard linear accelerator. Int J Radiation Oncology Biol Phys 21: 737–748

Correspondence: G. H. Hartmann, M.D., Department of Radiological Diagnostics and Therapy, German Cancer Research Center, D-69120 Heidelberg, Federal Republic of Germany.

Acta Neurochir (1994) [Suppl] 62: 101–104
© Springer-Verlag 1994

Quality Assurance for Non-Invasive Patient Fixation During Stereotactic Convergent Beam Irradiation

N. Hodapp, N. Nanko, F. Röhner, and **H. Frommhold**

Department of Radiation Therapy, Radiological University Clinics, Freiburg, Federal Republic of Germany

Summary

Using a non-invasive mask this patient fixation system for stereotactic radiotherapy allows one to perform fractionated irradiation. Measuring the statistical quantities of patient motion and positioning uncertainties and calculating its effect on a spherically symmetric dose distribution showed that there is no severe disadvantage in most cases. Only if small field-size, excentric target volume localisation and extreme proximity to an organ at risk coincides have the statistical effects to be taken into account. The greatest measured standard deviation for positioning uncertainty was 2.3 mm. Its effect on the dose distribution with a field size of 9.1 mm increases the diameter of the 80% isodose to about 115%.

Keywords: Stereotactic irradiation; head fixation system; quality assurance; standard deviations; effect on dose distribution.

Introduction

One of the main reasons for the high precision, which can be achieved with stereotactic single dose irradiation, is the rigid invasive fixation of the patient in the stereotactic ring. Such a fixation is scarcely applicable for fractionated irradiation. A non-invasive System would in that case be much more suitable. A number of different methods were developed for iteractive non-invasive Patient fixation. The most common systems use individually-shaped masks. In comparison with invasive fixation there are an increasing number of uncertainties involved in patient positioning. This may be caused by the movement of the patient during one irradiation and by differences in positioning between different sessions.

Our aim was to measure the extent of such variations and to calculate their influence on the dose distribution of a convergent beam technique with spherically symmetric dose distribution.

Methods and Materials

Equipment

Stereotactic convergent beam radiotherapy in Freiburg is carried out by a Philips SL75/20 Linear accelerator. Additional equipment according to the development of the German cancer research center[1]. This equipment includes a set for noninvasive patient fixation with individual masks.

Measurement of Movement and Positioning Uncertainties

In order to determine the positioning uncertainties, a special phantom head was made from silicon rubber. For localisation purposes, the phantom head contained 3 orthogonal wires through a point in the midst of the head, extending to the surfaces (Fig. 1). For this phantom, an individual mask was made in the usual way. Determination of positioning uncertainties was performed by the therapy simulator. The mask was attached to the simulator couch with the isocenter at the center of the mask. After that, the phantom was inserted into the mask. A pair of orthogonal radiographs in ventrodorsal and lateral projections was taken. The crossing- and endpoints of the wires and the centerline mark of the simulator were visible on the radiographs (Fig. 2). The pair of radiographs was repeated ten times. During that time, the position of mask and ring was kept constant with respect to the simulator isocenter. Between the pairs of radiographs the phantom head was removed from the mask and then repositioned. The co-ordinates of the central- and endpoints of the wire on the radiographs were read out with respect to the centerline mark of the simulator. For all seven wirepoints, the standard deviations of the mean co-ordinates were calculated.

Error Scrutiny

Two possible errors in the method, and their effect on the results were investigated. The error during the repositioning of the orthogonal gantry positions was determined by taking several orthogonal radiographs without removing the phantom. Possible read-out errors were determined by reading out the co-ordinates of the same radiograph several times or by comparing the values of the redundant co-ordinates.

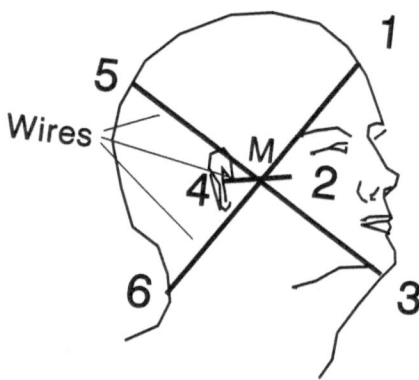

Fig. 1. Schematic drawing of the phantom head with wires and labelling of the measuring points

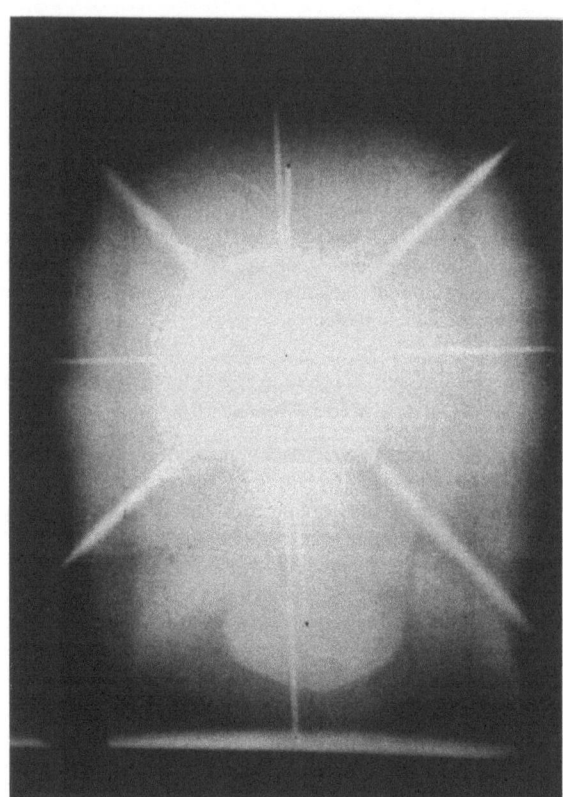

Fig. 2. Radiograph of the phantom head in antero-posterior direction with wires and field marks of the simulator

Effect on the Dose Distribution

The effect of the positioning uncertainties on the dose distribution was evaluated using a simplified model. With a therapy planning system (STP, Leibinger, Freiburg), the dose distribution of a stereotactic convergent treatment, consisting of six noncoplanar arcs, was calculated. The resulting dose distribution showed nearly spherical symmetry. This dose distribution was convoluted with the 3-D distribution of the positioning uncertainties, represented by a spherically symmetric Gaussian function. The standard deviations were kept within the range of the measured data. Due to the mentioned

simplifications, the following formulas[2] could be used:

$$\widehat{g_1(x)g_2}(y) = \frac{1}{(\sqrt{\pi}\beta)^3} \int_0^{2\pi} d\varphi \int_0^{\pi} d\vartheta \int_0^x c^2 dc \sin\vartheta$$

$$\cdot \exp{-\frac{1}{\beta^2}(r^2 + c^2 - 2rc\cos\vartheta)}$$

with

$$|x| = r \qquad |y| = c$$
$$|x - y| = r^2 + c^2 - 2rc\cos\vartheta$$

g_1 is a spherically symmetric function and g_2 a normalized 3-D Gaussian function with the standard deviation β.

Several substitutions lead to the one dimensional function:

$$\widehat{g_1 g_2}(r) = \frac{1}{r}[\widehat{G_1 G_2}(+r) - \widehat{G_1 G_2}(-r)]$$

with

$$G_1(c) = cg_1(c) \quad G_1(c) = 0 \quad for \ c < 0$$
$$G_2(r) = \frac{1}{\sqrt{\pi}\beta}\exp{-\left(\frac{r}{\beta}\right)^2}$$

Results

Movement and Positioning Uncertainties

Determination of the positioning uncertainties showed different results for the seven measuring points on the phantom head as well as for the three coordinate directions X (lateral), Y (longitudinal) and Z (anterior–posterior) (Fig. 3). Small standard deviations (SD) were calculated for point M in the midst of the head with a mean value for the three directions of 0.5 mm (Fig. 3). The greatest value of 2.3 mm showed Point 6 at the neck of the phantom. In most cases the longitudinal direction showed greater deviations than the others.

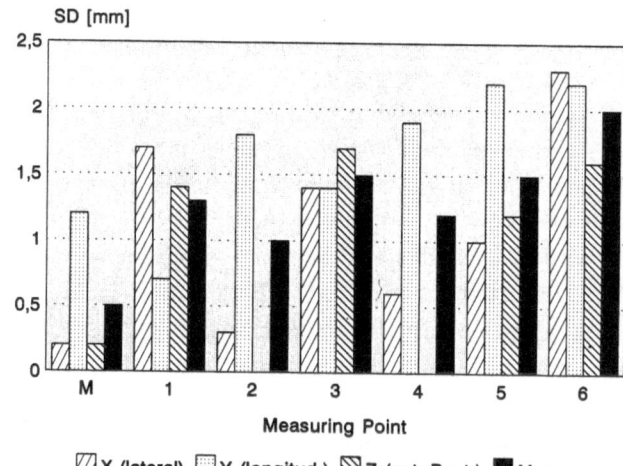

Fig. 3. Standard deviations from the mean value of the co-ordinates of the measuring points M and 1 to 6

Error Scrutiny

From the evaluation of repeated pairs of radiographs with the fixed phantom head, a precision of gantry repositioning with a SD of 0.3 mm resulted. The same value was found for the differences between the redundant co-ordinates. The repetition of reading out the deviation from the same radiograph showed a SD of 0.2 mm. This seems to be the limitation of this method.

Effect on the Dose Distribution

The diameter of the 80% Isodose changed depending on the SD of the positioning uncertainty (Fig. 4). For the smaller collimators with a field diameter of 3.1 and 9.1 mm, there is a nearly linear increase of the diameter of the 80% isodose up to the 1.23-fold respectively, the 1.15-fold value when the SD increases up to 2.5 mm. For the field diameters of 27.3 and 45.5 mm, a slight decrease of the 80% isodose diameter could be seen. The 80% to 20% distance increased for all field diameters with increasing SD (Fig. 5). For an SD of 2.5 mm, the amount of increase was 1.19 for a field

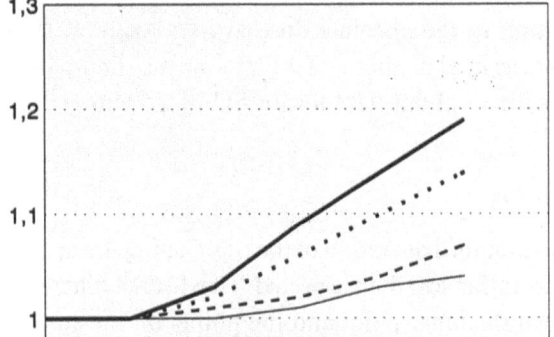

Collimator Diameter

— 3.1 mm

··· 9.1 mm

-- 27.3 mm

— 45.5 mm

Fig. 5. Dependence of the distance between the 80% and the 20% isodose on the standard deviation of the positioning uncertainties for different field sizes

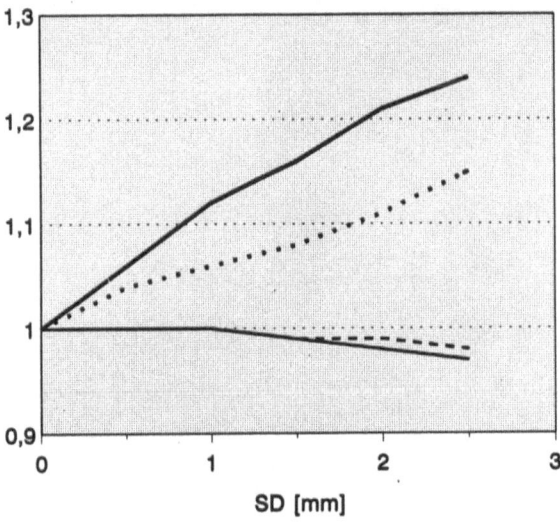

Collimator Diameter

— 3.1 mm

··· 9.1 mm

-- 27.3 mm

— 45.5 mm

Fig. 4. Dependence of the diameter of the 80% Isodose on the standard deviation of the positioning uncertainties for different field sizes

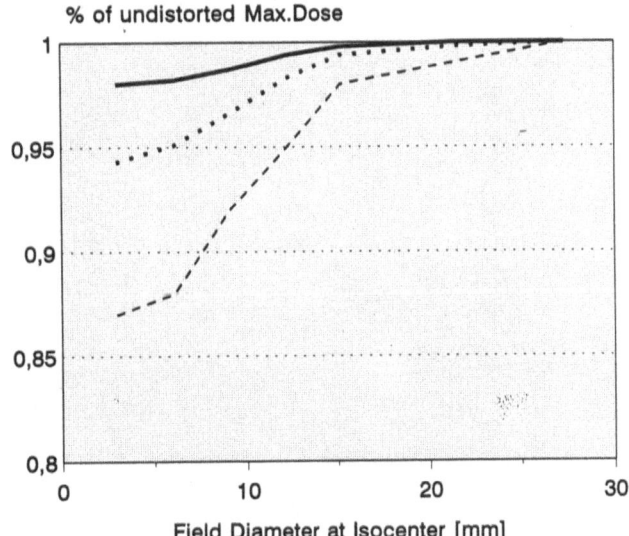

— SD = 1 mm

··· SD = 1.5 mm

-- SD = 2.5

Fig. 6. Relative Reduction of the absolute dose at the maximum depending on the standard deviation of the positioning uncertainties for different field sizes

diameter of 3.1 mm and 1.04 for 45.5 mm. The smearing effect of the positioning uncertainties also causes a reduction in the absolute dose at its maximum (Fig. 6). For the field diameter of 9.1 mm the maximum dose decreased to about 92% for an SD of 2.5 mm.

Discussion

The standard deviation of the positioning uncertainties was rather less than expected. The distinct difference between the inner point and the points on the surface suggests, that the possible motions of the head are mainly rotations around the midpoint. This means that the influence of the movement increases with decreasing distance of the target volume to the surface. The bigger SD in longitudinal direction can be explained with the missing fixation at the neck. This is also confirmed by the fact that the maximum value of the SD's is found for point 6 at the neck.

The effect of the positioning uncertainties on the dose distribution is at first glance surprising, as the 80% isodose diameter increases for small fields but decreases slightly for the larger field sizes. This can be explained by the shape of the radial dose profiles. Whereas the profile for the smaller field sizes is nearly Gaussian-shaped, the profiles for bigger field diameters are rather box-shaped. In spite of the fact that the resulting 1-D function for the disturbed dose profile is not a real convolution with a Gaussian function, it behaves in a similar way.

Only in the case of extreme proximity from target volume to an organ at risk, can the use of a mask, with the increasing distance between the 80% and the 20% isodoses be called into question. The decrease in absolute dose could be equalized by an adequate correction.

The measurements and calculations show that for the most target localisations and field sizes which are relevant in therapy, the positioning uncertainties, caused by the less rigid fixation in the mask, can be tolerated.

References

1. Hartmann GH, Schlegel W, Sturm V, Kober B, Pastyr O, Lorenz WJ (1985) Cerebral radiation surgery using moving field irradiation at a linear accelerator facility. Int J Radiat Oncol Biol Phys 11: 1185–1192
2. Hosemann R, Bagchi SN (1962) Direct analysis of diffraction by matter. North-Holland, Amsterdam, pp 69–70

Correspondence: Norbert Hodapp, Ph.D., Klinikum der Albert-Ludwigs-Universität Freiburg, Radiologische Klinik, Abteilung Strahlentherapie, Hugstetterstrasse 55, D-79106 Freiburg, Federal Republic of Germany.

Acta Neurochir (1994) [Suppl] 62: 105–110

Medial Thalamotomy with the Leksell Gamma Knife for Treatment of Chronic Pain

R. F. Young[1], **D. S. Jacques**[2], **R. W. Rand**[2], and **B. R. Copcutt**[2]

[1]Northwest Hospital Neuroscience/Gamma Knife Center, Seattle, WA and [2]Good Samaritan Hospital Neuroscience/Gamma Knife Center, Los Angeles, CA, U.S.A.

Summary

The authors describe 10 patients who underwent stereotactic medial thalamotomy with the Leksell Gamma Knife for treatment of chronic intractable pain. The pain was related to structural spinal disorders (4), postherpetic neuralgia (2), spinal cord injury (1), thalamic syndrome (1), anesthesia dolorosa of the face (1), and brainstem infarction (1). All patients had undergone extensive treatment with a variety of modalities prior to gamma thalamotomy. Nine patients underwent unilateral and one patient bilateral lesions. Magnetic resonance imaging (MRI) was used for target localization and the lesions were directed toward the intralaminar nuclei, the lateral portion of the medial dorsal nucleus, the centrum medianum and parafascicular nuclei. The lesions were made with radiation doses of 160–180 Gy using a 4 mm beam collimator and either a single isocenter (1 patient) or two isocenters (9 patients).

Follow-up MRI scans in all patients showed well localized lesions. Three patients experienced excellent pain relief, four had good pain relief and three were failures. No complications were seen in any of the patients. In the past gamma thalamotomy was used mainly for treatment of pain related to malignancies but our results indicate that it may also be a safe and effective treatment for pain of nonmalignant origin as well.

Keywords: Chronic intractable pain; thalamotomy; stereotactic medial thalamotomy; Leksell Gamma Knife; gamma thalamotomy; results.

Introduction

The actual role of stereotactic ablative brain lesions for the treatment of intractable pain is relatively limited[23,70]. Neurostimulation and opiate infusion techniques have largely replaced ablative brain lesions[71]. Nevertheless, there remains a small but definite group of patients who fail respond to less invasive methods. For these patients, stereotactic ablative lesions provide a suitable alternative[72].

Lesions in many locations have been tried in the past including the medial and lateral thalamus, the cingulum bundle, the mesencephalon and the brainstem[23,72]. Our own focus has been on the medial thalamus particularly the region of the intralaminar nuclei, medial dorsal nucleus, centré median, and parafascicular nuclei[70-72]. This region is thought to be the central relay of the paleospinothalamic input to the limbic and other higher systems which determine the affective and motivational responses to pain[1,2,3,7,11,13,19,20,30,32,40,44,46-48,56]. We have previously described spontaneous neuronal hyperactivity in this region in patients with chronic pain and have developed a radiofrequency lesioning technique designed to ablate such abnormally discharging neurons[55,72].

In an effort to reduce the invasive nature of the procedure, we have explored medial thalamotomy with the Leksell Gamma Knife, radiosurgical system for treatment of chronic pain in ten patients. We have expanded upon the earlier work of Leksell, Meyerson, and Forster who first reported so-called "gamma thalamotomy" for treatment of chronic pain[38]. We have tailored our lesion locations based on our experience using the open method previously referred to. The results are encouraging so far and this report describes our methods and results.

Materials and Methods

Ten patients with chronic intractable pain of a variety of etiologies (Table 1) were selected for gamma thalamotomy. All patients were presented the options of open stereotactic thalamotomy and deep brain stimulator (DBS) implantation alternatives. Extensive therapy, as appropriate, with medications, physical and psychological therapy, nerve blocks, neurostimulation procedures (spinal stimulation and DBS), spinal opiate infusion, and other ablative methods (dorsal

Table 1. *Gamma-Thalamotomy*. Patient population and results

Patient	Age	Pathology	Date	Follow-up (months)	Results
B.E.	71	spondylosis/osteoporosis	7/92	14	excellent
E.M.	83	failed spinal surgery	9/92	12	exc. → good
			3/93	6	good
S.D.	48	spinal cord injury	10/92	11	failure
M.L.	79	thalamic syndrome	11/92	4[a]	excellent
L.S.	68	post DREZ dysesthesias (postherpetic neuralgia)	12/92	9	failure
E.M.	75	postherpetic neuralgia	12/92	9	failure
J.V.	58	anesthesia dolorosa-face	12/92	9	good
M.B.	71	brainstem infarct	2/93	7	good
D.M.	56	failed spinal surgery	4/93	5	good
S.E.	78	failed spinal surgery	6/93	3	excellent

[a] Expired, unrelated cause.

Table 2. *Stereotactic Coordinates for Gamma-Thalamotomy*[a]

Isocenter	X	Y	Z
1	1	6 ant. P.C.	+2
2	10	9.5 ant. P.C.	+6

[a] Distances in millimeters X lateral, Y anteroposterior, Z superior to anterior commissure. AC posterior commissure. *PC* plane.

root entry zone lesions) had been explored in these patients prior to gamma thalamotomy.

Nine patients underwent unilateral lesions and one a bilateral lesion. There were a variety of causes of chronic pain (Table 1) with two patients considered to have purely nociceptive pain and five purely neuropathic pain, whereas three had both nociceptive and neuropathic components to their pains. All lesions were made with the Leksell Gamma Knife. Maximum radiosurgical doses of 160–180 Gy were used and were delivered in all patients using a 4 mm collimator. A single isocenter was used in one patient and two isocenters were used in all others. Target localizaton was by magnetic resonance image (MRI) scanning with the Leksell Model G stereo-

tactic frame and a *Phillips Gyroscan* 1.5T or Siemans *Magnatom 1.0T* MRI scanner [10,72]. The Schaltenbrand and Wahren Stereotactic Atlas, in conjunction with recent anatomical and physiological understanding of the thalamus, was used to obtain target coordinates based on our prior experience with radiofrequency thalamotomy[8,9,26,31,59]. The X, Y, and Z coordinates for the two isocenters are shown in Table 2. Our attempt was to reproduce as closely as possible the R-F lesions we had made previously[71,72]. Follow-up MRI scans were obtained at various intervals and follow-up periods have ranged from 3–15 months (mean 9 months).

Results

Our results are shown in Table 1. Patients were considered to have excellent, good, or unsatisfactory pain relief. Excellent pain relief included lack of narcotics utilization, 50% or greater reduction in pain intensity, and significant improvement in functional capabilities such as activities of daily living, leisure activities, or

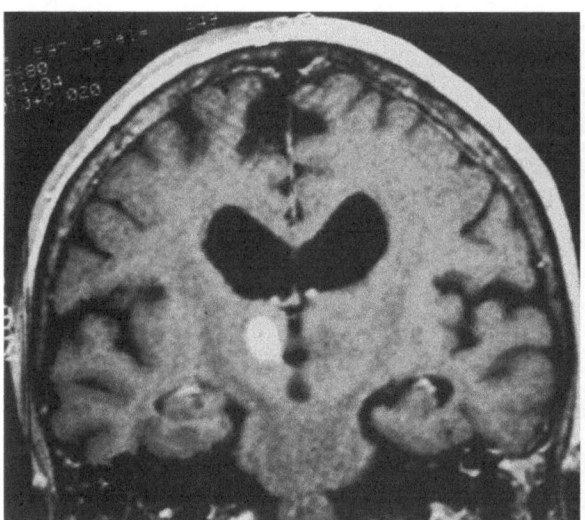 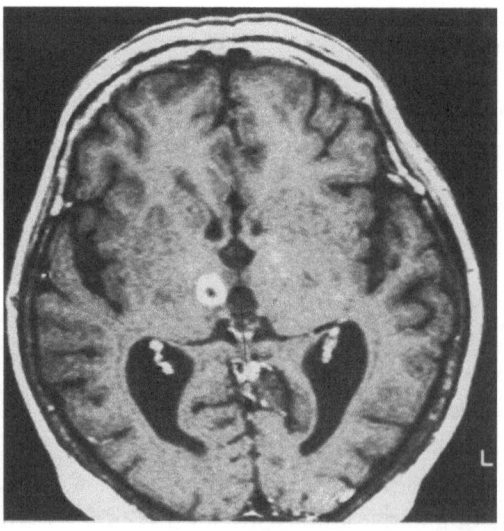

1   2

Fig. 1. Coronal T1 weighted MRI scan with gadolinium enhancement six months after gammathalamotomy in patient (EM)
Fig. 2. Axial T1 weighted MRI scan of same patient as Fig. 1

employment. Good pain relief included at least 50% pain relief, minimal narcotics use, and some improvement in functional capacity. All other results were considered failures.

Using these criteria three patients experienced excellent pain relief, four patients experienced good pain relief, and three patients were considered failures. Effects were usually evident within two to four weeks of the procedure. One patient who initially experienced excellent pain relief at about three months was placed in the good category subsequently due to increased pain intensity, although she did not use narcotic analgesics. Of the three patients who experienced excellent results two had pain of nociceptive origin and one had pain of neuropathic origin. Of the four patients with good results two had pain of neuropathic origin and two had pain with mixed neuropathic and nociceptive components.

No complications were experienced related to gamma-thalamotomy. Follow-up MRI scans (Figs. 1 and 2) demonstrated excellent lesion locations and lesion sizes compared to those previously made by R-F techniques. With contrast enhanced T1 weighed MRI scanning the lesions were oval in shape and exhibited a central low signal region which measured about 5×8 mm and an outer enhancing border which measured about 10×12 mm (Figs. 1 and 2). The lesion sizes appeared stable up to one year following the procedure. No evidence of perilesional white matter changes were seen in any patients.

Discussion

Tasker recently carried out an excellent review of his own experience and literature reports of prior experience with thalamotomy for pain control[62,63]. Regarding medial thalamotomy he identified 175 patients reported in the literature with an overall success rate of 46% for pain relief and with one author reporting 70% of patients successfully treated. In his own experience, Tasker reported 21 patients (some of whom also had additional lesions elsewhere) with 62% who had experienced some degree of pain relief. Our own experience with radiofrequency medial thalamotomy over the past five years (unpublished data) is similar to that of Tasker in that about 60% of our patients experienced pain relief. Tasker described a significantly lower success rate in the treatment of neuropathic pain than in the treatment of nociceptive pain. Our patient numbers and follow-up intervals are too short to make any comments on the efficacy of gamma thalamotomy in

these two pain types. It has been our experience and that of others that medial thalamotomy does not result in any alteration in sensation; that is there is no detectable loss of acute pain, tactile, thermal, vibratory, or kinesthetic sensation by the usual clinical assessment techniques and the patients do not complain of any sensory deficit.

Our most striking observation has been that medial thalamotomy reduces greatly the patient's attention to their pain. This effect appears specific for pain as there is no general reduction in attention or motivation in these patients. Afferent input to the medial thalamus via the multisynaptic paleospinothalamic tract and efferent connections between the medial thalamic nuclei and the cingulate and prefrontal cortical regions are well accepted[3,7,19,20,25,30,44-46,53]. More recently direct afferent input to this region has been demonstrated in both anatomical tracer studies of the spinothalamic pathway and electrophysiological studies in awake animals[5,11,12,13,32,40,41,51,56,67]. It has been suggested that the medial thalamus may participate in both discriminative and affective dimensions of pain[5,52]. Pain thresholds have been shown to be elevated following medial thalamic lesions on behavioral studies[47,48]. Prior reports of attempts to treat pain by radiosurgical ablative lesions are very few[4,18,38,60]. Steiner *et al.* made lesions in the ventromedial thalamus with the gamma knife in 52 patients with pain related to malignancies[4,60]. Several target points were used in a similar general location to our targets. Lesions were consistently seen at radiation doses of 160 Gy and the ideal dose was felt to be 170–180 Gy. Two-thirds of the patients described by Steiner *et al.* experienced early pain relief and 26 patients (50%) reported lasting relief[60]. The procedure was most effective for arm, shoulder, and facial pain and less effective for pain in the lower body and leg. The most effective lesions were located posteriorly near the posterior commissure and medially near the wall of the third ventricle[69]. The target coordinates used by Steiner *et al.* (X-8 to 12 mm lateral, Y-8 to 12 mm posterior to mid-commissural point, Z-0 to 5 mm above commissural plane) are similar although not identical to ours.

A major concern for functional neurosurgery using radiosurgical methods is the question as to whether or not functional targets can be sufficiently localized by anatomical techniques alone, without intraoperative physiological guidance[6,10,33,34,39,66]. Our prior extensive experience with functional neurosurgery using open stereotactic methods and anatomical, as well as physiological guidance for thalamic exploration and thalamotomy, convenced us that an atomical guidance with modern MRI scanning was sufficient[10,71-74]. As a matter of fact, there has been no reliable physiological signature of the medial thalamus although there certainly is such signature of the ventral posterior sensory nucleus[21,22,27]. Our description of spontaneous neuronal hyperactivity in medial thalamic structures in patients with chronic pain provides physiological guidance in some but not all patients since we were not able to record such activity in all patients[55]. There is usually no somatotopic organization within the medial thalamus, although stimulation may intensify the patient's preexisting pain or induce paresthesias in the contralateral face at high stimulus amplitudes, presumably from current spread laterally into the ventroposteromedial thalamic sensory relay nuclei from the face[72,74]. In addition, our prior experience with R-F thalamotomy using physiological guidance demonstrated a very consistent anatomical localization to the lateral portion of the dorsomedial nucleus, the intralaminar zone, and the centré median, and parafascicular nuclei[70,71,72,74]. Anatomical coordinate determination for our gamma-thalamotomies was based on this prior experience.

Our results with gamma-thalamotomy are very similar to those which we and others have reported using open stereotactic methods[14,15,16,24,28,37,41-43, 50,54,57,58,61,64,65]. Open stereotactic medial thalamotomy carries small but definite risks including intracranial hemorrhage and infections[29,62,63]. The later risks are not present with gamma thalamotomy. Neurological deficit from lesions in the medial thalamic area are in our experience rare but there are a number of reports of deficits including "peduncular hallucinosis," memory or speech deficits and contralateral neglect after injury to the medial thalamus although other authors report normal memory after damage to the medial thalamus[17,35,36,49,68]. We have so far experienced no complications either neurological or otherwise in our small patient population. Given the safety and efficacy we have demonstrated, it may be necessary to reconsider the place of thalamotomy in the treatment of chronic pain. It is considerably safer and less expensive in our experience than deep brain stimulator implantation for instance.

Our numbers are too small and our follow-up too short to determine whether nociceptive, neuropathic, or mixed pain syndromes will respond more or less favorably. We have had excellent and good responses in all these pain types but not uniformly. Only further experience can potentially refine the indications for and the place of gamma-thalamotomy in the spectrum of available pain therapies. We suspect that larger lesions and bilateral lesions may be required to achieve better pain relief and these approaches would carry a higher risk of neurological deficits.

Conclusions

Gamma-thalamotomy offers a less invassive alternative to stereotactic medial thalamotomy than does an open stereotactic procedure. The risks of hemorrhage and infection, although low, with open stereotactic procedures are obviated by gamma-thalamotomy. MRI guidance avoids the risk associated with ventriculography and as our follow-up scans show, lesion locations based on MRI scan localization are very accurate. The lesions produced by our technique are similar in size and location to lesions made by R-F methods with electrophysiological guidance. Our follow-up time is relatively short, however, and further follow-up will be required to determine the long-term efficacy of this technique but the results appear very promising at this point.

References

1. Albe-Fessard D, Kruger L (1962) Duality of unit discharges from cat centrum medianum in response to natural and electrical stimulation. J Neurophysiol 25: 3–20
2. Albe-Fessard D, Besson JM (1973) Convergent thalamic and cortical projections – the nonspecific system. In: Iggo A (ed) Handbook of sensory physiology, Vol II. Somatosensory system. Springer, Berlin Heidelberg New York, pp 490–560
3. Albe-Fessard D, Condés-Lara M, Sanderson, et al (1984) Tentative explanation of the special role played by the areas of paleospinothalamic projection in patients with deafferentation pain syndromes. In: Kruger L, Liebeskind JC (eds) Advances in pain research and therapy, Vol 6. Raven, New York, pp 167–182
4. Alexander E, Lindquist C (1993) Special indications: radiosurgery for functional neurosurgery and epilepsy. In: Alexander E, Loeffler JS, Lunsford LD (eds) Stereotactic radiosurgery. McGraw-Hill, New York, pp 221–225
5. Anderson KV, Mahan PE (1971) Increased pain thresholds following combined lesions of thalamic nuclei centrum medianum and centralis lateralis. Psychon Sci 23: 113–114
6. Birg W, Mundinger F, Mohadier M, et al (1985) X-ray and magnetic resonance stereotaxy for functional and nonfunctional neurosurgery. Appl Neurophysiol 48: 22–29
7. Bowsher D (1976) Role of the reticular formation in responses to noxious stimulation. Pain 2: 361–378
8. Bushnell MC, Duncan GH (1989) Sensory and affective aspects of pain perception: is medial thalamus restricted to emotional issues? Exp Brain Res 78: 415–418
9. Cesaro P, Mann MW, Moretti JL, et al (1991) Central pain and thalamic hyperactivity: a single photon emission computerized tomographic study. Pain 47: 329–336

10. Chodakiewitz JW (1991) Thalamotomy lesions: letter to the editor. J Neurosurg 75: 832–833

11. Craig, Jr AD, Linington AJ, Kniffki KD (1989) Cells of origin of spinothalamic tract projections to the medial and lateral thalamus in the cat. J Comp Neurol 289: 568–585

12. Dafny N, Reyes-Vazquez C, Qiao JT (1990) Modification of nociceptively identified neurons in thalamic parafascicularis by chemical stimulation of dorsal raphe with glutamate, morphine, serotonin and focal dorsal raphe electrical stimulation. Brain Res Bull 24: 717–723

13. Dostrovsky JO, Guildbaud G (1990) Nociceptive responses in medial thalamus of the normal and arthritic rat. Pain 40: 93–104

14. Fairman D (1966) Evaluation of results in stereotactic thalamotomy for the treatment of intractable pain. Confin Neurol 27: 67–70

15. Fairman D (1967) Unilateral thalamic tractomy for the relief of bilateral pain in malignant tumors. Confin Neurol 29: 146–158

16. Fairman D, Llavallol MA (1973) Thalamic tractotomy for the alleviation of intractable pain in cancer. Cancer 31: 700–707

17. Feinberg WM, Rapcsak SZ (1989) 'Peduncular hallucinosis' following paramedian thalamic infarction. Neurology 39: 1535–1536

18. Forster DMC, Leksell L, Meyerson BA, *et al* (1972) Gamma-thalamotomy in intractable pain. In: Janzen R, Keidel WD, Herz A, Steichele C (eds) Pain: basic principles-pharmacology therapy. Thieme, Stuttgart, pp 194–198

19. Giesler GJ, Menetrey D, Basbaum AI (1979) Differential origins of spinothalamic tract projections to medial and lateral thalamus in the rat. J Comp Neurol 184: 107–126

20. Giesler GJ, Spiel HR, Willis WD (1981) Organization of spinothalamic tract axons within the rat spinal cord. J Comp Neurol 195: 243–252

21. Gorecki J, Hirayama T, Dostrovsky JO, *et al* (1989) Thalamic stimulation and recording in patients with deafferentation and Central Pain. Stereotactic Funct Neurosurg 52: 219–226

22. Gucer G, Neidermeyer E, Long DM (1978) Thalamic recordings in patients with chronic pain J Neurol 219: 47–61

23. Gybels JM, Sweet WH (1989) Neurosurgical treatment of persistent pain. Thalamotomy. In: Gildenberg PL (ed) Pain and headache, Vol 16. Karger, Basel, pp 220–234

24. Hageman R, DeGrood MPAM (1970) Experiences with stereotactic treatment of intractable pain. Psychiatry Neurology Neurosurgery 73: 113–134

25. Hassler R (1972) The division of pain conduction into systems of pain sensation and pain awareness. In: Janzen R, Keidel WD, Herz A, Steichele C (eds) Pain: basic principles-pharmacology therapy. Thieme, Stuttgart, pp 98–112

26. Hirai T, Jones EG (1989) A new parcellation of the human thalamus on the basis of histochemical staining. Brain Res Rev 14: 1–34

27. Hirayama T, Dostrovsky JO, Gorecki J *et al* (1989) Recordings of abnormal activity in patients with deafferentation and central pain. Stereotact Funct Neurosurg 52: 120–126

28. Hitchcock ER, Teixeria MJ (1981) A comparison of results from center-median and basal thalamotomies for pain. Surg Neurol 15: 341–351

29. Hood TW, Yap JC (1981) A survey of infections in stereotactic surgery. Appl Neurophysiol 44: 314–319

30. Ishijima B, Yoshimasu N, Fukushima T, *et al* (1975) Nociceptive neurons in the human thalamus. Confinia Neurol 37: 99–106

31. Jones EG (1985) The thalamus. Plenum, New York, pp 607–645

32. Keyser V, Guilbaud G (1984) Further evidence for changes in the responsiveness of somatosensory neurons in arthritic rats: a study of the posterior intralaminar region of the thalamus. Brain Res 323: 144–147

33. Kelly PJ (1991) Thalamotomy lesions: response to letter to the editor. J Neurosurg 75: 833–834

34. Kondziolka D, Dolan EJ, Tasker RR (1989) Functional stereotactic surgery and stereotactic biopsy using a magnetic resonance imaging directed system. Results and comparisons to CT guidance. Presented at the 10th Meeting of the World Society for Stereotactic and Functional Neurosurgery. Maebashi, Japan

35. Kritchevsky M, Graff-Radford NR, Damasio AR (1987) Normal memory after damage to the medial thalamus. Arch Neurol 44: 959–962

36. Kritchevsky M, Graff-Radford NR (1989) Medial thalamus and memory: reply to letter to the editor. Arch Neurol 46: 483–484

37. Laitinen LV (1988) Mesencephalotomy and thalamotomy for chronic pain. In: Lundsford LD (ed) Modern stereotactic neurosurgery. Martinus Nijhoff, Boston, pp 269–277

38. Leksell L, Meyerson BA, Forster DMC (1972) Radiosurgical thalamotomy for intractable pain. Confin Neurol 34: 264

39. Lunsford LD (1988) Magnetic resonance imaging stereotactic thalamotomy: report of a case with comparison to computed tomography. Neurosurgery 23: 363–367

40. Ma W, Peschanski M, Ralston HJ (1987) Fine structure of the spinothalamic projections to the central lateral nucleus of the rat thalamus. Brain Res 414: 187–191

41. Mark VH, Ervin FR, Hackett TP (1960) Clinical aspects of stereotactic thalamotomy in the human in the treatment of chronic serve pain. Arch Neurol 3: 351–367

42. Mark VH, Ervin FR (1965) Role of thalamotomy in treatment of chronic severe pain. Postgrad Med 37: 563–571

43. Mark VH, Ervin FR, Yakolev PI (1971) Correlation of pain relief, sensory loss and anatomical lesion sites in pain patients treated by stereotaxic thalamotomy. Trans Am Neurol Assoc 86: 86–90

44. Marlbrug DL (1973) The effect on reaction of painful stimuli of lesions in the centromedian nucleus in the thalamus of the monkey. Intern J Neurosci 5: 153–158

45. McKenzie JS, Rogers DK (1981) Unit responses of intralaminar thalamus to midbrain and medullary stimulation and effects of conditioning caudate and hippocampal stimuli. Brain Res Bull 7: 345–352

46. Mehler WR (1966) Further notes on the center median nucleus of macague. In: Purpura DP, Yahr MD (eds) The thalamus. Columbia University Press, New York, pp 109–122

47. Mitchell CL, Kaelber WW (1966) Effect of medial thalamic lesions on responses elicited by tooth pulp stimulaton. Am J Neurol 210: 263–269

48. Mitchell CL, Kaelber WW (1967) Unilateral vs. bilateral medial thalamic lesions and reactivity to noxious stimuli. Arch Neurol 17: 653–660

49. Mori E, Yamadori A (1989) Medial thalamus and memory: letter to the editor. Arch Neurol 46: 482–483

50. Niizuma H, Kwak R, Ikeda S, *et al* (1982) Follow-up results of centromedian thalamotomy for central pain. Appl Neurophysiol 45: 324–325

51. Olausson B, Shyu BC, Rydenhag B (1989) Projection from the thalamic intralaminar nuclei on the isocortex of the rat: a surface potential study. Exp Brain Res 75: 543–554

52. Palestini M, Mariotti M, Velasco, *et al* (1987) Medialis dorsalis thalamic unitary response to tooth pulp stimulation and its conditioning by brainstem and limbic activation. Neurosci Lett 78: 161–165

53. Pearl GS, Anderson KV (1980) Response of cells of feline nucleus centrum medianum to tooth pulp stimulation. Brain Res Bull 5: 41–45

54. Richardson DE (1967) Thalamotomy for intractable pain. Confin Neurol 29: 139–145

55. Rinaldi PC, Young RF, Albe-Fessard D, *et al* (1991) Spontaneous

neuronal hyperactivity in the intralaminar thalamic nuclei of patients with deafferentation pain. J Neursurg 74: 415–421

56. Sadikot AF, Parent A, François C (1990) The centre médian and parafascicular thalamic project respectively to the sensori-motor and associative-limbic striatal territories in the squirrel monkey. Brain Res 510: 161–165

57. Sano K (1977) Intralaminar thalamotomy (thalamolaminotomy) and posteromedial hypothalamotomy in the treatment of intractable pain. Prog Neurol Surg 8: 50–103

58. Sano K, Yoshioka M, Ogashiwa M, *et al.* (1966) Thalamola-minotomy: a new operation relief of intractable pain. Confin Neurol 27: 63–66

59. Schaltenbrand G, Wahren W (1977) Atlas for stereotaxy of the human brain. Thieme, Stuttgart

60. Steiner L, Forster D, Leksell L, *et al* (1980) Gammathalamotomy in intractable pain. Acta Neurochir (Wien) 52: 173–184

61. Sugita K, Mutsuga N, Takaoka Y, *et al.* (1972) Results of stereotaxic thalamotomy for pain. Confin Neurol 34: 265–274

62. Tasker RR (1989) Stereotactic surgery. In: Wall PD, Melzack R (eds) Textbook of pain, 2nd Ed. Churchill Livingstone, Edinburgh, pp 840–855

63. Tasker RR (1990) Thalamotomy. Neurosurg Clin North Am 1: 841–863

64. Takaku A, Kwak R, Sakamoto T, *et al* (1973) Stereotactic thalamotomy for postherpetic central pain and muscular hyper-tonicity. Tohoku J Exp Med 85: 87–92

65. Tsubokawa T, Mariyasu N (1975) Follow-up results of centre median thalamotomy for relief of intractable pain. Conf Neurol 37: 280–284

66. Tomlinson FH, Jack CR, Kelly PJ (1991) Sequential magnetic resonance imaging following stereotactic radiofrequency ventra-lis lateralis thalamotomy. J Neurosurgery 74: 579–584

67. van Vulpen EHS, Verwer RWH (1989) Organization of projec-tions from the mediodorsal nucleus of the thalamus to the basolateral complex of the amygdala in the rat. Brain Res 500: 389–394

68. Watson RT, Valenstein E, Heilman KM (1981) Thalamic neglect. Possible role of the medial thalamus and nucleus reticularis in behavior. Arch Neurol 38: 501–506

69. Wennerstrand J, Ungestedt U (1970) Anatomical study of gamma-radiolesions. Acta Chir Scand 136: 133–137

70. Young RF, Modesti L (1985) Stereotactic ablative procedure for pain relief. In: Wilkins RH, Regachary SS (eds) Neurosurgery. McGraw Hill, New York, pp 2454–2457

71. Young RF (1988) Stereotactic methods in management of pain. In: Heilbrun MP (ed) Concepts in neurosurgery, Stereotactic neurosurgery. Williams and Wilkins, Baltimore, pp 149–160

72. Young RF (1992) Stereotactic surgical ablation for pain relief. In: Rengachary SS, Wilkins RH (eds) Neurosurgical operative atlas. Williams and Wilkins, Baltimore, pp 177–188

73. Young RF (1988) Functional stereotactic neurosurgery with magnetic resonance imaging guidance. J Mind Behavior 9: 263–272

74. Young RF (1993) Intracranial procedures for pain management. In: Apuzzo MLJ (ed) Brain surgery: complication avoidance and management. Churchill Livingstone, New York, pp 1497–1508

Correspondence: Ronald F. Young, M.D., Northwest Hospital Gamma Knife Center, 11560 North 115th Street, Suite G-5, Seattle, WA 98133, U.S.A.

Acta Neurochir (1994) [Suppl] 62: 111–113

Radiosurgery of Epilepsy. Long-Term Results

J. L. Barcia-Salorio[1,2], **J. A. Barcia**[1,2], **G. Hernández**[3], and **L. López-Gómez**[4]

[1] Servicio de Neurocirugía, Hospital Clinico Universitario, [2] Departamento de Cirugía, Universidad de Valencia, [3] Servicio de Terapéutica Fisica, Hospital Clinico Universitario, and [4] Servicio de Electroencefalografía, Hospital Clinico Universitario, Valencia, Spain

Summary

Based on experimental research, since 1982 until 1991 a series of 11 patients diagnosed as suffering from idiopathic focal epilepsy have been treated with stereotactic radiosurgery. Focus location was determined with cortical electrodes and confirmed by stereotactically placed deep electrodes.

Stereotactic radiosurgery was performed with photons from a cobalt source with a dose of 10 to 20 Gy, except in two cases in whom a betatron was used. The results were: complete cessation of seizures in four cases and a significant reduction in the number of seizures in five additional cases. Seizures began to decrease gradually after a period of three months of one year, except in two cases in whom there was an immediate response after treatment. In two cases there was no change. No complication related to the irradiation was recorded.

The gradual and delayed effect, obtained with low doses, may favour the hypothesis that non-descructive permanent structural changes, possibly related to the neuronal plasticity phenomenon, constitute the mechanism underlying these facts. Although the number of cases so far is too small, the absence of side-effects may make this bloodless method the one of choice specially in those cases in whom eloquent areas are involved.

Keywords: Epilepsy; radiosurgery.

Introduction

Several authors[5,8,11] have already observed that patients carrying epileptogenic intracranial lesions improved in the rate and intensity of their seizures after irradiation directed to cure the primary lesion, and that improvement occurred long before there was any sign of resolution of the lesion, if any. These observations increased with the development and applications of stereotactic radiosurgery[7]. However, up to 1982, there had been no attempt to directly treat the epileptic focus as such with radiosurgery, (in the case other treatable lesions explaining the occurrence of the seizures had been discarded.

Some considerations about the low dose the epileptogenic brain tissue surrounding the target volume would be receiving, and the results of experimental work with a model of chronic epilepsy in cats, directed the authors to attempt the irradiation of cases of focal idiopathic epilepsy with very low doses (10 to 20 Gy), in accordance with those normally used in radiosurgery and capable of producing tissue destruction.

This paper reports the results in a series of 11 cases, with a follow-up period ranging between two and 11 years.

Material and Methods

This series includes 11 epileptic patients (4 male, 7 female) who were treated with stereotactic radiosurgery at our institution from 1982 to 1991. Follow-up periods range between 127 and 28 months (mean: 75 months). Their ages ranged from 16 to 42 years old. The pre-operative symptomatic period varied from 3 to 24 years. We have excluded from this series five cases included in our first report[2], and diagnosed as epileptic psychosis, in order to have a more homogeneous group to evaluate the results. On the other hand, we could include and follow-up two patients of the first report who had been lost to follow-up.

Every patient was carefully studied to discard any primary treatable cause of the seizures. The pre-operative protocol included clinical and psychological studies, standard EEG, CT scanning, angiography in some cases and, in the most recent cases, MR imaging. Patients were considered as candidates for this programme only when more than two years of treatment with a single oral anticonvulsant drug and more than two years of treatment with a multidrug regime had elapsed, provided that the serum drug concentrations had been regularly monitored.

According to the results of the initial studies, patients were subjected to burr-hole electrocorticography. The technique consisted in introducing several uni- or multi-electrode probes through a single (or bilateral) burr hole into the subarachnoid space, and guiding them with the aid of radioscopical imaging to the problem areas previously selected by the non-invasive studies. The ECoG ictal and interictal recordings were carefully studied to determine the area of the cortex which was the origin of the seizures. This sometimes required the introduction of a new series of cortical electrodes directed to the problematic areas. The search for the most probable area where the focus could be located was guided by a computer-assisted method based on the mathematical model of dipole generators as has been previously reported[1].

When evidence existed that a certain cortical area was responsible of the epileptic activity, deep multicontact electrodes were stereotactically introduced to the area in order to accurately localize and estimate the size of the focus.

Those patients with a localized small focus received a radiosurgical session with a total dose of 10–20 Gy from a cobalt source, following a technique already described[2]. Only one patient received bilateral irradiation because of a right temporal focus and a contralateral kindling. Two patients with cortical foci of presumed greater extent were irradiated with electrons of 10–15 Mev from a 45 Me betatron, giving 10 Gy with only one entrance, and another patient received two fractions of 10 Gy from the cobalt source.

Patients continued receiving their anti-epileptic medication for one year after radiosurgery, and then it was progressively tapered off when possible.

Results

Of the eleven cases, four ceased to have seizures and are now medication free. In five additional cases, there was a marked reduction in the number of seizures. In two cases there was no change.

Seizures began to improve after a period ranging between 2.5 months and one year, and stabilization of the improvement ocurred progressively after three months to four years.

There were two exceptions to this general rule: in one case with up to 25 crises per day, and receiving toxic doses of anticonvulsants, there was a complete cessation of seizures, ocurring steeply during the 21 ensuing days after irradiation with 20 Gy. This patient reduced the medication suddenly, and the seizures occurred again with a frequency of one to five per day. After anticonvulsant stabilization, there has been an overall reduction of the crises to 12 per month. The other case had complete cessation of seizures for six days after radiosurgery, and then they returned again with less frequency and intensity than before, achieving a 75% reduction in seizure frequency.

No complications were observed, even in those cases in whom the focus was located near eloquent areas of the brain.

Discussion

As the use of stereotactic radiosurgery is gaining ground, the number of reports indicating the beneficial effects on seizures is increasing[4,7,10,12,13]. Furthermore[2], in addition to our report some have appeared about the application of radiosurgery specifically for

relief of epilepsy[6]. Although the number of cases already treated is too small to draw conclusions, some features about how radiosurgery affects seizures can be outlined: First, the doses used are very low (10–20 Gy). Maybe this is the reason for the absence of side-effects due to irradiation toxicity. Second, these low doses have proved effective for epileptogenic activity suppresion, so a selective effect over the epileptic neurons can be thought of. Third, the effects are delayed in time and appear progressively. In our series, seizures began to decrease after 2.5 months to one year, and stabilization of the improvement occurred progressively after three months to four years. In the case reported by Heikkinen et al.[6], frequency of seizures decreased two months after the treatment and disappeared after seven months.

All these features support the hypothesis that a long-term, structural effect is induced by irradiation on the epileptic focus. Experimental studies in a model of chronic epilepsy in the cat[3] suggest that this change is related to an effect on the local synaptic plasticity, probably associated with a decrease of the gliosis normally found in the focus, since the glia, specially the reactive one, is more sensitive to irradiation than the neurons. However, a direct effect on the neurons, preferentially on the pathologic ones, cannot be ruled out.

The main difficulty we have found in this series has been the correct localization of the epileptogenic focus, specially as the irradiated volume is very small. In fact, the two cases with poor results have been related to difficulties in locating the focus. In one of these cases, the target was selected according to an image of temporal gliosis seen on the MR image, instead of relying on the electrocorticographic findings. The failure in these cases reminds of the fact that the epileptogenic area is not located at the lesion, but in the cerebral tissue around it, and stresses the importance of obtaining a good electrophysiological localization. In the future, non-invasive localization procedures such as magneto-encephalography may be the ideal complement for this bloodless treatment method[10].

The lack of secondary effects achieved by this low-dose irradiation may indicate its use in foci located very close to eloquent areas of the brain.

References

1. Barcia-Salorio JL, Barcia JA, Ciudad J, *et al* (1987) Automatic calculation of epileptogenic focus location within the brain. Appl Neurophysiol 50: 600–603

2. Barcia-Salorio JL, Roldán P, Hernández G, *et al* (1985) Radiosurgical treatment of epilepsy. Appl Neurophysiol 48: 400–403

3. Barcia-Salorio JL, Vanaclocha V, Cerdá M, *et al* (1988) Response of experimental epileptic focus to focal ionizing radiation. Appl Neurophysiol 50: 359–364

4. DeRiu PL, Rocca A (1988) Interstitial irradiation therapy of supratentorial gliomas by stereotaxic technique. Long-term results. Ital J Neurol Sci 9: 243–248

5. Fabrikant JI, Lyman JT, Hosobuchi Y (1984) Stereotactic heavy-ion bragg peak radiosurgery for intracranial vascular disorders: method for treatment of deep arteriovenous malformations. Br J Radiol 57: 479–490

6. Heikkinen ER, Heikkinen MI, Sotaniemi K (1992) Stereotactic radiotherapy instead of conventional epilepsy surgery. A case report. Acta Neurochir (Wien) 119: 159–160

7. Heikkinen ER, Konnov B, Melnikov L, *et al* (1989) Relief of epilepsy by radiosurgery of cerebral arteriovenous malformations. Stereotact Funct Neurosurg 53: 157–166

8. Kjellberg RN, Davis KR, Lyons S, *et al* (1983) Bragg peak proton beam therapy for arteriovenous malformations of the brain. Clin Neurosurg 31: 248–290

9. Lance JW, Smee RI (1989) Partial seizures with visual disturbance treated by radiotherapy of cavernous angioma. Ann Neurol 26: 782–785

10. Lindquist C, Kihlström L, Hellstrand E (1992) Functional neurosurgery-a future for the gamma knife? Stereotact Funct Neurosurg 57: 72–81

11. Rossi GF (1985) Epileptogenic cerebral low grade tumours: effect of interstitial stereotactic irradiation on seizures. Appl Neurophysiol 48: 127–132

12. Steinberg GK, Fabrikant JI, Marks MP, *et al* (1991) Stereotactic helium Bragg-peak radiosurgery for intracranial arteriovenous malformations. Detailed clinical and neuroradiological outcome. Stereotact Funct Neurosurg 57: 36–49

13. Steiner L, Lindquist C, Adler J, *et al* (1992) Clinical outcome of radiosurgery for cerebral arteriovenous malformations. J Neurosurg 77: 1–8

Correspondence: Juan A. Barcia, M.D., Servicio de Neurocirugía, Hospital Clínico Universitario, Av. Blasco Ibáñez 17, 46010 Valencia, Spain.

Acta Neurochir (1994) [Suppl] 62: 114–117
© Springer-Verlag 1994

Application of Stereotactic Radiosurgery to the Head and Neck Region

C. Bajada, M. Selch, A. De Salles, St. Goetsch, G. Juillard, T. Solberg, and **R. Parker**

Department of Radiation Oncology, UCLA Medical Center, Los Angeles, CA, U.S.A.

Summary

Nasopharyngeal carcinoma recurrent following primary radiation therapy has been treated with surgery and reirradiation. Reirradiation is often limited by the tolerance of structures previously treated. Radiosurgery was used to boost the recurrent site while avoiding critical structures.

Seven patients were evaluated for treatment. Three patients met requirements for treatment. The lesions invaded the parapharyngeal region, the base of skull, cavernous sinus, cranial nerves, or carotid artery. Treatment included a radiosurgery boost utilizing multiple isocenters, noncoplanar arcs, and arc weighting, to yield a plan conforming to the tumors while avoiding critical anatomical structures.

The patients tolerated the procedure well with minor acute side effects. Follow-up included magnetic resonance imaging (MRI) and positron emission tomography (PET). Two lesions responded, and one had no significant change. One patient had a regional recurrence. Two patients had distance recurrence. Long term side effects include trismus, parotiditis, ear fullness, hemorrhage, and pain.

Radiosurgery may improve the local control rate of such lesions, however, with the severe long term complications of single fraction radiosurgery in the head and neck region this procedure may be more beneficial if the treatment is fractionated.

Keywords: Stereotactic radiosurgery; head and neck; carcinoma.

Introduction

Reirradiation of recurrent nasopharyngeal carcinoma to dose in excess of 60 Gray (Gy) results in 5 and 10 year survival rates of 45% and 39% respectively for patients with lesions confined to one or two walls of the nasopharynx $(T_1–T_2)$[8,23,24]. Lesions extending to the nasal cavity, oropharynx, and/or invading the base of skull or cranial nerves $(T_3–T_4)$[1] have a 5 year survival of 15%[23]. The tolerance of previously irradiated critical structures often prevents delivery of an adequate dose of further radiation therapy. A technique able to provide safe delivery of an effective radiation dose while sparing sensitive tissues may enhance the therapeutic ratio for this group of patients.

A 5 year survival rate of 40–45% has been obtained with combined transpalatal resection and radiation therapy[6,7,21]. However, the procedure is better suited for selected small lesions. Lesions extending to the base of the skull are difficult to completely resect[6,7,21]. Concomitant radiation therapy and chemotherapy for recurrent nasopharygeal carcinoma has been compared to the treatment with radiation alone, however, the results are controversial. Chemotherapy appears to decrease the incidence of distant metastases and to increase disease-free survival, however, no randomized trial has been conducted[4,19]. Tannock has reported high tumor remission but no increase is survival[18]. Afterloading intracavitary radiation has been used to add further local treatment, however, the dose distribution has limited the number of amenable tumors[20].

This report describes the application of linear accelerator-based stereotactic radiosurgery to the head and neck region. Delivery of single-dose radiation while sparing vital surrounding structures is shown to be possible. Radiosurgery techniques were used to treat three patients with recurrent nasopharyngeal carcinoma extending along the pharyngeal wall.

Materials and Methods

Patients

Seven patients were evaluated between August 1992 and November 1992 for radiosurgery boost following radiation therapy for recurrent nasopharyngeal carcinoma. The average time to recurrence was 122 months +/− 64 months. All patients were evaluated with an MRI scan, PET scan, and biopsy[3]. Four patients did not meet requirements for treatment. One lesion was too extensive, and was treated with interstitial therapy, one lesion was negative one PET scan and biopsy, one lesion was reported as hemorrhage on MRI and biopsy, and one patient medically was not a candidate for radiosurgery.

Three patients met requirements for treatment. The average volume of the lesions was 32.0 cc +/− 8.2 cc. Two lesions were parapharyngeal, one invaded the base of skull and the other invaded the carotid artery. The third lesion extended into the cavernous sinus.

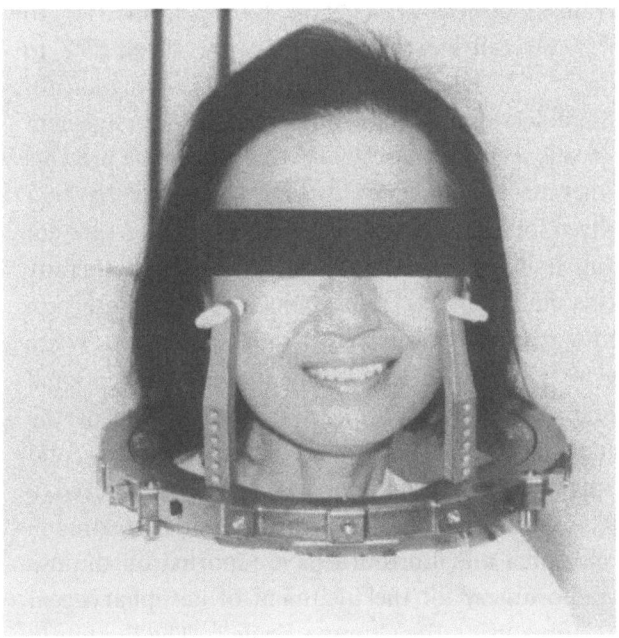

Fig. 1. Stereotactic BRW frame attached to the zygomatic and occipital bones allows for treatment to the head and neck region

Technique

A Brown–Roberts–Wells (BRW) (Radionics, Inc., Burlington, MA, USA) stereotactic frame was attached to the zygoma and occipital bone as shown in Fig. 1. The tumors were localized by CT and MRI.

Scans underwent volumetric and multiplanar reconstruction for detailed analysis of the tumor anatomical relationships. The stereotactic radiosurgery plan, Fig. 2, was developed using a Philips SRS 200 software system (Philips Medical Systems, Shelton, CN, USA). Radiation beams crossing the eyes and air cavities were avoided. When a proposed arc was observed to cross through an air cavity it was manually altered as in Fig. 3. Doses to critical structures were monitored (Table 1). The treatment was delivered by a Clinac 18 (Varian, Palo, Alto, CA, USA). The patients were discharged home the same day of treatment. Follow-up MRI and PET scans are performed at two month intervals.

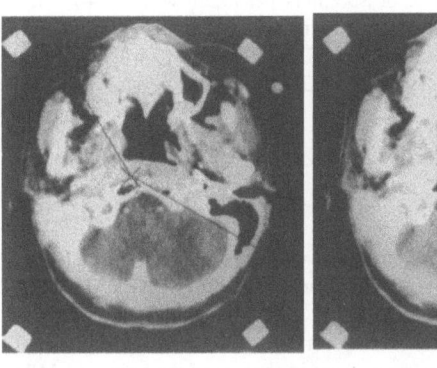

a   b

Fig. 3. Treatment with six isocenters and 21 noncoplanar arcs. Arcs were designed to avoid the air cavities. This prevents an overdose that can occur when photons pass through air cavities, which in this example would have caused an overdose in the brain stem. (a) An inappropriate arc, (b) modification of the arc to avoid air cavities

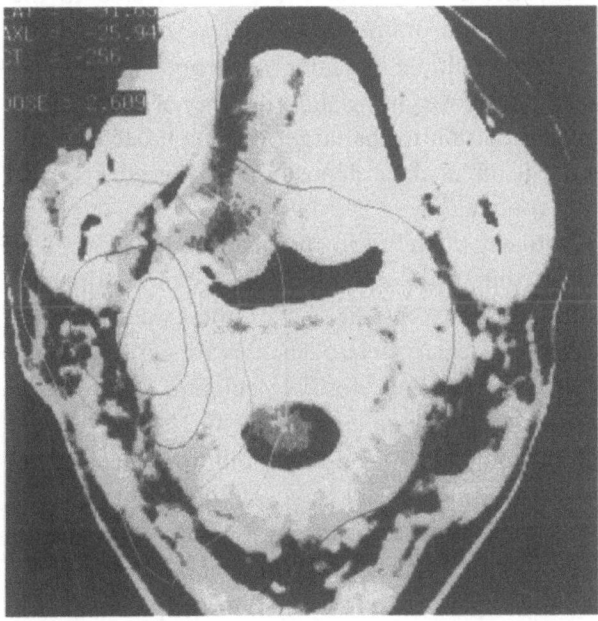

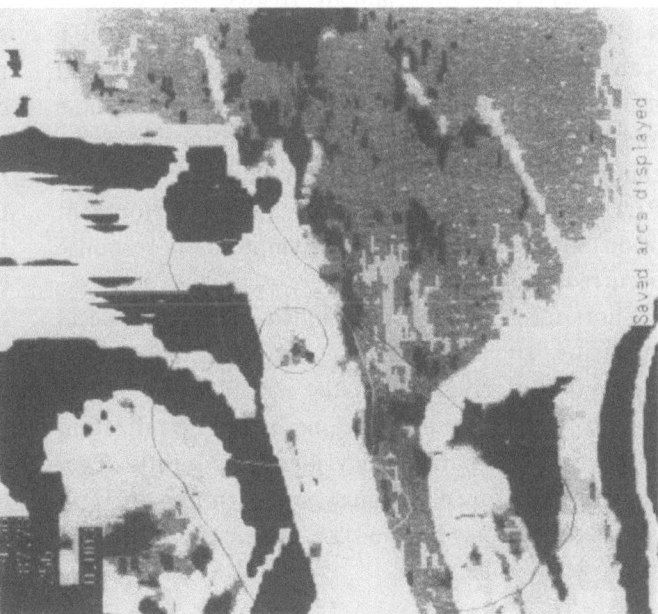

a   b

Fig. 2. (a) axial, (b) sagittal views of the treatment volume. The tumor was completely encompassed by the 50% isodose line. From the center of the isodose curves outward the lines represent 70%, 50%, 30%, 20%, and 10% for axial image and 70%, 50%, 20%, and 10% for sagittal image of the total dose prescribed to the lesion

Table 1 *Average Dose to Critical Structures Surrounding the Tumor*

Structure	Isodose line	Dose (cGy)
Spinal cord	10–30%	400–1200
Brain stem	0–10%	0–400
Carotid artery	30–50%	1200–2000
Mandible	10–50%	400–2000

Radiosurgery Planning

The average number of isocenters per lesion was 5.3 +/− 0.6, utilizing 20.3 +/− 0.6 arcs per treatment. The prescription dose was 20 Gy to an isodose line of 53.3% +/− 5.8% which yields a maximum dose 37.8 Gy +/− 3.9 Gy. Collimator sizes ranged from 20 mm to 32 mm.

Follow-up

All patients were followed with physical examination including flexible fiberoptic nasopharyngoscopy monthly. MRI and PET imaging was done at three month intervals. Response was defined as decrease in size of lesion and decrease in PET ratio. No significant change was defined as no increase in the size of the lesion on MRI imaging. Regional recurrence was appearance of lesion on PET or MRI scan outside of the prescribed treatment volume, within close proximity of the lesion. Distant recurrence occurred in the neck.

Results

Follow-up time ranged from 6–9 months (x = 7.3 +/− 1.5) for the three patients treated. Two patients had a response in the area treated on MRI and PET scan imaging. One of these patients had a regional recurrence outside of the prescribed treatment volume and in the neck. The third patient had no significant change in the lesion on MRI scan and had decreased PET scan ratios in the treated area with development of distant failure in the neck. Symptomatic response occurred in one patient.

Short term side effects included ipsilateral buccal mucositis, and ear fullness. Long term side effects included hemorrhage from the nasopharynx in one patient, which required packing and hospitalization to control. All patients developed parotiditis. Two patients developed trismus, one with pain and complete closure of the jaw requiring a feeding gastrostomy tube.

Discussion

Radiation therapy as primary treatment for nasopharyngeal carcinoma achieves a 5 year survival rate of 37% to 62%[2,5,9,14,15,22]. Local recurrence rates for advanced disease ($T_3T_4N_0N_+$) vary from 31% to 46%[2]. Overall local control rates vary from 56% to 69%[13,14,16]. Uncontrolled lesions cause significant cranial nerve palsy, pain, and epistaxis. Management of locally recurrent nasopharyngeal carcinoma presents a therapeutic challenge. Surgical resection is best utilized for limited stage recurrences[7,21]. Retreatment using fractionated external beam radiation therapy yields similar survival rates to that of surgical resection for limited stage disease, if doses greater than 60 Gy are given[8,23]. However, retreatment with conventional therapy includes anatomical structures such as the spinal cord, brain stem, mandible, carotid artery, and cranial nerves which may have already received a maximum dose of radiation in the initial treatment. Kondziolka and Lunsford have reported on the use of radiosurgery for the treatment of nasopharyngeal carcinoma using the Gamma Knife[11]. The limitation found with the Gamma Knife is that the interior extent of the tumor can not extend beyond the foramen magnum. The BRW radiosurgery system allows frame placement on the zygoma which can extend the inferior aspect of the treatment field to the level of the C5 vertebral body.

This pilot study shows the possibility of using radiosurgery for the treatment of recurrent nasopharyngeal carcinoma. The benefit of radiosurgery over boosting with interstitial brachytherapy appears to be better control over the dose delivered to the spinal cord and brainstem as well as a less invasive procedure. Multiple isocenters, noncoplanar arcs and differential arc weighting allow delivery of a high single dose of radiation to the target volume because of the rapid fall off in dose deposition at the edge of the target volume[10,12].

Treatment planning in the head and neck area is complex due to the optic structures and multiple air cavities. Beams crossing air cavities were avoided because low density heterogeneities are not accounted for in the current dose calculation algorithms. Treatment through an air cavity with 10 MV photons can lead to as much as a three-fold dose increase up to two centimeters outside of the field[17]. This miscalculation may lead to a critical overdoes of the spinal cord or brain stem. Avoidance of air cavities when treating head and neck tumors requires the use of multiple isocenters and differential arc weighting.

This report shows the feasibility of treating large T_4 lesions in the nasopharynx. The follow-up of these patients is too short to ascertain survival advantage with the treatment. The side effects, hemmorhage and trismus from single fraction therapy through the soft tissues of the head and neck region were severe. Stereotactic techniques in this region are ideal secondary to the spinal cord tolerance to radiation therapy, however, it would appear from the side effects seen in this pilot study that the dose should be fractionated. This would allow for a higher dose to the tumor bed to be given while limiting the dose to the surrounding critical structures. The development of fractionated stereotactic radiation therapy protocols may play an important role in the therapy of these tumors.

References

1. American Joint Committee for Cancer Staging and End Results Reporting (1978) Manual for Staging of Cancer. The American Joint Committee, Chicago
2. Bailet JW, Mark RJ, Abemayor E, et al (1992) Nasopharyngeal carcinoma: treatment results with primary radiation therapy. Laryngoscope 102: 965–972
3. Chaiken L, Rege S, Hoh C, et al (1992) Positron emission tomography with fluorodeoxyglucose to evaluate tumor response and control after radiation therapy. Abstract Int J Radiat Oncol Biol Phys 24: 172
4. Decker DA, Drelichman A, Al-Sarraf M, et al (1983) Chemotherapy for nasopharyngeal carcinoma. A ten year experience Cancer 52: 602–605
5. Dickson RL, Flores AD (1985) Nasopharyngeal carcinoma: an evaluation of 134 patients treated between 1971–1980. Laryngoscope 95: 276–283
6. Fee WE (1990) Nasopharyngeal carcinoma. Curr Opin Oncol 2: 585–588
7. Fee WE, Gilmer PA, Goffinet DR (1988) Surgical management of recurrent nasopharyngeal carcinoma after failure at the primary site. Laryngoscope 98: 1220–1226
8. Fu KK, Newman H, Phillipa TL (1975) Treatment of locally recurrent carcinoma of the nasopharynx. Radiology 117: 425–431
9. Hoppe RT, Goffinet DR, Bagshaw MA (1976) Carcinoma of the nasopharynx: eighteen years experience with megavoltage. Cancer 37: 2605–2612
10. Kaplan ID, Adler JR, Hicks WL, et al (1992) Radiosurgery for palliation of base of skull recurrences from head and neck cancer. Cancer 70: 7: 1980–1984
11. Kondziolka D, Lunsford D (1991) Stereotactic radiosurgery for squamous cell carcinoma of the nasopharynx. Laryngoscope 101: 519–522
12. Kooy HM, Nedzi LA, Loeffler JS, et al (1991) Treatment planning for stereotactic radiosurgery of intracranial lesions. Int J Radiat Oncol Biol Phys 21: 683–693
13. Mesic JB, Fletcher GH, Goepfert H (1981) Megavoltage irradiation of epithelial tumors of the nasopharynx. Int J Radiat Oncol Biol Phys 7: 447–453
14. Meyer JE, Wang CC (1971) Cancer of the nasopharynx: factors influencing results of therapy. Radiology 100: 385–388
15. Monench HC, Philips TL (1972) Carcinoma of the nasopharynx: review of 146 patients with emphasis of radiation dose and time factors. An J Surg 124: 515–518
16. Schabinger PR, Reddy S, Hendrickson FR (1985) Carcinoma of the nasopharynx: Survival and patterns of recurrence. Int J Radiat Oncol Biol Phys 11: 2081–2084
17. Solberg TD, Holly FE, Wallace RE, et al (1992) Small field dose perturbation by heterogeneous material. Med Phys 19: 791
18. Tannock I, Payne D, Cummings B, et al (1987) Sequential chemotherapy and radiation for nasopharynx cancer: absence of long term benefit despite high rate of tumor response to chemotherapy. J Clin Oncol 5: 629–634
19. Teo PT, Ho JHC, Choy DD, et al (1987) Adjunctive chemotherapy to radical radiation therapy in the treatment of advanced nasopharyngeal carcinoma. Int J Radiat Oncol Biol Phys 13: 679–685
20. Teo P, Tsao SY, Leung SF (1989) Afterloading intracavitary radiation treatment of nasopharyngeal carcinoma: description of a technique and preliminary treatment results. Acta Oncol 28: 525–527
21. Tu GY, Hu YH, Xu GZ, Ye M (1988) Salvage surgery for nasopharyngeal carcinoma. Arch Otolaryngeal Head neck Surg 114: 328–329
22. Vikram B, Strong EW, Manolatoss S, et al (1984) Improved survival in carcinoma of the nasopharynx. Head Neck Surg 7: 123–128
23. Wang CC (1987) Re-irradiation of recurrent nasopharyngeal carcinoma treatment techniques and results. Int J Radiat Oncol Biol Phys 13: 953–956
24. Wang CC, Shultz (1966) Management of locally recurrent carcinoma of the nasopharynx. Radiology 86: 5: 900–903

Correspondence: Cynthia Lee Bajada, M.D., Department of Radiation Oncology, UCLA Medical Center, 200 Medical Plaza, B-265, Los Angeles, California 90024, U.S.A.

Acta Neurochir (1994) [Suppl] 62: 118–123
© Springer-Verlag 1994

Stereotactic Radiotherapy: A Technique for Dose Optimization and Escalation for Intracranial Tumors*

D. C. Shrieve, N. J. Tarbell, E. Alexander III, H. M. Kooy, P. McL. Black, S. Dunbar, and **J. S. Loeffler**

Stereotactic Radiotherapy/Radiosurgery Center, Brigham and Women's Hospital, Children's Hospital, Joint Center for Radiation Therapy and the Departments of Radiation Oncology and Surgery (Neurosurgery), Harvard Medical School, Boston, MA, U.S.A.

Summary

Stereotactic radiosurgery offers the ability to treat relatively small volume intracranial lesions with single fraction, high dose radiotherapy while sparing surrounding tissue due to rapid fall off of dose outside of the treatment volume. Conventional radiotherapy takes advantage of the sparing effects of dose fractionation, but includes relatively large amounts of normal brain in the treatment volume the tolerance of which is dose-limiting. For some intracranial lesions it may not be optimal to treat with large single fractions due to tumor location or size. Conventional fractionated radiotherapy may not be optimum in all cases due to the necessary inclusion of normal structures. Through the development of relocatable head frames, the precision of stereotactic techniques and the biologic advantages of fractionation may be combined in stereotactic radiotherapy (SRT).

We report on the treatment of 68 patients with intracranial lesions using a dedicated stereotactic linear accelerator to deliver SRT between June 1992 and June 1993. SRT was used either in order to optimize dose distribution and spare normal tissues in patients with excellent prognosis or in order to increase the dose to tumor while keeping doses to normal tissues below tolerance levels in patients with poorer prognosis (dose escalation). Histologies treated included meningioma, low grade astrocytoma, pituitary adenoma and acoustic neuroma. The most common treatment sites were the parasellar region and cavernous sinuses. Most patients (79%) had surgical debulking prior to SRT. 10–12 patients were treated daily. Patient positioning using relocatable stereotactic frames was highly precise.

Acute and subacute side effects were minimal and radiographic responses have been similar to those expected with conventional radiotherapy. There have been no marginal failures or cranial neuropathies reported. Neurocognitive and neuroendocrine follow up will provide important information regarding the advantages of SRT over conventional radiotherapy. In addition, further patient accrual and follow up will provide information regarding rates and patterns of recurrence following SRT.

Keywords: Stereotactic radiotherapy; brain tumors; radiosurgery.

*This work is sponsored in part by a grant from the National Institute of Health (NIH 1P2ONS3110-01).

Introduction

Radiotherapy (RT) plays a central role in the treatment of intracranial neoplasms. Although some central nervous system (CNS) malignancies are focal in nature, the majority infiltrate the surrounding brain parenchyma[10]. Conventional radiation fields, therefore, must include not only the tumor bed (tumor volume) but also tissue felt to be at risk for microscopic disease. Additional normal tissue volume must be included to allow for uncertainty in tumor definition and inconsistency in daily treatment set up (target volume). A significant volume of normal tissue is therefore included in the irradiated volume using standard techniques. Because of this, the tolerance of the normal brain parenchyma and its vascular and supportive structures limits the dose of radiation that may be safely delivered. Potential long-term effects of cranial RT include permanent cranial nerve damage, hypothalamic-pituitary dysfunction, loss of memory and deficits in intellectual ability[9,18]. White matter tends to be more sensitive to the effects of RT than gray matter, and young children (less than two years of age), in whom myelination is incomplete, are known to be at greater risk than adults[2,6]. Late effects appear in a predictable manner in terms of daily RT dose, total dose and volume of tissue irradiated.

The use of stereotactic radiosurgery (SRS) to reduce the volume of normal tissue irradiated in patients with benign, radioresponsive tumors (e.g., pituitary adenoma, craniopharyngioma, acoustic neurinoma, meningioma, optic glioma) has been advocated. Recent clinical experience with SRS indicates that the risk of normal tissue complications following SRS is closely correlated with the size and location of the target volume[13,14]. The tolerance of the optic nerve, for example, is 800–1000 cGy. Hearing loss can be expected when a greater than 1 cm segment of cranial nerve VIII receives >1500 cGy[4]. Severe complication rates of >35% have been reported following radiosurgery for benign meningioma[3].

Through the delivery of multiple small daily doses (fractionation) both acute and late normal tissue effects of RT may be kept to a minimum. With conventional fractionation schedules (180–200 cGy per day), total doses of up to 6000 cGy are well tolerated for limited intracranial fields. Sheline *et al.*[16] have shown that frank radiation necrosis is a function of total dose and fraction size with threshold doses of approximately 4500 cGy in 10 fractions; 6000 cGy in 35 fractions; and 7000 cGy in 60 fractions, respectively. Thus, small volumes, low daily doses, and multiple fractions decrease the overall incidence of late effects associated with conventional external beam therapy.

Fractionated RT administers a high cumulative dose to the target volume in multiple treatments extending over several weeks. Compared to single large doses of radiation (i.e., radiosurgery), fractionation spares both early (e.g., tumor) and late (e.g., normal brain) responding tissues; that is, larger total doses are required to achieve a given effect as the number of fractions is increased. However, the magnitude of this sparing effect of fractionation is much larger in late responding tissues than in early responding tissues. Fractionation magnifies the difference between normal and tumor tissue response to radiation and allows a higher effective *tumor* dose to be delivered for the same level of risk to *normal brain*[19].

Until recently, the precision of conventional RT has been limited by inadequate diagnostic definition of tumor volumes, lack of sophisticated treatment planning systems, and unreliable patient immobilization devices. CT and MRI scans now provide much improved definition of CNS neoplasms and treatment planning systems that utilize the three dimensional information provided by these imaging studies are available. These technological advances allow for the precise administration of radiation dose to the target without delivering significant dose to surrounding normal structures. The availability of these technologies has led to stereotactic radiosurgery (SRS, the delivery of a single large radiation dose to a small volume) becoming increasingly accessible to brain tumor patients and their physicians. With SRS, normal tissue effects are minimized by the inclusion of the minimum amount of normal tissue in the high dose volume.

For some primary intracranial neoplasms, neither the irradiation of large volumes of normal tissue with conventional RT nor the delivery of a single large radiation dose with SRS seem optimal. It is now possible to combine the advantages of conventional fractionation with the accurate and focal distribution of radiation achieved with SRS in a treatment technique referred to as stereotactic radiotherapy (SRT). The following describes the technique used to deliver SRT and the early experience with SRT at the Brigham and Women's Hospital.

Methods and Materials

A dedicated stereotactic facility opened at the Brigham and Women's Hospital (BWH) in June 1992. Between June 1992 and June 1993 68 patients have completed therapy with SRT. A modified form of the original Gill Thomas Frame[5], the GTC III frame, (Radionics Inc., Burlington, MA) was used for SRT. Stabilization of the head was provided by an acrylic oral appliance individually constructed for each patient. The appliance is amalgamated into a plastic tray which attaches either directly to the anterior portion of the base ring or to a metal extender plate of which there are three sizes to accommodate various head diameters. Posterior support was provided by an individually molded silicon head-rest fixed to a plastic tray, which fits over the occipital protuberance and firmly attaches to the base ring by two upright aluminium bars. The anterior portion of the base ring slides forward and is locked into place by bilateral locking rods. Once the base ring is locked, it is secured to the head by one posterior and two lateral Velcro straps; the anterior portion of the strap system is constructed of spandex which conforms to the frontal region. The GTC III is easily mounted within 2 to 3 minutes and is well tolerated. Thus far, the frame has been used on adults and children ages 6 and above. With added experience and modifications, there has been improved versatility in fitting the frame to anatomic variations. Even edentulous patients can be accommodated.

In order to assure reproducibility, once the frame is securely fit, a depth confirmation helmet is placed onto the base ring and a set of 25 helmet-to-scalp measurement is obtained. These are repeated at subsequent fittings and before daily treatment for comparison to the baseline measurements. Reproducibility of individual measurements between fittings is within 0.5 mm.

Children under 6 years of age, generally require anesthesia for treatment planning and daily stereotactic therapy. In order to provide full access to the airway in the event of desaturation or aspiration during treatment, fixation by means other than a dental appliance is required (Boston Children's Frame, BCF). A set of plastic ear plugs is custom fashioned for each patient and attached to the base ring by means of an upright bar. An individually molded silicon form of the glabellar-nasion region is held in place by an aluminum face mask. This is also attached to the halo by the lateral bars, and provides further stabilization of the head position. The modified base ring is also compatible with the depth confirmation helmet and verification of repositioning is based on multiple sets of scalp measurements with the same accuracy used for the standard GTC frame.

Following custom frame-fitting, patients undergo a CT scan with the frame and fiducial markers in place. In addition, MRI information may be merged with the CT information using image fusion techniques. This is especially crucial in cases of low-grade, non-enhancing astrocytomas and acoustic neuromas, which are not well evaluated by CT.

The X-Knife version 2 software is used for planning (Radionics, Burlington, MA). Treatments were delivered with a Varian series 600 SR prototype linear accelerator (6 mV) (Varian, Palo Alto, CA). Each daily treatment was delivered in multiple non-coplanar arcs. Circular collimators ranging in diameter from 5–50 mm are available. Cumulative doses ranged from 4500 to 6000 cGy using conventional fraction sizes of 180 to 200 cGy using 6 MV photons. Tumor volumes ranged from 0.57 to 38.7 cc (median 8.2 cc) and were treated with 17.5 mm to 50 mm collimators. To avoid significant tumor dose inhomogeneity, one isocenter was used for each patient and normalization ranged from 90–95%.

Patients treated for histologies that are well controlled by standard doses of radiotherapy entered the dose optimization arm, intended to limit the volume of normal tissue irradiated. Those treated for histologies with five year control rates of 50% or less were entered on the dose escalation arm. The dose escalation study allows for a 10% increase in dose for the first two years of the study. For example, low grade astrocytomas receive 6000 cGy rather than the standard 5400 cGy.

Endpoints of particular interest are neuroendocrine function, cranial neuropathies and patterns of failure for the dose optimization arm and survival and patterns of failure for the dose escalation arm.

Results

Sixty-eight patients have completed treatment. A total of 1876 treatment fractions have been delivered. Patients ranged in age from 9 months to 76 years. The most common histologies were meningioma (17), low grade astrocytoma (15) and pituitary adenoma (13) (Table 1). The most common treatment sites were the parasellar and cavernous sinus regions (31) and brainstem (7) (Table 2). Fifty-four patients (79%) were treated following surgical debulking.

Sixty-three patients were treated using the modified GTC III frame while 5 children were treated using the BCF. More than 2000 sets of helmet-to-scalp measurements (>45,000 individual readings) have been made on treatment patients as well as volunteers. Reproducibility of these measurements is within 0.5 mm (H. Kooy, personal communication).

45/68 (66%) were treated on the dose optimization arm, 16/68 (24%) on the dose escalation arm, and the remaining seven patients were treated off study for various reasons. Many of these patients were initially considered for or referred for SRS. The reasons for using SRT rather than SRS were the following: location only – 23 patients, volume only – 19 patients, both volume and location – 26 patients.

The radiographic response following SRT has been similar to that seen following conventional fractionated RT (Table 3, Fig. 1). Since most benign tumors (e.g., meningiomas, pituitary adenomas) respond slowly to RT, many years of follow-up will be needed to determine rates of control in these tumors and comparison with patterns of failure seen following standard RT. There have been no marginal recurrences seen to date.

Acute toxicity has been minimal. Temporary alopecia occurred in 5 patients with superficial tumors; minor headache and fatigue was reported by 16 patients. Among 28 patients with tumors within the cerebellar-pontine angle or cavernous sinus, there have been no

Table 1. *Histologies Treated with SRT*

Histology	Number of patients
Astrocytoma	20
Meningioma	16
Pituitary adenoma	14
Acoustic neurinoma	4
Craniopharyngioma	5
Germinoma	2
Oligodendroglioma	2
Retinoblastoma	1
Malignant teratoma	1
Chordoma	1
Rhabdomyosarcoma	1
Endodermal sinus tumor	1
Total	68

Table 2. *Location of 68 Lesions Treated with SRT*

Location	Number of patients
Parasellar	23
Cavernous sinus	8
Brainstem	7
Cerebellar-pontine angle	5
Thalamus	5
Clivus	5
Deep white matter	5
Motor cortex	5
Orbit	3
Pineal region	2
Middle ear	1
Total	68

Table 3. *Radiographic Response Following SRT*

Response	Number of patients
Stable	47
Decreased	15
Not evaluable	4[a]
Increased	2[b]
Total	68

[a] Patients had no radiographic evidence of tumor at time of SRT.

[b] Patients with pilocytic astrocytoma had enlarging cyst formation, but decreased enhancing tumors volume. Subsequently both cysts have decreased in size.

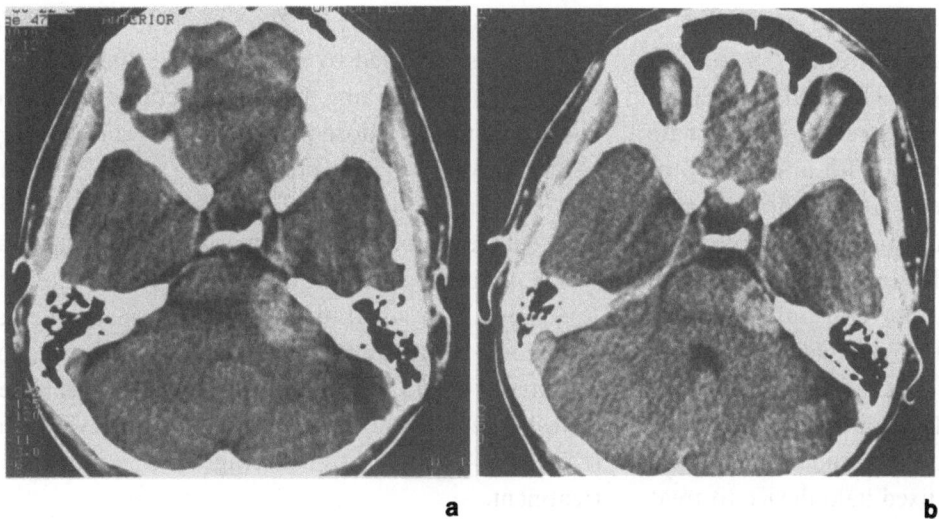

Fig. 1. Mri scan of patient with acoustic neurinoma recurrent following surgery. (a) At time of SRT and (b) 1 year following SRT

new cranial neuropathies with a median follow-up of 9 months.

Discussion

A key component of SRT is a reliably precise relocatable immobilization device. There are several relocatable frame systems currently available. The Laitinen head frame is based on fixation by means of ear plugs and a nasion support[12]. A study by Hariz et al.[8] has shown a high degree of reproducibility using this device for stereotactic biopsy and for fractionated therapy limited to 2 to 5 treatments. Delanes et al.[1] used the Laitinen device and also reported accurate relocatability. The authors found that in relation to a hypothetical intracranial target, differences in scalp measurements between separate mountings were within 1 mm. The Gill-Thomas II frame is another non-invasive, well tolerated option which provides accurate repositioning[5]. The aluminium base ring, developed at the Neurosurgical Unit of The National Hospital, London, is stabilized by an oral appliance and is compatible with the BRW neurosurgical frame. In testing the frame for use, Graham et al.[7] found mean anterior to posterior and mean lateral displacements of 1 mm with multiple repositionings on phantoms and volunteers. The device can be positioned within a reasonable time, worn without significant complaints, and easily adapted for individual use at reasonable cost. In addition to being accurately repositioned, the authors further commented that the Gill-Thomas frame is considerably less labor intensive than conventional cellulose acetate casts.

We have used the GTC III frame and the BCF (in children requiring anesthesia) to successfully treat 68 patients with SRT. These frames provide reproducible relocation, are easily mounted in 2–3 minutes and are well tolerated by adults and children over 6 years of age. Daily helmet-to-scalp measurements provide an assessment of each frame positioning to ensure treatment accuracy. Our measurements are in agreement with those of Graham et al.[7], indicating a relocation accuracy of 1 mm, well within the tolerance required.

A small number of institutions are currently treating patients with fractionated irradiation using stereotactic techniques. The vast majority of the published experience, however, utilizes unconventional fractionation schemes of 500–800 cGy fractions (hypofractionation). The primary reason for the investigators doing this type of fractionation was the lack of both an available dedicated radiation facility and non-invasive relocatable stereotactic frames. Normal tissue tolerance is unknown using these hypofractionation schemes and should be considered highly experimental at this time. Prolonged placement of the stereotactic halo provides immobilization in some cases. Other centers are using either the Laitinen or Gill Thomas frame. The experiences and follow up thus far, however, are limited and results preliminary.

Several authors report their experience with protracted use of the invasive stereotactic halo. Souhami et al.[17] also used protracted base ring placement and report on 15 patients treated from May 1987 to August 1989. Histology of the lesions included 7 low grade astrocytomas, 2 meningiomas, and one each of the following: craniopharyngioma, chordoma, subepen-

dymoma, grade III astrocytoma, GBM, and heman-
gioblastoma. Doses administered were prescribed to
the 90% isodose line and ranged from 3780 to 4550
in fractions of 630 to 750 cGy. The field size varied
from 15 to 30 mm. Patients were treated on alternate
days during a two week period. With a follow up of
28 months, 12 of the 15 patients treated showed rapid
improvement clinically within 2 to 3 months following
treatment. Radiographic reduction of tumor size was
more protracted, occurring on average at 7 months.
Patients reportedly adapted to extended halo placement. Although the results are preliminary, the authors
conclude that SRT is a well tolerated approach that
warrants further investigation. Schwade *et al.*[15] used
prolonged placement of the fixed halo device to treat
24 patients between January 1983 and June 1987. The
lesions treated included: 8 pituitary adenomas, 7 low
grade astrocytomas, 4 craniopharyngiomas, 2 glioblastomas, 1 mixed astrocytoma, and 2 lesions of
unknown origin. The doses delivered ranged from
360–6000 cGy in 12 to 31 fractions. The mean treatment time with the invasive frame in place was 40 days
(range 19 to 58 days). With follow up of 7 to 49 months,
15 patients were alive without complications or evidence of disease. Six patients were alive with residual
or recurrent disease 11 to 29 months after treatment.
One patient was alive, but blind presumably secondary
to radiation-induced optic neuropathy. No significant
complications involving the halo were noted. The
patients adapted well to prolonged halo placement.

Delannes *et al.*[1] reported on treatment of 21 patients
from April 1988 to June 1989, using the Laitinen frame.
Of the lesions treated, 15 were benign including 8 AVMs;
the remainder were malignant, including 2 low grade
astrocytomas. Benign and low grade lesions received
3000 cGy in a three week period; neurinomas received
5000 cGy in 5 weeks, and 5500 cGy was administered
to meningiomas over 5 1/2 weeks. The dose per
fraction ranged from 180 to 250 cGy prescribed to 90%
isodose line. The authors report a high degree of
accuracy in both spatial target location and also in
dose delivered to the target volume.

The Gill Thomas frame is being used for fractionated
stereotactic radiotherapy at the Royal Marsden Hospital. Two studies fully describe the non invasive head
fixation system and report on 22 patients treated
with a total of 78 fractions using this device[5,7]. Patient
tolerance is excellent and reproducibility extremely
accurate. Laing *et al.*[11] also reported on a Phase I/II
study of recurrent glioma. Twenty two patients with
unifocal lesions (19 high grade, 3 low grade) were

treated initially with conventional external beam therapy
ranging from 4000 cGy in 20 fractions to 6000 cGy in
33 fractions, followed by stereotactic technique using
the Gill Thomas Frame. Five Gy fractions were used
and the cumulative dose was escalated from 2000 cGy
to 5000 cGy. Doses were prescribed to the 90% isodose
line. The target volume which ranged from 1 cc to 93 cc
included the tumor and a 2 cm margin. Median survival
was 9 months with follow up of 3 to 35 months.
Regression of residual disease was seen in 7 patients.
Functional status was stable in 86% and 75% of
patients at 4 and 6 months, respectively. Steroid re-
sponsive deterioration was seen in 5 patients who had
received > 4000 cGy at an average of 5 months after
treatment.

The series of patients reported on here represents
the experience with SRT at the BWH over the initial
12 months of operation of the dedicated stereotactic
radiotherapy facility. Treatment of these patients has
been integrated into the "routine" daily schedule of
the radiotherapy department. Due to the availability
of the relocatable frames and the dedicated linear
accelerator, up to 10 patients are treated each day.
The accelerator remains available for the one or two
daily radiosurgery cases. The availability of SRT has
created a new and challenging treatment option for
the radiation oncologist and neurosurgeon presented
with a patient with an intracranial tumor. It is felt
that SRT should be limited in use to tumors meeting
the following criteria: 1) Clear radiographic definition
by CT or MRI; 2) relatively small tumor volume; 3)
non-invasive or non-infiltrating. For tumors that are
infiltrative (e.g., malignant astrocytoma) or have a
propensity for neuraxis dissemination (e.g., medulloblastoma), SRT could be considered as a boost for
regions of gross residual disease following conventional
RT to a larger field.

The decision to use stereotactic radiotherapy rather
than radiosurgery can be difficult and controversial.
Tumor volume and location within the intracranial
space are the most important parameters used in this
decision analysis. Specific factors that are considered
in this decision process at the BWH are the following:
1) lesions located less than 5 mm or intrinsic to relatively
sensitive CNS structures (e.g. retina, sensory cranial
nerves including chiasm and optic pathways, brain
stem, motor cortex, speech areas), 2) spherical tumor
volumes with a greatest diameter of 3 cm or more
particularly if located in deep white matter regions, 3)
tumor histologies (e.g. retinoblastoma, craniopharyngioma) that have historically been well controlled with

conventional radiotherapy, but associated with late brain or soft tissue toxicity, and 4) tumor histologies (e.g. acoustic neurinoma, large base of skull meningioma) that have historically been well controlled with radiosurgery, but associated with subacute brain or cranial nerve injury. Our experience to date indicates that by fractionating stereotactic radiotherapy, less subacute and probably less late radiation damage is seen versus radiosurgery.

Stereotactic techniques are not intended to replace large field radiotherapy in the treatment of widely infiltrating or seeding tumors. The developments discussed above have paralleled the recent progress that has been made in conformal radiotherapy techniques for non-intracranial sites (3-D planning, non-coplanar arc therapy, dynamic field shaping). While the ultimate benefits of these novel techniques for our patients will take many years to determine, it is clear that conventional radiotherapy techniques may no longer be the optimal treatment available for a large subgroup of our patients with intracranial tumors.

In summary, the BWH SRT program utilizes a dedicated stereotactic linear accelerator and relocatable head immobilization to treat 10–12 patients each day in addition to 1–2 SRS patients. This compares favorably to existing proton facilities. Significant acute and subacute effects of therapy have not occurred. Mild fatigue and temporary alopecia has been seen in a minority of patients. Radiographic response to SRT appears similar to that seen with conventional RT. No new cases of cranial neuropathy (including hearing loss) has been reported with median follow-up of 9 months. No cases of marginal failure (disease recurring or spreading just outside the target volume) have occurred. Prospective long term neurocognitive and neuroendocrine studies are ongoing and will be required to assess if SRT offers advantages over conventional RT in terms of decreasing morbidity related to loss of endocrine function and intellect in children requiring radiotherapy to intracranial sites.

References

1. Delannes M, Daly NJ, Bonnet J, Sabatier J, Tremoulet M (1991) Fractionated radiotherapy of small inoperable tumors of the brain using a non-invasive stereotactic frame. Int J Radiat Oncol Biol Phys 21: 749–755
2. Ellenberg L, McComb JG, Siegel SE (1987) Factors affecting intellectual outcome in pediatric brain tumor patients. Neurosurgery 21: 638–644
3. Engenhart R, Kimming BN, Hover KH, Wowre B, Strum V, Kaick G, Wannenmacher M (1990) Stereotactic single high dose radiation therapy of benign intracranial meningiomas. Int J Radiat Oncol Biol Phys 19: 1021–1026
4. Flickinger JC, Lunsford LD, Linskey ME, *et al* (1992) Gamma knife radiosurgery for acoustic tumors: Four year results and multivariate analysis of treatment techniques. Int J Radiat Oncol Biol Phys 24: 128
5. Gill SS, Thomas DG, Warrington AP, Brada M (1991) Relocatable frame for stereotactic external beam radiotherapy. Int J radiat Oncol Biol Phys 20: 599–603
6. Glauser TT, Packer RJ (1991) Cognitive deficits in long term survivors of childhood brain tumors. Child Nerv Syst 7: 2–12
7. Graham JD, Warrington AP, Gill SS, Brada M (1991) A non-invasive, relocatable stereotactic frame for fractionated radiotherapy and multiple imaging. Radiother Oncol 21: 60–62
8. Hariz MI, Henriksson R, Lofroth P, Laitinen LV, Saterborg N (1990) A non-invasive method for fractionated stereotactic irradiation of brain tumors with a linear accelerator. Radiother Oncol 17: 57–72
9. Jenkins JS, Gilbert CJ, Ang V (1976) Hypothalamic-pituitary dysfunction in patients with craniopharyngiomas. J Clin Endocrinol Metab 43: 394–399
10. Kelly PJ, Daumas-Duport C, Kispert DB, Kall BA, Scheithauer BW, Illig JJ (1987) Imaging-based stereotaxic serial biopsies in untreated intracranial glial neoplasms. J Neurosurg 66: 865–874
11. Laing RW, Warrington AP, Graham J, Brada M (1992) Fractionated external beam stereotactic radiotherapy (SRT) for recurrent glioma. Int J Radiat Oncol Biol Phys 24: 11
12. Laitinen LV, Liliequist B, Fagerland M, Eriksson AT (1985) An adapter for computer tomography-guided stereotaxis. Surg Neur 23: 559–566
13. Marks LB, Spencer DP (1991) The influence of volume on the tolerance of the brain to radiosurgery. J Neurosurg 75: 177–180
14. Nedzi LA, Koy HM, Alexander E, III, Svensson G, Cheng C-W, Mannarino EG, Loeffler JS (1991) Variables associated with the development of complications form radiosurgery using a standard linear accelerator. Int J Radiat Oncol Biol Phys 21: 591–599
15. Schwade JG, Houdek PV, Landy HJ, Bujnoski JL, Lewin AA, Abitbol A, Serago CF, Pisciotta VJ (1990) Small field stereotactic external beam radiation therapy of intracranial lesions: fractionated treatment with a fixed hal immobilization device. Radiology 176: 563–565
16. Sheline GE, Wara WM, Smith V (1980) therapeutic irradiation and brain injury. Int J Radiat Oncol Biol Phys 6: 1215
17. Souhami L, Olivier A, Podgorsak EB, Villemure JG, Pla M, Sadikot AF (1991) Fractionated stereotactic radiation therapy for intracranial tumors. Cancer 68: 2101–2108
18. Thomsett MJ, Conte FA, Kaplan SC, Grumbach MM (1980) Endocrine and neurologic outcome in childhood craniopharyngioma: review of effect of treatment in 42 patients. J Pediat 97: 728–735
19. Withers HR (1985) Bilogical basis for altered fractionation schemes. Cancer 55: 2086–2095

Correspondence: Dennis C. Shrieve, M.D., Ph.D., Department of Radiation Therapy, Brigham and Women's Hospital, 75 Francis Street, Boston, MA 02115, U.S.A.

Subject Index

Jeremy C. Ganz

Gamma Knife Surgery

A Guide for Referring Physicians

1993. 45 figures. XVII, 163 pages.
Soft cover DM 69,–, öS 485,–
ISBN 3-211-82476-6

Radiosurgery has become an established technique, with more than 15000 patients treated world-wide, most of them in the last five years. Yet, there is much uncertainty in the general medical community as to the nature, advantages and limitations of the method. This uncertainty provokes unnecessary debate between colleagues and is a source of avoidable stress to patients.

This book provides an account of the scientific basis of radiosurgery and describes its current applications in respect of the only well established radiosurgical device, the Leksell Gamma Knife. The book assumes the general medical knowlegde of a newly qualified medical practitioner.

There are three sections. The first outlines the rationale for radiosurgery and the principles of stereotaxy, radiophysics and radiobiology. The middle section, consisting of a single chapter, describes what a potential patient may expect to experience. In the final section, the current applications are gone through, one by one, indicating what can and what cannot be achieved. The book is intended for neurologists, neurosurgeons, internists, otolaryngologists, oncologists, ophthalmologists, general practitioners, medical students and anyone else who might wish to refer a patient to or advise a patient about Gamma Knife radiosurgery.

Prices are subject to change without notice

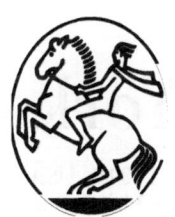

Springer-Verlag Wien New York

Sachsenplatz 4–6, P.O.Box 89, A-1201 Wien · 175 Fifth Avenue, New York, NY 10010, USA
Heidelberger Platz 3, D-14197 Berlin · 3-13, Hongo 3-chome, Bunkyo-ku, Tokyo 113, Japan

B. L. Bauer, D. Hellwig (eds.)

Minimally Invasive Neurosurgery II

1994. 110 figures. VIII, 116 pages.
Cloth DM 150,–, öS 1050,–
Reduced price for subscribers to "Acta Neurochirurgica":
Cloth DM 135,–, öS 945,–
ISBN 3-211-82593-2

(Acta Neurochirurgica, Supplement 61)

In 1992 the Editors published the first volume of Minimally Invasive Neurosurgery (MIN I) which described the current state of the art in this rapidly developing field of neurosurgery and reported first clinical experiences with these new technologies. The subject of MIN II is limited to endoscopic anatomy, technical devices and surgical management of disorders suitable for endoscopic procedures. The indications and approaches in different diseases are still highly preliminary and longterm results are not yet available. The clinical value and the benefit to the patients treated with these new techniques must still be proven against the well established standards of microsurgery. This volume presents a critical update of neuroendoscopy.

B. L. Bauer, D. Hellwig (eds.)

Minimally Invasive Neurosurgery I

1992. 113 partly coloured figures. VII, 98 pages.
Cloth DM 150,–, öS 1050,–
Reduced price for subscribers to "Acta Neurochirurgica":
Cloth DM 135,–, öS 945,–
ISBN 3-211-82321-2

(Acta Neurochirurgica, Supplement 54)

Prices are subject to change without notice

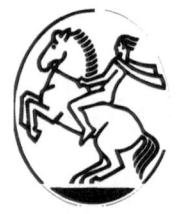

Springer-Verlag Wien New York

Sachsenplatz 4–6, P.O.Box 89, A-1201 Wien · 175 Fifth Avenue, New York, NY 10010, USA
Heidelberger Platz 3, D-14197 Berlin · 3-13, Hongo 3-chome, Bunkyo-ku, Tokyo 113, Japan